T0123041

Imaging and
Imagining the Fetus

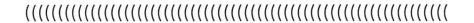

Imaging and
Imagining the Fetus
The Development of Obstetric Ultrasound

Malcolm Nicolson
and
John E. E. Fleming

The Johns Hopkins University Press
Baltimore

© 2013 The Johns Hopkins University Press
All rights reserved. Published 2013
Printed in the United States of America on acid-free paper
9 8 7 6 5 4 3 2 1

The Johns Hopkins University Press
2715 North Charles Street
Baltimore, Maryland 21218-4363
www.press.jhu.edu

Library of Congress Cataloging-in-Publication Data

Nicolson, Malcolm, 1952–
   Imaging and imagining the fetus : the development of obstetric
ultrasound / Malcolm Nicolson and John E. E. Fleming.
      p. ; cm.
   Includes bibliographical references and index.
   ISBN 978-1-4214-0793-7 (hdbk. : alk. paper) —
ISBN 1-4214-0793-0 (hdbk. : alk. paper) — ISBN 978-1-4214-0824-8
(electronic) — ISBN 1-4214-0824-4 (electronic)
   I. Fleming, John E. E. (John Eric Edgcumbe), 1934– II. Title.
   [DNLM: 1. Donald, Ian, 1910–1987. 2. Ultrasonography,
Prenatal—history—Scotland. 3. Ultrasonography, Prenatal—
instrumentation—Scotland. 4. Diffusion of Innovation—Scotland.
5. Fetal Diseases—diagnosis—Scotland. 6. History, 20th Century—
Scotland. 7. Politics—Scotland. WQ 11 FS2]
618.3'207543—dc23   2012017646

A catalog record for this book is available from the British Library.

*Special discounts are available for bulk purchases of this book. For more
information, please contact Special Sales at 410-516-6936 or specialsales@
press.jhu.edu.*

The Johns Hopkins University Press uses environmentally friendly
book materials, including recycled text paper that is composed of at
least 30 percent post-consumer waste, whenever possible.

To the memory of John's parents, Eric E. and Emilie M. Fleming

To John's children, Alan, Rachel, and Peter, and to his grandchildren, Hannah, whom we never knew, Rhona, and Benjamin

And to Catherine and Eilidh Nicolson, who were fortunate enough never to need much assistance from the technologies of modern obstetrics

Contents

Acknowledgments

We have been engaged in this work for what seems like an inordinate amount of time and have acquired many substantial debts over the years. We are particularly happy to acknowledge the support of Professor Iain T. Cameron. Following his appointment to Glasgow University as Regius Professor, he initiated collaboration between the Department of Obstetrics and Gynaecology and the Centre for the History of Medicine, and generously sponsored this project in its early stages. Also deserving of special thanks is Dr. Ian Spencer, whose work as Research Assistant was instrumental in getting the project going. Ian did much of the initial groundwork and skillfully conducted a number of key interviews.

This book would not have been possible without the cooperation of the Donald family. Mrs. Alix Donald made a large number of her late husband's papers available to us and shared her recollections of many of the key episodes in Ian Donald's career. Dame Alison Munro provided us with valuable insights into her brother's character and early life, and she allowed us to quote from her account of the family's time in South Africa. We also benefited from much moral and practical support and advice from Donald's daughters, Tessa Eide, Caroline Wilkinson, Christina Sargent, and Margaret Weston.

We owe a significant debt to all who were willing to speak to us and our voice recorders about their experiences with Ian Donald, Thomas G. Brown, and ultrasound: Wallace Barr, Dugald Cameron, Stuart Campbell, Winnie Childs, Robert Chivers, Jack L. Crichton, Alexander D. Christie, John Crofton, Bernard Donnelly, Thomas C. Duggan, Brian W. Fraser, Angus J. Hall, Malcolm MacNaughton, John MacVicar, W. Norman McDicken, Margaret B. McNay, John Rennie, Hugh P. Robinson, Robert E. Steiner, Bertil Sundén, John Julian Wild, James Willocks, and Maureen Young. A special mention should be made of Tom Brown, who patiently submitted to being interviewed several times, and who read and made extensive comments on a draft version of the book. We also benefited from conversations with Usama Abdulla, Alan D. Cameron, Christopher R. Hill, Hylton B. Meire, Debbie Nicholson, Phillip Rhodes, Clive Ross, Alastair Tough, Peter N. T. Wells, and Charles R. Whitfield. Our cooperation with Professor Tilli Tansey, then of the Wellcome Institute, resulted in a Wellcome Witness Seminar, ably chaired by Angus Hall, from which we learned a great deal. Jean Hyslop, Lydia Marshall, and Jonathan R.-B. Powell assisted us in many ways throughout our researches, as did the staff of Media Services, University of Glasgow. Professor Jack Boyd and his colleagues in the Department of Veterinary Anatomy enabled us to reenact Donald's earliest experiments, which was an invaluable exercise. We are grateful to all who participated in the reenactment.

Mike Barfoot, Margaret McNay, Morrice McRae, Andrew Pickering, Andrew Wear, Lawrence Weaver, and John Wilkinson all read drafts of the book. Their careful and scholarly scrutiny of our text saved us from many errors of fact and interpretation and much infelicity of expression. Neither they, nor any of the above-mentioned, necessarily endorse the book in its entirety, and all mistakes remain our responsibility.

We are grateful for the professional assistance of the archivists of the University of Glasgow, the University of Minnesota, the Yorkhill Hospitals, the American Institute for Ultrasound in Medicine, the Wellcome Library, the Royal College of Obstetricians and Gynaecologists, and the NHS Greater Glasgow and Clyde Health Board, and of the curators of the Hunterian Museum and the Glasgow Museums. In the course of our work on the history of ultrasound, we regularly gave research presentations to academic audiences, too many to enumerate. We have gained from all the comments and suggestions we received on those occasions.

We also greatly benefited from our association with the Johns Hopkins University Press. We thank an anonymous reader for an attentive and perceptive examination of earlier drafts and many helpful suggestions for improvement. Jackie Wehmueller, Sara Cleary, and Linda Strange patiently and professionally guided us through the production processes.

John Fleming wishes particularly to thank Tom Brown for offering him a job, in 1962, to work on ultrasound, and later entrusting him with the Bedtable Scanner; Dr. Patricia Morley, who in 1984, while President of the British Medical Ultrasound Society, suggested to him that he consider forming a historical collection on behalf of the Society; Professor Charles R. Whitfield, who lent his support to that enterprise; and Horace E. B. Lakin, schoolteacher, "a fine and generous man who taught me far more than simply woodwork."

Our research was generously supported by a Project Grant and other monies from the Wellcome Trust, without which this book would not have been possible. We also received valuable financial support from the British Medical Ultrasound Society.

Note on Sources

Since we undertook the primary research for this book, the Donald Papers and the British Medical Ultrasound Society (BMUS) Historical Collection Papers have both been transferred to the care of the Archivist to the NHS Greater Glasgow and Clyde Health Board and are housed in the Mitchell Library, Glasgow. Detailed indexed listings have been prepared: HB112 British Medical Ultrasound Collections and HB110 Prof. Ian Donald Papers. We have provided file numbers, and the individual documents to which we refer should be readily findable. Transcripts of our interviews are available from the Centre for the History of Medicine, University of Glasgow.

Imaging and
Imagining the Fetus

CHAPTER ONE

Introduction

Historiographies of Obstetrics

Visualizing the internal structures of the living body is a characteristic and defining feature of modern medicine.[1] Several new imaging technologies were invented in the second half of the twentieth century, with ultrasound, computerized tomography, and magnetic resonance imaging being the most famous examples.[2] Of these three, diagnostic ultrasound was the first to be invented and, arguably, has had the greatest clinical utility. Ultrasonic imaging has also had a momentous social impact because it can visualize the fetus.

Fifty years ago, the unborn human being was hidden, enveloped within the female abdomen, away from the medical gaze. The fetus made its presence known largely by its effects on the pregnant woman's body, and many of its activities and characteristics were understood by doctors only through the medium of her verbal testimony. Imaged by the ultrasound scanner, the developing human being became, for the first time in its history, a clinical entity, a patient in its own right. Ultrasonography has comprehensively revealed the fetus, its age and state of development, whether it is single or twinned or more, its problems and imperfections. What is more, the fetus has acquired a public presence, a social identity. It now features in family photograph albums, pictured apparently as casually as a toddler on the beach. The fetus has even appeared in advertisements (fig. 1.1), for cars, jobs, and soft drinks.[3] Some commentators argue that these images from within the gravid uterus have changed "the very experience of pregnancy."[4] They have certainly played a central role in the abortion debate.[5] The present volume is intended to be a contribution to the history of the ultrasound scanner—as a technological innovation, as a clinical tool in obstetrics, and as an artifact of profound cultural significance.

The latter half of the twentieth century saw a transformation in the British way of birth.[6] Before 1950, most confinements took place in the mother's home, the laboring woman attended by a midwife or her family practitioner, or

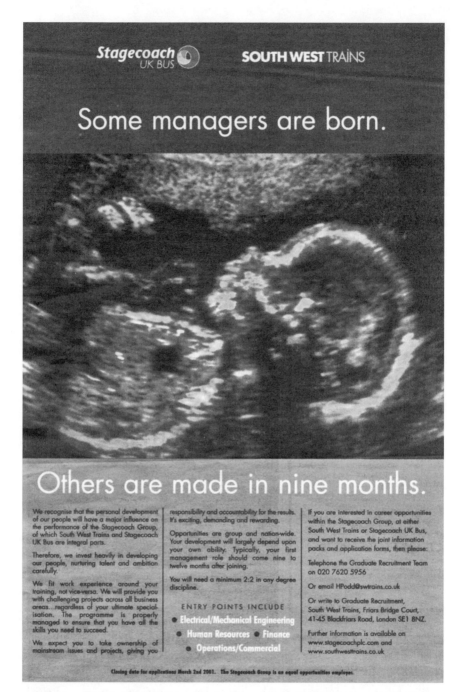

Figure 1.1. This advertisement, from February 2001, exemplifies how ultrasound images have become part of common experience. *Reproduced from color original courtesy of Stagecoach Group*

both. In the majority of cases, there was little significant medical input, apart from the administration of analgesia. However, in the decades following the setting up of the National Health Service in 1948, this situation changed. By the 1970s, most births were taking place in a hospital. Pregnancy and parturition were now routinely supervised by specialist obstetricians. The invention and diffusion of the ultrasound scanner occurred contemporaneously with these developments—the initial experiments in Glasgow took place in 1956, and the scanner had become widely deployed within the British hospital system by 1975. By the end of the century, ultrasound machines were ubiquitous in maternity clinics throughout the developed world.[7] This synchronism between the diffusion of the new technology and the increased frequency of hospital confinement is not wholly a coincidence. The ultrasound scanner was both a major agent for and a potent symbol of the medicalization of childbirth.

Reproduction and the medical practices that surround it are essentially contested domains, and two broadly opposing versions of the history of obstetrics can be discerned. According to some authors, the story of obstetrics is that of a long march from darkness into light. Thus Philip Rhodes, a distinguished professor of obstetrics, began *A Short History of Clinical Midwifery* with a description of the "ignorance" of Ancient Mesopotamia and ended it with an expression of enthusiasm for the clinical possibilities afforded by the artificial induction of labor.[8] By contrast, Jo Murphy-Lawless, a radical feminist midwife, introduced her account of "the history of obstetric thinking" with a paean of praise to the traditional birthing practices of the Bolivian Andes and concluded with the hope that similar womanly wisdom was, after centuries of neglect by the male-dominated medical profession, finally being rediscovered in her native Ireland.[9]

A similar dichotomy may be observed in attitudes to the ultrasound scanner. Few critics of modern obstetrics would be as dismissive of scientific medicine as is Murphy-Lawless. Nevertheless, to many feminist commentators, the medicalization of childbirth and, in particular, the increased use of a technological device to visualize the fetus have become issues of serious concern. To its proponents, the ultrasound scanner is a safe, reliable, and indispensable aid to diagnosis. But others argue that its development has been driven, not by the ostensive concern to improve the clinical care of women, but by the technological enthusiasms of doctors and engineers, not to mention the commercial interests of manufacturers.[10] Moreover, some consider that the primary role given to a machine in the clinical consultation expresses a prioritization of technical over humane values within the culture of hospital obstetrics.[11] It is also asserted that the safety of the diagnostic modality remains unproven.[12] Thus the history of the ultrasound scanner is central both to the development of modern medical technology and to the articulation of a concerted critique of that technology.

The history of diagnostic ultrasound is a large subject. Even in the 1950s, several groups of researchers were engaged in the development of the modality—in the United States, Europe, and Japan, as well as in the United Kingdom.[13] We have not attempted to provide a comprehensive account of this work, which took place across a number of medical specialties. Rather, the present book explores one of the principal strands of innovation that led to the modern ultrasound scanner, that which took place in the West of Scotland and, in particular, in hospitals associated with the University of Glasgow—namely, the Western Infirmary, the Glasgow Royal Maternity Hospital, and the Queen Mother's Hospital—and on the premises of Kelvin Hughes Ltd. (later known as Smiths Industries).

We tell the story of the development of the diagnostic scanner around the work of Ian Donald, who, as Regius Professor of Midwifery at Glasgow University from 1954 to 1976, led the team of clinicians and engineers who established pulse-echo ultrasound as a useful clinical modality within gynecology and obstetrics. Donald's early life is examined, as is his education at St. Thomas's Hospital Medical School. We discuss the low professional status of obstetrics and gynecology when he entered the specialty and explore the efforts of his mentors to raise that status and to ensure better care for pregnant and laboring women. We follow the development of his clinical and research interests and his involvement with a variety of medical technologies, not only ultrasound. In particular, we emphasize that Donald's research deployment of diagnostic imaging sprang from his seeking to address specific and pressing clinical issues. More broadly, we contend that his interest in diagnostic imaging followed from his commitment to a particular clinical tradition, one that valued the clinico-anatomical method and the postmortem examination.[14] Having received an excellent training in pathology at St. Thomas's, Donald was accustomed to trying to understand disease in structural terms. We argue that he sought to use imaging technologies to discern the physical attributes of health and disease within the living body, as he had been taught to scrutinize them within the dead body.

While our main focus is on the program of research and development (R&D) with which Donald was directly involved from the mid-1950s onward, we also survey earlier attempts to employ ultrasound diagnostically. In particular, we explore the work of Douglass Howry, in Denver, and John Julian Wild, in Minneapolis.[15] It is important to have a full account of these endeavors, for two reasons. First, without an awareness of earlier accomplishments, one cannot properly situate the achievement of the Glasgow team. Second, despite the ingenuity of their designs, the prototype scanners invented by Howry and Wild must be regarded as failed innovations. They did not lead to sustained technical development or significant clinical application. The Glaswegian initiative, by contrast, triumphed magnificently on both counts. Why the earlier innovations failed and the later one succeeded is an intriguing issue, upon which we hope to shed some light.

Ian Donald was not only a pioneer of ultrasonography. He was one of the leading academic obstetricians of his generation. His work on diagnostic imaging cannot be seen in isolation from his clinical concerns or from his wider professional, social, and moral commitments. He was, for instance, a vigorous campaigner against the 1967 Abortion Act. The connections between Donald's interest in fetal imaging and his political activism will be scrutinized, for they reveal the cultural meanings that quickly became attached to the ultrasonic image of the fetus, as well as the wider social status of obstetric knowledge.

A fascinating aspect of the story of diagnostic ultrasound is that Professor Donald did not work alone. The invention and development of the scanner was a crucial meeting point between clinical medicine, technological innovation, and commercial enterprise. We give particular attention to the creative input of Thomas (Tom) Graham Brown, the project's principal engineer and the man who designed and built the first contact scanner.

Tom Brown's place in the history of the ultrasound scanner is a central feature of our narrative, for several reasons. First, the crucial input of engineers to medical innovation is often underrated or even ignored, and Brown has suffered somewhat in this regard. Second, there is an abundance of historical studies of doctors, but fewer detailed treatments of the careers of engineers, particularly those who worked principally in nonacademic environments, as Brown did. The world of manufacturing R&D, of patent applications and commercial feasibility studies, is a strange, unexplored one to most historians of medicine. Yet the R&D departments of engineering and electronics companies have arguably had as important a role in the development of modern health care as have the hospital clinic and the laboratory. Brown is, moreover, a major figure in his own right. He might reasonably be compared with Alan Blumlein, who made important contributions to the development of radar and invented stereo sound reproduction, among much else. Blumlein is one of the few engineers working in a commercial environment whose careers have received detailed historical examination. The attention lately paid to him has considerably enhanced historians' understanding of this important category of technological innovator.[16] We hope that our exploration of Brown's key role in the invention of the ultrasound scanner will similarly help to illuminate the part played by engineering innovation in the history of medical technology. The contributions of a number of Donald's other colleagues, both engineers and clinicians, are also investigated.

The ultrasound scanner first became a useful clinical instrument in the late 1950s. Its underlying principles and much of its hardware were derived from sonar and radar and from equipment devised initially for the nondestructive testing of military and industrial equipment. Diagnostic ultrasound was a product of the revolution in electronic technologies that followed the Second World War, what Stuart Blume termed the *demobilization* of technology.[17] The development of the ultrasound scanner is part of the large-scale technological and social transformation that led eventually to electronic devices—color television and the personal computer, for instance—becoming commonplace objects, not only in hospitals and clinics, but also in our homes and workplaces. However, the early history of obstetric ultrasonography is also specific to particular localities. The instrument that Brown and Donald used in their first investigations—the industrial flaw detector—was available to them because Glasgow was, in the 1950s, a major center of shipbuilding and related industries. An inheritance from heavy engineering can be readily discerned in the shape and size of the first ultrasound scanners to be commercially marketed. These early machines were, in a word, Clyde-built.

At first, the ultrasound scanner was a useful tool of diagnosis only within the research environment in which it was devised. Diagnostic ultrasound provided an entirely novel way of seeing the body, exposing its cavities and soft tissues to the medical gaze in an unprecedented manner. The images that the first scanners produced were difficult to read, even for the clinicians directly involved in their production. The original prototypes, although effective instruments, were relatively crudely put together, and their use required supervision by skilled engineers. We investigate how the machines became easier to use and how the ability to interpret ultrasound images, and confidently base clinical decisions on the evidence they provided, was gradually acquired.

We follow the development and early diffusion of the ultrasound scanner from its first research applications in the 1950s to its widespread acceptance as an instrument of routine clinical investigation in the 1970s. Adoption of the technology beyond the West of Scotland initially happened largely through personal contacts and the movement of trained staff, many of whom retained supportive links with Glasgow. We also elucidate the process of black-boxing, whereby detailed knowledge of how the scanner worked was no longer essential for its effective use.[18] Few of us understand how our computers work, but we can still do our word processing effectively. By the late 1960s, many of the personnel who used the ultrasound scanner clinically had a similar relationship to this diagnostic technology. Scanners could be found in a large variety of medical settings, routinely used by staff who did not know, and did not need to know, anything beyond the basics of the underlying physics or electronics.

When the first contact scanner was built, its mechanism was housed in an unadorned gray metal box, betraying the technology's industrial and military antecedents. By the late 1970s, the ultrasound scanner had become a medical white good, a standardized commodity in a mass marketplace.[19] The gleaming pale enamel of its outer casing now bore the badges and logos of one or other of the major electronics manufacturers. We follow the design and development of the first commercial machines by Kelvin Hughes Ltd., by its successor company, Smiths Industries, and by Nuclear Enterprises Ltd.

(((((This book is structured around a particular historiographic agenda, but we have chosen not to interrupt the flow of the narrative with theoretical digressions or engagement with the work of other scholars. Thus it is incumbent upon us to outline here, at the outset, our historiographic stance. As already noted, the present volume is intended as a contribution to the history of medical technology and to the history of medical imaging. It is also a study of several interrelated medical and engineering careers. But, first and foremost, we have written it as a detailed exploration of the development of medical and technological practice.

Our analysis is broadly cognate with that of current work in the social construction of technology (SCOT).[20] However, as recently emphasized by several scholars, scientific research is essentially heterogeneous; it necessarily involves the combination of the social with cognitive, material, and economic factors.[21]

Accordingly, we have studied the development of obstetric ultrasound as a particular sequence of complex interactions between physical entities (sound waves, piezoelectric crystals, potentiometers, and the like), the biological substrate of the human body, and human actors from a variety of backgrounds and with diverse skills and interests.

While any process of research is underway, the nature of the phenomenon under study is uncertain, as indeed is the future direction, not to mention the success or failure, of the project as a whole. In our account of the development of the ultrasound scanner, we have tried to recreate that feeling of inherent uncertainty, of the pioneering participants not knowing where the process of investigation and experimentation is leading, not being sure how the next problem is to be solved. Andrew Pickering describes the trajectory of research as typically following a pattern of *modeling, resistance,* and *emergence.*[22] The investigator sets goals in the light of what he or she already knows and wishes to achieve (modeling), designs experiments to move toward the accomplishment of these goals, routinely fails to accomplish them (experiences resistance), attempts to accommodate this failure by defining modified goals and designing new experiments, again fails to accomplish them, or perhaps partially succeeds, and so on. In the course of these endeavors, in solving these problems, the researcher may veer into unexpected areas of investigation and stumble upon wholly unforeseen phenomena. Pickering's term *emergence* invokes the sense in which scientific research entails the unfolding of genuine novelty. In our account of the work of Brown, Donald, and their colleagues, we attempt to follow Pickering's tripartite schema. We believe that this is a fruitful way to reconstruct the scientist's interaction with his or her subject matter, as it happened— before the end point is known, while scientific practice is being freshly reconstructed, day to day and moment by moment.

As a clinical professor in a Scottish medical school, Ian Donald had many advantages, such as considerable freedom of action and easy access to patients. Yet, as the leader of a successful biomedical research team, Donald needed to have at his command more than clinical material and engineering expertise. He also had to be an effective manager and mentor, because the junior doctors who provided an essential supply of scientific person-power had to be convinced that involvement with his projects would be advantageous for their careers. Donald also needed to ensure continuing support for his work by building interpersonal networks—within the medical and engineering communities of Glasgow and its environs, with senior members of the university, and within the specialty of obstetrics and gynecology, both nationally and internationally. Most of all, Donald's project required funding. It could not have been sustained through its difficult early stages without the visionary commitment and financial backing of William Slater, deputy managing director of Kelvin Hughes (fig. 1.2). We document Slater's key role in supporting and encouraging Brown, as well as the part played by Donald's other major providers of funding.

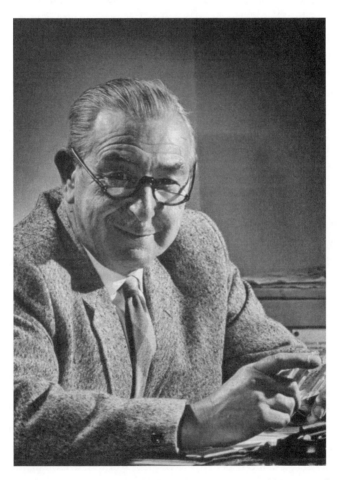

Figure 1.2. Mr. W. T. Slater, Kelvin Hughes Deputy Managing Director, whose responsibilities included the factories in Glasgow, Barkingside, and Basingstoke, from sometime before 1951 until 1966—by which time the Diasonograph (see chapter 7) had been designed and a dozen delivered to hospitals in the United Kingdom, United States, and Iraq. *Reproduced with permission of the British Medical Ultrasound Society (BMUS) Historical Collection*

We emphasize the importance of contingency in the story of diagnostic ultrasound in Glasgow. Donald's first contact with Brown, for instance, was entirely unplanned but was crucial to the success of the research enterprise. A number of such lucky accidents are described in the following chapters—Donald had a happy knack of meeting the person he needed at the time when he or she was most required. Without a fortuitous sequence of happenstances and coincidences, Donald's later career, and Brown's, would have turned out very differently. Though the development of diagnostic ultrasound was indeed structured by the broad historical contexts of postwar scientific medicine—such as the electronics revolution, the commodification of medical technology, and the medicalization of childbirth—events in Glasgow were not narrowly determined by these larger trends. The story of obstetric ultrasound is essentially a micro-narrative, a story of particular groups and individuals, of local and specific plans, actions, and events. The devil, as always, is in the detail, and we have not flinched from a dense reconstruction of the minutiae of the processes of research and dissemination. As John Pickstone put it, "to understand how medicine has changed, we have no alternative but to study the real, messy, contested and complex debates by which, over time, some procedures were accepted in preference to others."[23]

Following scientific inquiry through its trajectory of modeling, resistance, and emergence and its various contingencies permits a symmetrical handling of social and material factors and elides any analytical distinction between them. In our view, this is an important attribute of an adequate historiography of biomedicine. As already argued, the challenge facing the historian is to employ forms of analysis that do not prioritize either the material or the social, or any other aspect of the research process, but instead follow all the heterogeneous elements that are intermingled in unexpected and unpredictable combinations, to achieve that temporary stability of practice that is deemed a research result.

Our approach might be termed *posthumanist*, in that we work with the assumption that the rigid dichotomy that social scientists, including historians, have traditionally made between the natural world and human society is an unhelpful one.[24] The distinguished theorist Donna Haraway has eloquently called attention to the way in which our bodies exist at the interfaces between the social, the biological, and the technological—hence the attention she pays to what she calls *cyborgs*, entities in which human bodies and machines are inextricably interconnected.[25] Following Haraway, we are here centrally concerned with the mutual and reciprocal interactions between and among human bodies and material objects, both natural and technological. It is out of such interactions that our modern conceptualization of the fetus and of pregnancy has emerged.

A methodological commitment to a posthumanist agenda may seem incongruent in the context of a volume that also aspires to be a study of careers in research, a genre necessarily centered on human individuals. But we would claim that the posthumanist program, with its symmetrical handling of the natural, the social, and the technological, allows us to provide a more precise and convincing account of the origins of human actions, by placing them in their fullest context.

For all its value as a research heuristic for historiography, however, we must acknowledge that posthumanism cannot provide a complete understanding of the significance of any particular ultrasound scan. To most observers, lay or clinical, when confronted by the image of a specific fetus, the physical means by which that image was generated and the route by which the technology was developed are largely, if not wholly, irrelevant. As noted above, many feminist commentators have regarded the ultrasound scanner with suspicion, stigmatizing imaging technology as an impersonal, mechanical intrusion into the intimate realm of childbearing. With the rise of "third-wave" feminism, however, a cautiously less hostile attitude toward fetal imaging may be discerned. Many pregnant women (and their partners) have become enthusiastic about the possibilities of an imaginative engagement with their fetuses through the medium of the ultrasound screen. The fetus may itself have become a cyborg, but its emotive significance is not thereby diminished, as we explore in our final chapter. Images of the fetus may be produced by machines, but they live vividly in the human imagination.[26]

CHAPTER TWO

Diagnostic Ultrasound before Thomas Brown

Ultrasonic echolocation has its origins in the military and industrial contexts. We describe in this chapter the more important of the early attempts to adapt the technology for medical purposes.[1] We investigate the problems and difficulties—biological, physical, electronic, social, and organizational—that confronted the pioneers of diagnostic ultrasound, and outline the modality's state of development before Tom Brown and Ian Donald entered the field. Particular attention is given to Douglass Howry in Denver and John Wild in Minneapolis, since study of their work reveals instructive similarities to and differences from the approach taken by Brown.

The ears of a healthy young human can detect sound over a range of frequencies, from about 30 Hz to about 20 kHz. Thus, by convention, sound of frequency greater than 20 kHz is termed *ultrasound*. The medical ultrasound scanner works by echolocation. Echolocation technologies (sonar and radar are other examples) transmit pulses of energy from known positions and in known directions and detect returning echoes.[2] In the case of diagnostic ultrasound, a pulse of high-frequency sound is sent into the body. Some of that sound energy is reflected back from the body's internal surfaces, and the time taken for the echoes to return to the transmitter is measured. If the speed of sound in tissue is known, the distance between the transmitter and the surface that produced the echo can be determined. From these basic pieces of information (position of source, direction, and distance), an image of the interior of the body can be built up.[3]

Ultrasound pulses are generated and received by a transducer with a piezoelectric element.[4] In obstetrics and gynecology, frequencies of 3 to 10 MHz are typically used. With such high frequencies, the pulses can be very short and confined to a small-diameter beam, thereby producing images that reveal fine detail.[5] There is a practical upper limit to the frequency that can be employed, however, as the absorption of sound energy increases with frequency and hence the depth of effective penetration into tissue is reduced.

The scientific study of sound beyond the range of human hearing began toward the end of the nineteenth century. In his classic text *The Theory of Sound*, published in 1877, Lord Rayleigh developed mathematical characterizations of a wide range of acoustical phenomena, including the relationships between frequency and reflection, diffraction, and absorption.[6] In April 1912, shortly after the sinking of the *Titanic*, Lewis Fry Richardson, a British applied mathematician, patented a method of locating icebergs at sea by sending out pulses of sound and detecting the incoming echoes.[7] However, Richardson was unable to secure a commercial sponsor to allow him to develop his ideas. He worked on the project intermittently for many years, but his invention was never deployed. Just before the outbreak of the First World War, his friend Maurice Wilson advised him to approach the Admiralty: "It would be extraordinarily useful to the country just now for our fleet to be able to detect the presence of other boats and particularly submarines." But Wilson added, "Perhaps you feel you would not like to lend your aid to the method of warfare."[8] He was right on both counts. A Quaker and a pacifist, Richardson refused to be involved in any research that had a direct military application. For the next forty years, however, the development of ultrasonic echolocation would be intimately linked with military research and deployment.

In the second decade of the twentieth century, the imminent prospect of war stimulated the navies of Western Europe and the United States to explore methods of protecting ships from the increasing threat of the submarine. In 1915, Constantin Chilowsky, a Russian engineer living in Switzerland, suggested that echolocation could be an effective method of detection, if a sound signal of sufficiently high frequency were used. Chilowsky's idea was quickly taken up by the French physicist Paul Langevin.[9] By 1916, Chilowsky and Langevin, working together and in cooperation with the French Navy, had demonstrated that it was possible to detect submerged objects by using ultrasound beams of about 40 kHz.[10] Two serious problems remained to be solved, however, before an ultrasonic antisubmarine system could be put into military service. First, ultrasound had to be generated at an intensity that would permit echolocation over operationally useful distances. Second, a reliable means had to be found for recognizing the relatively weak returning echo.

Langevin ingeniously utilized the piezoelectric effect to solve these problems. In 1878, William Thomson (later, Lord Kelvin), at the University of Glasgow, had postulated that electric polarization was intrinsic to many crystalline substances.[11] In 1880, Pierre and Jacques Curie observed that when mechanical pressure was exerted across a crystal, an electric potential was produced between the two sides.[12] The following year, Gabriel Lippman predicted the existence of the reverse effect, whereby application of an electric charge to a crystal produced mechanical deformation. This property was quickly confirmed experimentally by the Curies. Working with specially prepared crystals, they established the complete reversibility of electrical and mechanical deformations.

Langevin, who had been a student of Pierre Curie, exploited the finding that when an alternating voltage is applied at an appropriate frequency to a piezoelectric crystal, mechanical vibrations are produced, which propagate through the surrounding medium as sound waves. In April 1917, he built an ultrasonic transmitter that incorporated a slice of quartz. Using a thermionic valve-oscillator, the crystal was made to resonate at 150 kHz. The results were spectacular. In trials in a laboratory tank, "fish placed in the beam in the neighbourhood of the source were killed immediately, and certain observers experienced a painful sensation on plunging the hand in this region." Sea trials with a less powerful transmitter, running at 40 kHz, began in February 1918.[13]

Langevin's transmitter was designed to emit short, heavily damped pulses of ultrasound. The shorter the pulse, the easier it is to distinguish the returning echoes from the outgoing signal. Langevin thought it should also be possible to use the piezoelectric effect to receive as well as transmit ultrasound. Incoming sound waves would mechanically distort the quartz crystal, producing an electric charge and hence a voltage across the electrodes. Initially, he was unable to detect the very small potentials generated. However, while Langevin was working on antisubmarine echolocation, the French Army's signal corps, the Radiotélégraphie Militaire, was engaged in an intensive program of research and development in the field of radio communication.[14] By 1917, exploiting the innovation of the triode valve, the corps had built a very sensitive, high-frequency radio amplifier, the R6. Later in the same year, the R6 was made available to Langevin, which enabled him to build a practical piezoelectric receiver and recognize faint ultrasonic echoes.

Drawing on the French research, British and American military engineers began to build similar antisubmarine systems from 1918 onward. The first sonar (*s*ound *n*avigation *a*nd *r*anging) echolocation set was fitted into a Royal Navy vessel in 1922. In peacetime, Langevin applied his echolocation expertise to another important maritime problem: measuring the depth of the sea. He showed that, by bouncing an ultrasonic pulse off the seabed, the depth of water under a ship could be accurately determined. In the 1920s, a civilian version of the Langevin echo sounder was marketed commercially by the Marconi Company.[15]

Ultrasonic echo sounders were also developed by the Royal Navy, in cooperation with Henry Hughes and Son, a London-based company specializing in marine navigational equipment. In 1931, Henry Hughes was licensed to produce echo sounders for the civilian market.[16] Donald Sproule, one of the company's senior engineers, invented a recording device that showed the ocean floor as a black outline.[17] Sproule's innovation had some unexpected but marketable capabilities. It could detect shoals of fish, for instance. The Henry Hughes echo sounder became the focus of some public interest in 1935, when it was used to locate the wreck of the *Lusitania*.[18]

Gradually, the staff of the naval research establishments of France, Britain, and the United States built up expertise in the physics and technology of ultrasound. Much fundamental work, theoretical and practical, was done on the design of ultrasonic transducers. The use of oscilloscopes allowed a more detailed characterization of the echo signal.[19] With the diffusion of echolocation technology outside the military sector and its development by commercial companies such as Marconi and Henry Hughes, civilian engineers became interested in finding new, nonmilitary applications of ultrasound.

(((((Between the wars, the biological effects of ultrasound also became an important focus of scientific investigation. Frank Hopwood, working in Britain, and Robert Wood and Alfred Loomis, in the United States, confirmed Langevin's observation that exposure to powerful ultrasonic beams could have deleterious consequences. Ultrasound was also observed to have more specific effects on biological materials. Ultrasonic irradiation could heat tissue, and the internal structure of cells might be disturbed by thermal currents set up in cytoplasm. Ultrasound could also release dissolved gases from body fluids, producing bubbles or blisters. E. Newton Harvey described these and related phenomena in an authoritative survey, published in 1930.[20]

In the 1930s, several attempts were made to find medical applications for ultrasound's biological effects. Germany, for example, saw a great vogue for treatments based on the ultrasonic heating of tissue. Ultrasound therapy became vaunted as a "cure-all for anything from cancer to *Violinspielerkrampf.*"[21] Most of these therapeutic applications had little scientific or clinical rationale. As a result, medical ultrasound gained, in some quarters, a somewhat unsavory reputation.[22] We must note here the fundamental difference between how ultrasound was used in these early medical applications and its subsequent use for imaging. In the therapeutic context, ultrasound is a means of conveying energy to tissue; a continuous beam of sound is generally used. By contrast, in imaging techniques, as in marine echolocation, short pulses of ultrasound are employed solely to gather information.

In the late 1930s and early 1940s, investigators first began to examine the possibility of applying the information-gathering capabilities of ultrasound to medical diagnosis. The earliest pioneers were André Dénier, a French inventor who had known Paul Langevin, and Karl Theodore Dussik, an Austrian psychiatrist and neurologist. However, both Dénier and Dussik rejected echolocation in favor of techniques based on transmission ultrasound. Their innovations were unsuccessful and are somewhat outside the main line of development that led to the acceptance of diagnostic ultrasound as a clinically useful modality. Nevertheless, the reasons these men gave for rejecting echolocation are worth examining for the light they shed on the difficulties of working with ultrasound within body cavities. The direction of their research also reveals the cultural expectations then prevalent within medicine as to what a diagnostic image should look like.

In the mid-1930s, working at the Metropolitan State Hospital in Massachusetts, Dussik had become interested in the diagnosis of brain tumors.[23] The principal diagnostic imaging technique then available, X-radiography, had proved to be of limited utility in localizing cerebral pathology. The brain is, to a substantial extent, shielded from X-rays by the highly absorbent bones of the skull. Moreover, the difference in radiopacity between normal and pathological brain tissue—unless a tumor is calcified—is generally too small to provide adequate contrast on an X-ray plate. Visualization can be improved by injecting high-contrast medium into the cerebral arteries or the ventricles, but such procedures are inconveniently invasive and can be uncomfortable, even dangerous, for the patient.[24] While in the United States, Dussik learned of the use of pulse-echo ultrasound to locate shoals of fish. On returning to Austria in 1937, to take up a post at the University Klinik in Vienna, he began to investigate whether ultrasound might be used to improve the diagnostic localization of brain disease.[25]

At the outset of his investigations, Dussik made a strategic decision to reject pulse-echo techniques. He wished to emulate X-radiography and produce two-dimensional images.

> Because of the complicated structure of animal tissue, it would be impracticable to use an echomethod, such as used in detecting . . . schools of fish in the ocean. Besides, I thought that visualisation of differences of attenuation could bring us real pictures, in some sense similar to the way, in witch we can read an X-ray picture. On the contrary the echomethod would us give complicated curves, which would be . . . inconvenient for clinical use. Thus the invention of a trans-mitting method, suitable for use in medicine seemed to be preferable.[26]

The X-ray image was, of course, the exemplar of diagnostic imaging at this time.

In deciding to work with transmission ultrasound, Dussik was following the example of recent developments in the industrial application of ultrasound. In the interwar period, some attempts had been made to use transmission ultrasound to detect cracks or other flaws in castings and other metal arti-facts.[27] The principle of transmission ultrasound is closely analogous to that of X-radiography. In an X-ray machine, a beam of radiation is directed from a source, on one side of the target, toward a recording device, generally a photo-graphic plate, on the other side. Parts of the target object absorb X-rays more readily than others, and thus radiation shadows are cast on the plate. Similarly, in a transmission flaw detector, piezoelectric transmitters would be placed on one side of the target and receivers on the other and a beam of continuous ultra-sound sent between them. Cracks in metal, being highly reflective of ultrasound, would reveal their presence by the sonic shadow they cast on the receiving transducer.

In 1945, Dussik became the head of a private hospital in Bad Ischl, Austria. Around this time, his brother, Frederich, a physicist, began to cooperate with him in his ultrasound research. They constructed an instrument in which the patient's head was positioned between two transducers. A continuous beam of ultrasound was scanned along one side of the head, and the ultrasonic energy arriving at the receiver, on the other side, was detected and amplified. The intensity of the incoming signal was registered by means of a neon light, the brightness of which was proportional to the received energy. The light moved, reproducing the scanning motion of the ultrasound beam across the other side of the target, and its luminous intensity was recorded on a photographic plate. (This scanning system has some basic resemblance to television, in which Frederich Dussik had done development work.)[28] Thus the Dussiks' apparatus created two-dimensional patterns of light and dark that matched the spatial variation in the intensity of ultrasound transmitted through the head.

The Dussik brothers dubbed their technique "hyperphonography." In the late 1940s, they published a number of images that they claimed were visualizations of the cerebral ventricles. They asserted that these images were, potentially at least, practical aids to the diagnosis of brain disease, allowing the presence of space-occupying masses in the cerebrum to be inferred from distortion of the ventricles. The Dussiks also claimed that their technique had, on one occasion, directly visualized a tumor.[29]

Karl Dussik rejected echolocation because he thought it would not provide pictorial images comparable to those provided by X-radiography. André Dénier, by contrast, saw possible advantages in employing a pulse-echo technique, in that more detailed information could be obtained from the study object. There was a technical difficulty, however. When a pulse-echo method is used, the receiving transducer must be in close proximity to the transmitting transducer. Under these circumstances, the receiver picks up the transmission pulse as well as the returning echo. This was not an insurmountable problem in marine applications; owing to the large distances involved, there was a relatively long time interval between the outgoing and incoming signals. But medical pulse-echo ultrasound would necessarily have to be done at close range, and the interval between the transmission pulse and the returning echoes would be very short. Dénier could not conceive of a practical method of reliably distinguishing the returning echo with the electronic equipment available to him. It would be, he wrote, "like listening for a cricket in a bombardment." Accordingly, he concentrated on developing a transmission system.[30] Dénier's work attracted little interest outside France, and even there, only for a short time.

In the late 1940s, a German electronics company, Siemens, began to explore the commercial potential of Dussik's technique. This work was led by Reimer Pohlman, an important pioneer of industrial ultrasound, and was based in the company's research laboratory at Erlangen.[31] In 1948, an investigative team from the U.S. Army visited Dussik's institute in Bad Ischl, and a report on his ultrasound work was sent to the Acoustics Laboratory at the Massachusetts Institute of Technology (MIT).

(((((In the 1930s, as the Second World War approached, the nondestructive testing of metal fabrications, such as the wings of aircraft or welds in ships' hulls and boilers, was identified as a matter of national importance.[32] The use of X-rays was not practical in many military or industrial settings. Moreover, X-radiography had proved to be not wholly effective in detecting very fine cracks. In the United Kingdom, the Iron and Steel Research Council asked its Alloy Steels Research Committee to advise on the matter. A Hair-Line Crack Sub-Committee was formed, under the chairmanship of an eminent metallurgist, Professor Cecil H. Desch. In November 1939, it was decided to investigate the possibility of employing "supersonic waves" for industrial purposes.[33]

The use of audible sound to test metal, glass, or ceramics for flaws is traditional. If one taps a china cup, a clear ring indicates that no gross defect is present. A cracked cup does not resonate. The wheels of railway rolling stock were checked in a similar manner. But only relatively large imperfections can be detected in this way. Defects smaller than the wavelength of audible sound do not impede the transmission of sound waves and thus do not prevent the test object from resonating. Also, audible sound provides little information on the location of flaws. Desch concluded that the shorter wavelengths of ultrasound offered the possibility for both detecting and localizing fine irregularities.

Desch knew of the involvement of Henry Hughes Ltd. in the development of marine ultrasonic systems, and in 1940 he invited the company to assist the Hair-Line Crack Sub-Committee in its investigations. Much of the experimental work sponsored by the subcommittee was undertaken in the Research Division of Henry Hughes, under the direction of Donald Sproule. Initially, the engineers at Henry Hughes experimented with transmission techniques.[34] These methods were, however, found to be quite insensitive, even at very high power outputs. Not until 1942, when Sproule began to investigate the potential of a pulse-echo technique, did real progress begin. Sproule applied his experience of, as he put it, "echo-sounder principles to sounding in a solid sea."[35] He knew that, unlike X-rays, ultrasonic waves tended to be strongly reflected at the boundaries between different media.

The suggestion that pulse-echo ultrasound could be applied to the detection of flaws in metal was not original to Sproule. It was first made in 1928 by the Russian engineer Sergei Sokolov.[36] Sokolov's idea could not be implemented in the 1920s, however, because equipment capable of producing high-frequency, short-duration ultrasonic pulses was not available.[37] By the 1940s, improved oscillators had been developed for use in radar, and these could readily be adapted for use with ultrasonic transducers. Moreover, radar R&D had transformed the oscilloscope from a laboratory instrument for the characterization of waveforms to a precision tool ideally suited to the measurement of very small time intervals.[38] The transit time of the signal could be ascertained accurately even when pulse-echo techniques were used at close quarters.

In July 1943, Sproule and his colleagues demonstrated a working prototype of a pulse-echo flaw detector. The apparatus used two separate probes. One transmitted heavily damped pulses of ultrasound from a quartz crystal transducer resonating at 2.5 MHz. Returning echoes were detected by a similar transducer element in the second probe. The probes were moved by hand across the test area to locate defects. The amplitude of the returning echo was simply plotted against time on an oscilloscope screen. The resulting image was a distinctive spike, or series of spikes, the height of each spike being proportional to the strength of the echo received. The distance of the spike along the screen's x-axis represented the elapsed time between firing of the initial pulse and reception of the echo and thus indicated how deep the flaw was within the test object. This form of display became known as *A-scan* or *A-mode*.[39]

Sproule's work remained classified for the duration of hostilities, but Henry Hughes Ltd. was allowed to supply prototype flaw detectors to industrial and scientific customers. As was later discovered, a very similar device had been invented, entirely independently, by Professor Floyd Firestone at the University of Michigan. Firestone had been granted a secret patent for his Supersonic Reflectoscope in 1942. The only substantial difference between the British and the American machines was that, whereas the Henry Hughes flaw detector used two probes, Firestone's model used only one.[40] When the war was over, Firestone, Desch, and Sproule were able to publish accounts of their investigations.[41] In 1946, Henry Hughes began the commercial production of the first of a series of pulse-echo metal flaw detectors, the Mark (Mk) I. In 1947, Henry Hughes amalgamated with the Glasgow firm of Kelvin Bottomley and Baird to form Kelvin & Hughes Ltd.[42]

Subsequent refinements led to flaw detectors that operated at higher frequencies and with shorter pulse durations, resulting in finer resolution. In the early 1950s, the availability of new amplifiers with high input impedance, low noise, and wide bandwidth—again, a spin-off from the radar industry—enabled engineers to improve sensitivity. Interest in the military applications of ultrasound also led to the discovery that some ceramic materials are highly efficient converters of electrical into mechanical energy. These piezo-ceramics, produced by sintering metallic oxide powders, were relatively easy to manufacture, and their electrical properties could be precisely tailored to specific applications.[43] Transducers made from barium titanate, the first of these new materials to be put to practical use, exhibited vastly improved performance over their quartz equivalents and stimulated much interest in finding new applications of ultrasound technology.

(((((Shortly after the war, several investigators realized, simultaneously and independently, that the new pulse-echo devices might have medical diagnostic potential. One of the first of these was Floyd Firestone. As Benson Carlin, an associate, recalled, "You know Firestone, himself, [word missing] that it might be used. Firestone used to point it [the probe of the Reflectoscope] on his leg and say, 'See, you might be able to find things in the body.' "[44] Neither Firestone nor any of his immediate colleagues took up this idea for further investigation, however. In Hamburg in 1946, Dr. Netheler of the scientific instruments manufacturer Eppendorf, in cooperation with Professor Hansen of South Lübeck Hospital, thought of using pulse-echo ultrasound in the noninvasive investigation of the liver.[45] But Netheler and Hansen were unable to secure funding to develop their idea, and it remained merely a research proposal.

In 1948, in an article in the American hobbyist magazine *Audio Engineering*, S. Young White, a well-known engineer and inventor, noted that pulse-echo equipment could now be assembled quite cheaply. The flood of cheap war-surplus electronics parts on the market after the Second World War, mostly developed for radar, had made electronics a considerably less expensive, more accessible, and more interesting hobby. War-surplus variable-pulse generators retailed for about $100.[46]

Young White suggested that the problem of paralysis, whereby the receiving ultrasound transducer was knocked out of action for a few microseconds by the magnitude of the transmission pulse, could be solved by fitting a short water-filled tube in front of the probe. He concluded that pulse-echo ultrasound might potentially be useful in diagnosis.

> Feed the assembly into a [oscillo]scope . . . Apply this to your leg and obtain a reflection from the bone . . . and you will have a nice tool for work on the body. It will locate bullets, which are an ideal type of load. Some tumours should give reflections which will appear on the screen. If pus or other matter forms between the skull and the brain, it should also show up as a reflecting layer . . . If you can co-operate with the medical people in your vicinity, many of these simple things and the obvious modifications they suggest have a chance of really helping the medical researcher who has almost an infinity of problems to contend with. It is possible that by concentrating on one line of work you would be able to . . . give medicine a tool it really needs, and have all the fun of discovery at the same time.[47]

Young White did not claim to have done any biological investigations himself. Indeed, his remarks on the application of pulse-echo methods to the diagnosis of brain disease indicate that he did not fully appreciate the technical problems associated with these procedures. Nevertheless, he conveyed to his readers the strong impression that using ultrasound to investigate the structure of the human body was technically feasible and would be medically worthwhile.

By the time Young White's article was published, cooperative research along the lines he was suggesting, between medicine and engineering, was already underway. The American electronics company RCA was the world's largest manufacturer of domestic radio sets and, during the war, had become a major supplier of radar and sonar equipment to the U.S. armed forces. In the late 1940s, the company encouraged its research staff to develop new commercial applications that would exploit the technical expertise they had acquired while working on war-related projects. In the laboratory of RCA's subsidiary company in Argentina, engineer R. P. McLoughlin and physician G. N. Guastivino chose to investigate the potential of pulse-echo ultrasound for locating foreign objects in human tissue. In 1949, they published a paper describing a prototype apparatus, dubbed LUPAM (localizador ultrasonoscopico para aplicaciones medicas).[48]

LUPAM was very similar in construction to an industrial flaw detector. Like the Reflectoscope, it produced A-scan images. McLoughlin and Guastivino's paper features an A-scan of an excised kidney in which a stone had been embedded. An echo spike from the stone can be clearly seen. The paper also reproduces an A-scan of a human forearm in which the reflections of the two bones can be distinguished. McLoughlin and Guastivino were not content with this mode of presentation, however. Toward the end of their paper, they suggested that it should be possible to render the information gained by pulse-echo more accessible by presenting it in a different format, similar to the two-dimensional form of display known as plan position indicator (PPI), which had been developed for radar.[49] In PPI, echoes are displayed as bright dots at a position corresponding to their point of origin. (PPI is explained more fully in chapter 6.) Radar operators could thus view on their cathode-ray screens a pictorial representation of the landscape swept by their scanner, and they could follow the virtual movement of planes or ships across it.[50] Similar two-dimensional formats had been devised for use with sonar.[51] McLoughlin and Guastivino proposed that PPI could be adapted for diagnostic imaging. Their paper provides a rough sketch of what such a two-dimensional image, in this case of a human forearm, might look like. They did not claim to have built a machine capable of processing information in this way, but with the technical resources at RCA's disposal, it would surely have been possible to construct such a device, had a determined attempt been made.

McLoughlin and Guastivino had begun a process of innovation that might well have led, under different circumstances, to the development of a diagnostically useful ultrasonic scanner. They had a clear and explicit aim—namely, the invention of a two-dimensional imaging system based on the pulse-echo principle. But no further development of the LUPAM project seems to have taken place. RCA's management evidently decided to direct its corporate strategic R&D funding in other directions.[52]

(((((By the time McLoughlin and Guastivino's report was published, several other groups of researchers had begun to investigate the diagnostic potential of ultrasound. Three of the most important research programs were based in the United States. Douglass Howry and his colleagues in Denver employed pulse-echo techniques, as did John Wild and his colleagues in Minneapolis. However, given the more direct links between the Glasgow work and that of Howry and, especially, Wild, we will leave a description of the work undertaken in Denver and Minneapolis until later in this chapter. Here we focus on the third American group, based at MIT, in Cambridge, Massachusetts.

The laboratories of MIT had been a key site for military R&D during the Second World War.[53] They played a major role, for instance, in the Allied radar program.[54] Owing to its strategic importance, radar became a focus of intense investment of resources and scientific expertise, in Britain, Germany, and the United States, from the mid-1930s onward. The rate of refinement of the technology was remarkable. In 1940, radar sets were bigger than garden sheds; by 1945, many were the size of small suitcases and could be fitted into aircraft.[55] The demand for more sophisticated radar equipment was an enormous stimulus to the development of electronic components. The design and manufacture of cathode-ray tubes, oscilloscopes, amplifiers, valves, and signal-processing circuits, to name only a few, were greatly improved as a result. An electronics industry, formidable in size and diversity, developed to service the intense demand for electronic equipment and instrumentation.[56]

In the decades after the war, MIT retained its position as the preeminent center for research in electronics and related fields. In 1949, the institute's Acoustics Laboratory embarked on a major program of diagnostic research, jointly with Massachusetts General Hospital. The aim of the project, funded by the United States Public Health Service, was to improve the diagnosis of brain disease.[57] Finding a safe and noninvasive means of localizing brain tumors was the Holy Grail of medical imaging in the immediate postwar period. Improvements in equipment and technique had enhanced the ability of surgeons to operate effectively and safely on brain tissue. The more precisely the position of a tumor could be determined before surgery, the less destructive the procedure was likely to be and the better the potential outcome for the patient. Conventional X-radiography was, as already noted, of limited utility in localizing cerebral pathology—hence the strong interest in the development of alternative diagnostic methods. Richard Bolt, director of MIT's Acoustics Laboratory, assembled a strong team of researchers. Theodor Hueter, an engineer, was recruited from Siemens's Erlangen laboratory, where he had trained with Pohlman and gained considerable experience of both industrial and biological applications of ultrasound.[58] The MIT staff worked in cooperation with Thomas Ballantine and George Ludwig, surgeons at the Massachusetts General Hospital.

Ludwig had already undertaken some pioneering experiments with ultrasound as a diagnostic modality. He had served as a medical officer in the U.S. Navy's Medical Research Institute in Bethesda, Maryland. With his naval experience, Ludwig was well aware of the "successful application of ultrasonic pulse techniques and the echo-ranging principle to underwater detection and ranging and to the localization of flaws in metal."[59] He was prompted to investigate whether an analogous pulse-echo technique might be applicable to medical diagnosis. Accordingly, he acquired a Firestone Reflectoscope and secured the assistance of F. W. Struthers, a technician in the Naval Research Laboratory.

As the focus for their research, Ludwig chose the problem of the detection of gallstones. There was a good clinical reason for this decision. In the investigation of the gallbladder, as for the brain, existing imaging techniques were only partially helpful. Ordinary X-ray films of the abdomen could confirm a clinical diagnosis of gallstone in less than 20 percent of cases. With the excellent equipment available to them in the Naval Research Laboratory, Ludwig and Struthers conducted an elegant series of in vitro measurements of the "acoustic impedance mismatch at a tissue-gallstone interface" to determine how much energy might be reflected from a gallstone in situ. Encouraged by their results, they proceeded to embed human gallstones in isolated muscle tissue and in the gallbladders of living dogs. In both cases, strong echoes were received from the implanted calculi.[60]

Ludwig concluded that, in principle, the in vivo detection of gallstones was possible. There were technical problems, however. The Reflectoscope provided only A-scan images, and Ludwig and Struthers found interpretation of the echo spikes difficult because of the numerous "transient smaller signals returning from this area."[61] Moreover, because of the large difference between the acoustic impedance of gas and tissue, gas in the gut acted as an almost perfect sonic reflector, shielding underlying organs from ultrasound. Ludwig became convinced that the gastrointestinal tract would have to be cleared of gas before detection of gallstones by ultrasound in an intact abdomen would be feasible. This was, he feared, a major obstacle to the clinical utilization of the technique. Nevertheless, Ludwig did envisage some possible diagnostic applications for an ultrasonic probe. On occasion, after removing the gallbladder, a surgeon might be unsure whether further calculi remained in the common bile duct. Ludwig suggested that a probe might be devised to enable an intraoperative yet noninvasive examination of the duct. Such a tool might also aid in the location of foreign bodies in wounds.

Ludwig did not continue to investigate the possibilities of visualizing the contents of the gallbladder. Instead, he chose to join with Bolt at MIT to aim at a much greater prize: the localization of brain disease. Ludwig also ceased to work with the Reflectoscope, having come to the conclusion that pulse-echo ultrasound did not hold much promise as a tool for detecting neoplasms,

especially in the brain. He had already done several experiments using a transmission technique, and it was to transmission ultrasound that Ludwig and his
new collaborators at MIT turned in their search for a diagnostic method applicable to the brain.

For the MIT team, there were several reasons for deciding to work with
transmission ultrasound. Ludwig's in vitro measurements seemed to indicate
that the difference in acoustic attenuation between brain tissue and ventricular
fluid was considerable.[62] The cerebral ventricles should cast strong sonic shadows. While at Siemens, Hueter, like Ludwig, had experimented with the application of pulse-echo techniques to animal tissues and had also found the resulting "Reflectoscope reflectograms" (A-scans) difficult to interpret.[63] The team
also had the example of the Dussik brothers' work on which to base its initial
research program. Bolt, Ballantine, and Hueter visited Bad Ischl to consult
with K. T. Dussik in October 1949 and were encouraged by what they saw.[64]
But perhaps the most important influence on their decision was what Hueter
was later to term the "visualization paradigm."

> Medical diagnosticians at that time envisioned "ultrasonograms" that would re-
> semble the familiar roentgenograms, hopefully with better contrast and delinea-
> tion of the soft tissues. Clearly, they were not looking for complex pulse reflec-
> tion trains on an A-scope, but for a two-dimensional . . . rendering of internal
> body topography, for an analogue to the X ray.[65]

For Hueter and his colleagues, as for Dussik, transmission ultrasound had the
considerable virtue of apparent similarity to X-radiography; it appeared to
offer the possibility of pictorial representation of structures within the skull.
Most clinicians wanted two-dimensional diagnostic images resembling the
X-radiographs and anatomical diagrams they had been trained to interpret in
medical school.

With the benefit of hindsight, it might appear odd that the MIT group, unlike
McLoughlin and Guastivino, did not seriously consider the possibility of constructing two-dimensional images from pulse-echo information, in a manner
analogous to PPI. MIT was a major center of radar and sonar research, and by
the late 1940s, both these pulse-echo technologies could supply two-dimensional
images. Furthermore, the difficulty in extrapolating from X-radiography to
transmission ultrasound was already well understood in the industrial context.
As Sproule had pointed out in 1946:

The analogy with X-rays breaks down . . . in a number of ways and this accounts for the meagre success claimed for the above method [transmission ultrasound]. X-rays are not refracted or reflected appreciably from the boundary of a solid or liquid medium whereas supersonic rays are generally reflected and refracted heavily. This simple difference is of great importance in the practical application of supersonic waves to the detection of flaws. For instance, suppose that we wish to scan a sheet of steel . . . in a liquid bath . . . the coefficient of reflection at the liquid solid interface will be so high that the energy due to direct transmission from the transmitter to the receiver will be small in comparison with the energy which has suffered multiple reflections between the parallel surfaces of the sheet or between the surfaces of the sheet and the walls of the bath . . . [A] flaw . . . is completely obscured by these multiple reflections.[66]

The bony vault of the skull was to prove similar, acoustically speaking, to the walls of an industrial water bath. And there was another potential problem with examining the head by ultrasound, one that had no parallel in the industrial situation. In the medical context, transducers could not be placed directly against the study object, the brain. They had to be placed on the outside of the head, so the ultrasound beam had to pass through the bones of the skull, which strongly reflect, refract, and absorb sound energy.

The Acoustics Laboratory at MIT, however, was riding a wave of technological optimism. Throughout the war years and into the postwar era, MIT's scientists had swept all before them in the successful development of radar and other advanced electronic systems. Doubtless, no problem seemed beyond them. Bolt was in charge of the most lavishly equipped acoustics laboratory in the world. He had assembled an impressive team of scientists, doctors, and engineers. He had seen what Dussik seemed to have achieved with transmission ultrasound, and it is understandable that he should have considered that, with the greatly superior resources at their disposal, his team could do better still.[67] Bolt was not unaware of the problems posed by the skull. But, as Yoxen remarks, the highly accomplished electronic engineers at MIT were not likely to be easily daunted by the challenge of extracting a meaningful signal from within a high level of noise.[68] They were confident that they could provide what the clinicians wanted—a shadowgraph capable of displaying detail in soft tissue.

By 1950, the MIT engineers had built a working test apparatus that incorporated the latest piezo-ceramic transducers and other refinements of Dussik's prototype.[69] In 1953, however, their program of investigation was subjected to devastating criticism. As noted above, researchers working for Siemens were also investigating the diagnostic potential of transmission ultrasound. W. Güttner and his colleagues had come to the conclusion that variations in the thickness of the skull would mask any changes in the intensity of transmitted ultrasound produced by the soft tissue of the brain.[70] They demonstrated that images virtually identical to Dussik's hyperphonographs could be obtained if an empty skull were used as the target object, instead of an intact head. Dussik's images were evidently not visualizations of the ventricles but artifacts, produced by the variable absorption of the skull bones. In 1954, the MIT group confirmed Güttner's findings, acknowledged the force of his argument, and announced the end of their research on transmission imaging.[71]

The vanquishing of MIT's aspirations by Siemens can be seen as a victory for one diagnostic technology over another, as a triumph, indeed, for the dominant technology in the field over an emerging rival. Alongside its interest in ultrasound, Siemens was a major manufacturer of X-ray equipment. Owing to major investments in R&D by Siemens and its competitors, the sensitivity and accuracy of X-radiography was improving rapidly in the 1950s. Güttner's argument was essentially that X-ray techniques, despite their undoubted limitations when applied to the head, were getting better at brain visualization and had greater potential than the ultrasonic alternative. Bolt effectively conceded the point when he checked the accuracy of his ultrasonograms against X-ray images and found the former wanting in comparison with the latter. By the mid-1950s, there were also other possible solutions to the difficult problem of locating brain tumors—notably, tracer techniques using radioactive isotopes and scintillation counters. To many commentators, ultrasound seemed to possess neither the advantage of being the established diagnostic method nor, any longer, that of being at the cutting edge of innovation.[72] Güttner's disparagement of the potential of ultrasound in brain imaging was, it should be noted, quite general. From measurements of the reflection coefficient at the interface between brain tissue and cerebrospinal fluid, he concluded that pulse-echo techniques would be no more successful than transmission ultrasound in localizing the ventricles.[73]

Despite abandoning the diagnostic project, the MIT group remained active in basic ultrasonic research into the 1960s.[74] Much of their work, such as the measurements of dosage and the velocity of sound in soft tissue, was of considerable value to other investigators, but their withdrawal from diagnostic research was the end of attempts to use transmission ultrasound for imaging purposes.

(((((Despite improvements in X-radiography and other diagnostic techniques, the enormous clinical demand for improved diagnosis of brain disease remained substantially unmet. By the time the MIT group withdrew from the field, several other workers had taken up the challenge of trying to localize cerebral pathology with ultrasound. Some of the most active centers for diagnostic ultrasonic research, from the late 1940s onward, were in Japan. In 1949, Rokuro Uchida, a physicist working with Kenji Tanaka, professor of surgery at the Juntendo University, Tokyo, modified an industrial flaw detector for medical research. Uchida and his colleagues investigated the use of pulse-echo ultrasound in the diagnosis of intracranial lesions.[75] In 1956, and again in 1957, Japanese investigators presented papers at medical ultrasound conferences in the United States.[76] Uchida and his compatriots met many of the leading American ultrasound investigators. Despite these contacts, the Japanese work was largely ignored in the West. A major review of cerebral applications of diagnostic ultrasound published in 1963 failed to make any mention of work done outside Europe and the United States. It was not until the 1980s that a full appreciation of the pioneering investigations undertaken in Japan appeared in English.[77]

Work on the localization of brain pathology was also underway in England. In the late 1940s, Professor Valentine Mayneord had become interested in the diagnostic possibilities of ultrasound.[78] Mayneord was Head of the Department of Physics as Applied to Medicine at the Institute of Cancer Research, Royal Cancer Hospital, London.[79] R. C. Turner, an electronics engineer in Mayneord's department, began work with a Henry Hughes Mk IIb flaw detector. By 1950, he was able to elicit an echo from the midline of the brain and to demonstrate that this echo could be displaced from its normal position by space-occupying lesions in either cerebral hemisphere. Turner showed his results to several clinicians, including Wylie McKissok, a neurosurgeon. McKissok was very interested in Turner's findings but did not envisage any immediate clinical application. However, he introduced several visiting clinical colleagues to Turner, notably Lars Leksell, chief neurosurgeon at the University Hospital in Lund, Sweden.[80]

Leksell was particularly interested in the identification and localization of traumatic brain damage, especially intracranial hemorrhage, the early recognition of which is crucially important in the management of head injuries.[81] He knew that a subdural hematoma often displaces the midline, but this deviation could not be detected by existing clinical methods with the skull intact. Intrigued by Turner's findings, Leksell borrowed a Kelvin and Hughes Mk IIb flaw detector from a company that undertook nondestructive testing for the Swedish ship-building industry. Initial clinical trials were wholly unsuccessful.

Two years later, Leksell discovered that two of his colleagues at Lund, the cardiologist Inge Edler and the physicist Hellmuth Hertz, had acquired a Siemens flaw detector to investigate its potential in the diagnosis of heart disease. In December 1953, Leksell was faced with a clinical emergency: a baby boy who had suffered a head injury and was in a deepening coma. The case presented Leksell with a critical problem in differential diagnosis. The coma might be the result of diffuse cerebral edema, in which case surgical intervention would be futile and probably detrimental. Alternatively, it might be a consequence of intracranial bleeding, in which case immediate surgical intervention was the best, if not the only, hope for the child's survival. Clinical and radiological examination could not provide reliable guidance. Leksell borrowed Edler's instrument to try, once again, to detect any deviation of the midline. This time the technique seemed to work. A midline echo was detected that seemed to be consistently displaced to the left. A burr hole made in the right side of the child's skull revealed a large hematoma. This was successfully removed and the child survived.

Inspired by this success, Leksell subsequently bought a Kelvin and Hughes flaw detector. On a number of occasions over the next two years, he was able to identify midline shifts caused by subdural hematoma or hygroma. He also recognized a case of traumatic pneumocephalus (air in the cerebral ventricles), which was later confirmed by X-ray. Leksell published four case histories in 1956.[82] However, even working with children, whose skulls are thinner and less calcified than those of adults, Leksell found it difficult to obtain consistent results, and only occasionally were they diagnostically useful. Reverberations within the cranial vault proved a formidable obstacle to the application of pulse-echo ultrasound to detecting midline shifts in adults.[83]

Meanwhile, Edler and Hertz were continuing their research into cardiac applications of pulse-echo ultrasound. At the time, the two principal tools used in investigation of the heart were the stethoscope and the electrocardiograph. Both these diagnostic modalities monitored function rather than structure directly. X-radiology was useful in cases of gross enlargement or abnormality but could not reveal fine anatomical or pathological detail, such as the presence of small tumors (myxomas) or the precise extent of damage to a valve. It was also difficult to assess the extent of mitral regurgitation. Thus, for the heart, as for the brain, its constitution and ailments challenged the diagnostic technology of the 1950s.

Using their flaw detector, Edler and Hertz were able to recognize consistent echo patterns coming from the heart, one of which they took to be produced by the motion of the anterior atrial wall.[84] Edler compared the shapes of these echoes in healthy individuals with those of patients with hearts enlarged by mitral stenosis, and he found that variations in echo correlated well with the severity of stenosis as revealed during surgery. He came to rely on A-scan ultrasound in the diagnosis of mitral stenosis and began to study other motion patterns of the heart. Edler's cardiac work was not published until 1954 and, initially, was little known outside Sweden.[85] By this time, however, both he and Leksell were using pulse-echo examinations routinely in their clinical work. The academic medical community in Lund was developing a collective interest in and acceptance of ultrasound as a valid diagnostic modality. As we shall see in chapter 7, this degree of familiarity with the technology would make Lund-based doctors particularly receptive to future developments in ultrasonic diagnosis.

At London's Royal Cancer Hospital, work was continuing on the localization of brain tumors, using their Mk IIb flaw detector.[86] This instrument had two transducers, one transmitting and the other receiving. This arrangement was inconvenient for cranial applications. Positioning a single probe optimally on the curved and uneven surface of the skull was difficult enough; positioning two probes successfully was often an impossible feat of ambidextrous manipulation. Turner thought that for investigations at short range within the skull, a single transducer system would be preferable. Initially he attempted to modify his flaw detector to accept a single probe, but the results were not satisfactory. The decision was made to design a new instrument specifically for brain work, with a very narrow, light probe and a single piezo-ceramic transducer. Development work continued, under Mayneord's auspices, at the Institute for Cancer Research throughout the 1950s. The new instrument was not made public until 1960, and the first clinical trials were published in 1961.[87]

(((((In the early 1950s, in addition to the work being undertaken at MIT, two major programs of research into the diagnostic potential of ultrasound were underway in the United States, one led by Douglass Howry and the other by John Wild. Of the two, Wild was the first to publish his results. For the purposes of our present discussion, it is convenient to turn our attention initially to Howry.

Douglass Hamilton Howry was born in Montana in 1920.[88] While training as a radiologist in the mid-1940s, at the Medical School of the University of Colorado in Denver, he became aware of the limitations of X-radiology in the diagnostic imaging of major organs such as the liver and pancreas. Information that could have been of crucial assistance to therapy was often revealed only at autopsy. Shortly after qualifying in 1947, Howry developed an interest in the potential of ultrasound to improve the visualization of soft tissue. With the help of Roderic Bliss, an electrical engineer, he built a pulse-echo apparatus, along lines similar to those suggested by Young White. Howry's machine incorporated an Air Force surplus amplifier, an oscilloscope built from a hobbyist kit, and the power source from his record player.[89] With this homemade equipment, Howry obtained strong echoes from within the body. He quickly realized that these A-scan images contained a great deal of information—but not in the form he wanted: "The complexity of the sound-reflecting structures produces echoes which are so numerous and variable that . . . consistent results are difficult to obtain."[90] Howry was not interested in trying to interpret abstract patterns of blips on an oscilloscope screen. As Koch emphasizes, Howry's "unwavering goal" was to make "a better X-ray."[91] As a trained radiologist, he sought, as he put it, to achieve a "true image similar to a roentgenograph or photograph."[92] One of his co-workers recalled that Howry was "intent on producing an image comparable to the fixed and stained . . . sections in *Gray's Anatomy*."[93] Howry described his ambition as the creation of ultrasonic images "in a manner comparable to the . . . sectioning of structures in the pathology laboratory." He hoped, in other words, to produce two-dimensional representations in which the body parts were portrayed in accurate spatial relation to one another and in their correct proportions.[94]

At the beginning of his interest in ultrasound, Howry briefly experimented with transmission ultrasound, but he quickly came to appreciate the problems inherent in using the technique for diagnosis, particularly around bony structures.[95] Two-dimensional visualization with ultrasound in a manner strictly analogous to X-ray shadowgraphs did not seem feasible. By the late 1940s, however, other visualization exemplars were available. Methods for producing two-dimensional images by echolocation had been developed for radar applications, notably PPI.

In 1948, Howry began to collaborate with Carl Spaulding, an engineer with considerable experience of radar. Spaulding and Howry concluded, on theoretical grounds, that pulse-echo ultrasound could supply useful two-dimensional images if the target objects were scanned from several directions. By 1950, working again with Bliss and with another engineer, Gerald Posakony, Howry had built his first two-dimensional scanner, the Somascope.[96] To eliminate air and thus ensure good acoustic coupling between transmitter and target, the Somascope's ultrasonic probe was placed in a water tank. A single transducer acted as both transmitter and receiver. The target object was placed at the far side of the tank from the probe. The probe, driven by an electric motor, swept back and forth in an arc around the target, emitting very short ultrasonic pulses at a rate of more than a thousand per second. As the transducer was in constant motion, each new pulse followed a slightly different pathway from the previous one. The returning echoes were displayed as spots of light on an oscilloscope with a long-persistence screen. The brightness of each spot was proportional to the amplitude of the echo it represented, and the position of the spots on the screen corresponded to the point of origin of the echoes in the scanned area. Thus a two-dimensional, cross-sectional image of the target was produced that could be either viewed on the screen or photographed (the form of display known as *B-mode* or *B-scan*).[97] B-mode is similar to PPI but with the transducer moving around the scanned area instead of rotating around a fixed point.

The Somascope produced readily interpretable images of simple, inanimate test objects such as a cup or a condom filled with water. It could locate foreign bodies, such as nails and pieces of plastic, embedded in a lump of liver. However, its images of anatomical structures, such as an extirpated gallbladder or the intact forearm of one of the investigators, were crude and blurred. Far from emulating *Gray's Anatomy*, Howry's early images required labels cross-referencing structures to an anatomical diagram if they were to be deciphered correctly.[98] Moreover, the Somascope's water tank was too small to accommodate any biological object larger than an upper limb.[99] Accordingly, Howry was unable to undertake diagnostic work with this machine. As late as 1955, he presented clinical application as a hope for the future, as the "ultimate use" of the technology.[100] Nevertheless, the images produced by the Somascope were good enough to encourage Howry to persevere with further development.

In 1951, Howry began to work under the auspices of Joseph Holmes, a physician and the director of the Medical Research Laboratory at the Veterans Administration (VA) Hospital in Denver. Holmes secured funding from the VA to support the development of an ultrasonic instrument that could be used clinically. By 1953, with the collaboration of engineers from the University of Denver's Institute of Industrial Research, Howry had constructed an improved version of the Somascope, the M2.[101] Despite the explicit directive of the funding body to develop a diagnostic instrument, the improvements incorporated in the M2 related more to the apparatus's image-producing capability than to its clinical applicability.

A further improved version of the Somascope, the Mark IV, followed shortly.[102] Its water tank was derived from the gun turret of a B-29 bomber and was large enough to hold a human subject. Moreover, the probe could now complete an arc of 360 degrees around the target. Howry introduced other important refinements, notably what he termed *compound circular scanning*, in which the probe had a double motion: as it traveled steadily around the circumference of the tank, the probe also moved rapidly backward and forward.[103] Ultrasound is most strongly reflected when it strikes a reflective surface perpendicularly. Compound scanning produced more 90-degree hits and thus better echoes. The echoes of the same reflective surface from different angles of the probe were integrated as precisely as possible on the oscilloscope screen, providing a clearer image.

Despite Howry's design refinements, reverberation of pulses through the water and off the sides of the tank and the water surface continued to produce artifacts in the final image. Howry sought to overcome the effect of the reverberations by prolonged scanning at high intensity. As a result, the making of an image required the subject to sit motionless in a bath of hot, degassed water for up to forty-five minutes while scanning took place—an ordeal to which ill, frail, or elderly patients could not be reasonably subjected. Moreover, in his determination to extract the greatest possible image definition from the system, Howry insisted that the water in the tank be heavily salted to render its acoustic characteristics as similar as possible to those of tissue. This meant that patients with open wounds, such as those who had recently undergone surgery, could not be scanned.[104] The briny water also created engineering problems, as the machine's components had to be made resistant to corrosion.[105]

Many of the pictures obtained with the Mark IV Somascope were magnificent technical achievements. Particularly notable are some very detailed cross-sectional images of the normal human neck, which have been reproduced many times.[106] Howry also achieved visualization of some pathological abnormalities in the body cavities of patients with extensive metastatic neoplasms, the ultrasonic findings being confirmed on autopsy. Nevertheless, although Howry and Holmes appealed to their clinical colleagues to send them patients to scan, the Mark IV Somascope, like its predecessors, had little or no recognized clinical utility.[107] Throughout the 1950s, indeed, Howry's attention remained fixed on exploring every means of improving the resolution of the ultrasound image. By 1957, he had produced some marvelous pictures and gained considerable recognition from his professional colleagues. He received, for instance, the Gold Medal Award for Outstanding Research from the American Medical Association and the Medal of Honor of the Radiological Society of North America.[108] But he still had not convincingly demonstrated to his peers that his invention had real diagnostic value.

Howry's continued, almost obsessive drive for further refinement of the ultrasound image eventually frustrated his engineers and his funding patrons, both of whom wished to see machines built for clinical service.[109] The Denver team was not able to publish an account of an unequivocally successful diagnostic application until 1959, and even then only in the relatively minor areas of edema and ascites.[110] It was into the 1960s before a machine suited to hospital use was finally built.[111] Howry left Denver in 1962 to resume his career as a radiologist at the Massachusetts General Hospital; he died in Boston in 1969.

(((((John Julian Wild was born in Kent, England, in 1914 and graduated in medicine from the University of Cambridge in 1942.[112] He spent two years as a surgical registrar at University College Hospital (UCH), London. (In the British system, a registrar is a middle-ranking hospital doctor, above house officer but below consultant.) Later in the Second World War, he practiced surgery at Miller General Hospital, Greenwich, and at North Middlesex Hospital, before joining the Royal Army Medical Corps. On demobilization in 1946, he emigrated to the United States, taking up an appointment as a postdoctoral surgical fellow at the University of Minnesota. Despite the surgical fellowship, Wild's ambition on leaving Britain was to give up surgery and become a full-time clinical scientist. He had already undertaken some important basic research, having elucidated the lifecycle of the protozoan parasite *Trichomonas vaginalis*. And he had greatly admired the clinical science he had seen undertaken by Harold Himsworth and his colleagues at UCH. He had also come to the conclusion that he was not temperamentally suited to routine clinical work.[113]

As well as being a trained surgeon and an experienced researcher, Wild was an inventor of considerable ingenuity and enthusiasm. During the war, for example, he had responded to petrol rationing by successfully modifying his motorcycle to run on gas generated by a solid-fuel burner built into the sidecar.[114] Early in his medical career, he began applying these skills and interests to clinical problems. While working in Greenwich, he had become concerned with the problem of intestinal stoppage and subsequent distension due to build-up of gas in the bowel, a frequent complication among bomb-blast victims in London during the Blitz. Wild developed a device to facilitate intubation of the bowel, patenting his invention in 1944.[115] His intention when he arrived in Minnesota was to do further work on intestinal obstruction. However, while in Minneapolis, he began to appreciate more fully that two (at least) distinct clinical entities were implicated in the interruption of intestinal motility, one caused by mechanical blockage and the other by factors intrinsic to the physiological functioning of the bowel.[116] He postulated that these two conditions might be differentiated by determining the thickness of the bowel wall around the point of obstruction.

One evening in the spring of 1949, at a cocktail party in Minneapolis, Wild was introduced to a physicist, Dr. Finn J. Larsen of the Research Division of Honeywell, the electronics manufacturer. During the war, while working for the Navy, in cooperation with MIT's Radiation Laboratory, Larsen had designed an ultrasonic radar trainer.[117] The navigational radar system of an aircraft was simulated by replacing the radar transmitter and receiver with an ultrasonic transducer and "flying" the transducer over a model landscape submerged in a water tank. The ultrasound trainer was an important invention in the context of the war because, before its introduction, basic training in air-to-ground navigation by radar had to be done while airborne, an expensive and resource-intensive procedure. To optimize miniaturization, the ultrasound transducer in the trainer operated at the relatively high frequency of 15 MHz.

On hearing of Wild's research interest, Larsen suggested that the pulse-echo ultrasound equipment in the trainer might be applicable to the problem of measuring the thickness of bowel wall. He had noticed that his fingers produced ultrasonic echoes when placed in the path of the ultrasound beam.[118] A radar trainer had recently been installed at the Naval Air Station at Wold-

Chamberlain Field, near Minneapolis, and Larsen was able to secure access for Wild to this facility.

In his initial series of experiments with the trainer, Wild received considerable assistance from the engineer in charge, Donald Neal. A small metal container was devised into which the quartz transducer, removed from its tank, could be fitted. The container was open at one end and was filled with water, the materials to be tested being placed across the opening. The first specimen that Wild and Neal examined was a section of small intestine from a freshly killed dog. Wild found that different echoes were received when the intestine was arranged in one, two, or three layers. These investigations were done in A-mode, but Wild was immediately intrigued. Wild and Howry were, at this time, unaware of each other's ultrasound investigations, but Wild later contrasted his attitude to A-scan images with that of Howry and other early investigators.

> Howry was not a . . . clinician, he was not a . . . biologist so he felt that A-scan echoes were horseshit and no use to him and I, on the other hand, when I . . . saw them, I thought it was a bloody miracle, the challenge to get something out of them. That was the same with Ludwig and Struthers. They found these echoes coming out of their crude machines too confusing to bother with.[119]

Next, Wild examined the first fresh human specimen that came to hand, a piece of stomach removed from a patient with a carcinomatous ulcer. Wild found that he could detect differences between the A-scan echoes from normal and cancerous tissue. Moreover, he was surprised to note that he could trace the infiltration of the cancerous tissue into the normal stomach wall, even where no changes were visible on the surface of the specimen. This immediately suggested to him that pulse-echo ultrasound might be of value in the detection of in situ tumors, at least in accessible portions of the gastrointestinal tract. Again, Wild's approach contrasted with that of the Denver-based investigators. If Howry's Somascope had been used in the detection of tumors, they would have been identified by their disturbance of "the gross structure of the body, as in X-radiology."[120] Wild, on the other hand, sought to recognize cancerous tissue directly by identifying what he considered to be its distinctive ultrasonic properties. Wild quickly wrote and sent off his first paper on diagnostic ultrasound, which duly appeared in *Surgery* in February 1950.[121]

To allow the active scanning of specimens, Wild and Neal built a moveable probe. The quartz crystal was fixed into a small cylinder that could be filled with water and sealed with a thin rubber membrane. The Ultrasonoscope, as it was called, was connected to the amplifier of the radar trainer by long, flexible cables, allowing the device to be placed directly against the skin or against the surface of an exposed organ. Late in 1949, Wild used this equipment to examine an entire brain, removed immediately after death. A large mass was palpable in the right frontal lobe. Wild was again able to note clear differences in the A-scan appearance of the neoplasm and of normal brain tissue. Moreover, by using the echoes of the known tumor as a comparison, he located a further tumor in the thalamic region, which was neither visible nor palpable but the presence of which was later confirmed when the brain was sectioned.[122] These startling observations on brain and stomach tissue set Wild off on a long program of research into the use of ultrasound for the detection of early cancer.

The transducer that Wild used in these early experiments vibrated at 15 MHz, a much higher frequency than that used by other early investigators. Howry, for instance, worked with a crystal oscillating at 2 MHz. Wild had not deliberately chosen this frequency; it was simply the frequency of the equipment that happened to be at hand. It was fortuitous that, with its short wavelength, ultrasound at 15 MHz gave clear echoes and very good definition—hence its advantages in characterizing the fine structure of tissue. On the other hand, the disadvantages of very high frequency are relatively short penetration and thus very little depth of field. To obtain clinically useful information about the condition of the intestinal wall, the probe would need to be situated directly within the lumen of the gut. In other words, diagnostic ultrasound would have to become a variety of endoscopy. Wild did not consider this an insuperable problem. In fact, he suggested the construction of such a probe in his first paper on ultrasound.[123] Based on his experience with intestinal intubation, Wild's initial working assumption was that ultrasonic investigation of the gut would be by the rectal or esophageal route. There was, however, a design constraint on an ultrasonic intestinal probe that did not apply to a tube devised to alleviate blockages: the necessity, as Wild saw it, to incorporate a water barrier between the transducer and the target tissue. Wild assumed this essential partly to ensure good acoustic coupling and partly because the type of transducer used in the radar trainer generated a considerable amount of heat. If it were introduced into living bowel, it would have to be cooled in some way. Wild's early papers therefore envisaged an intestinal ultrasonic transducer contained within a water-filled balloon. This requirement posed a substantial obstacle to the immediate application of ultrasound as a diagnostic tool for intestinal investigations.

Wild prided himself on the breadth of his interests in biology and medicine and had no intention of confining himself to gastroenterology.[124] He looked around for other fields in which to use the Ultrasonoscope and soon realized that it might be readily applied to the diagnostic investigation of the breast. In this application, depth of field would not be a seriously limiting factor. Moreover, since the transducer would remain outside the body, the size or temperature of the probe would be less important. But Wild faced an obstacle to developing this field of inquiry. The admission of civilian women to a U.S. Naval base was strictly forbidden. He and Neal resorted to smuggling their subjects into Wold-Chamberlain Field under cover of darkness. Despite these suboptimal working conditions, a paper describing the successful tissue characterization of two breast lesions appeared in the *Lancet* in March 1951.[125]

On the basis of these early successes, Wild secured a grant from the National Cancer Institute (NCI) of the National Institutes of Health (NIH) to explore the clinical potential of pulse-echo ultrasonic diagnosis. He was now able to recruit an assistant, John Reid, a newly graduated electrical engineer who had previously worked as a radar technician in the Navy.[126] The NCI funding also enabled Wild to build a new ultrasound machine, thus freeing him from the inconveniences of using the naval trainer, access to which was becoming more problematic with the outbreak of the Korean War. Complications loomed, however. Wild was having difficulties in the Department of Surgery at the University of Minnesota. He was not being allowed to devote himself solely to clinical research as he had hoped, and his relationship with his head of department, the well-known and controversial gastrointestinal surgeon Owen Wangensteen, was deteriorating.[127] Wild was effectively denied laboratory space in his own department. He solved the problem by designating his house a research institution, and so, as Reid recalled, "we proceeded to build the clinical machine out of primarily war surplus radar parts in his basement."[128]

Initially, Wild was content to pursue his diagnostic investigations with an A-mode display. However, one of Reid's teachers in the Department of Electrical Engineering suggested that they might think of experimenting with two-dimensional visualization using a scanning probe and a brightness-modulated (B-mode) display. Wild and Reid had soon modified their existing equipment to achieve what they called "two-dimensional echography." On the screen of the new apparatus, dubbed the Echograph, each returning echo was represented by the brightness of a spot on the vertical time-base deflection. Hence the echoes from a probe held stationary against the target produced a vertical line of spots of varying brightness—"one-dimensional echography," as Wild now termed it.[129] If the probe were moved across the study object, vertical lines would follow one another in a horizontal series across the oscilloscope screen, thus forming a two-dimensional profile of the echoes produced in a single plane of the study object. Wild compared one-dimensional echography to the visualization of a single needle biopsy and two-dimensional echography to a graph made from the results of a large number of adjacent needle biopsies. The latter technique might also be compared to imaging of the seabed obtained from the echosounder of a moving ship.

Wild and Reid tried out their new system on a patient hospitalized with recurrence of a myoblastoma in the left thigh. By comparing echograms from both legs, they were able to display, albeit rather crudely, the position of the tumor. As Reid described it, "We were able to make our system work, make the first scanning records in the clinic, and mail a paper off to *Science* . . . within the lapsed time of perhaps ten days."[130] Their preliminary statement of results was accepted by *Science* late in 1951 and published in February 1952. This paper contained the first two-dimensional ultrasound image to appear in the medical press. Wild and Reid were thus able to claim priority over Howry and Bliss, whose first account of their more elaborate system was published a few weeks later.[131]

Later in 1952, Wild and Reid published another paper that contained the first two-dimensional echograms of breast tissue.[132] Wild argued that it was possible, by calibrating his equipment on the normal breast, to determine whether a lesion in the abnormal breast was malignant or benign. The second publication described a series of twenty-one cases in which substantial agreement was achieved between preoperative ultrasonic diagnosis of malignancy and postoperative histological determination. Wild hypothesized that cancerous tissue returned more echoes than normal tissue because of the greater concentration of cell nuclei in a rapidly dividing tumor.

Wild was soon able to move the project to St. Barnabas Hospital in downtown Minneapolis, which greatly increased the number of available breast cancer patients. He developed considerable experience in comparing his ultrasonic examination of breast lumps with histological findings on biopsy. Wild and Reid recorded some impressive diagnostic coups at this time. In May 1953,

Mrs. M.J. complained of a pain in her left nipple, of only five days' duration. A statement by her examining clinicians, Drs. J. H. Strickler and C. O. Rice, recorded that "examination of the breast revealed a slightly enlarged, slightly indurated, reddened left nipple, as compared to the right."[133] She had no palpable lump in her breast and no distortion of, or discharge from, the nipple. The preliminary diagnosis was an infection, and she was referred to ultrasound investigation merely as a precaution. Wild and Reid located what they thought was a typical carcinoma, 7 mm in width, under the nipple.[134] A surgeon was unable to confirm the presence of the tumor by palpation even when its precise location was indicated to him, but the ultrasonic finding was shortly confirmed by biopsy. This case was presented at a meeting of the Minnesota State Medical Association in St. Paul later in the same month and won Wild and Reid the conference prize. Strickler and Rice put on record their appreciation.

> Needless to say, the clinician and surgeon involved in this case were amazed at the accuracy of the echograph studies . . . Although one might tend to underestimate the value of a single instance, it should be pointed out that such a demonstration in a case where clinical evidence was far in favor of a benign lesion, and in which the clinical evidence was in error, is to us much more impressive than had the diagnosis been made in several cases where the clinical diagnosis would have been obvious.[135]

In another case, a nurse at St. Barnabas, unaware that Wild and Reid were working only with patients with suspected breast disease, requested an ultrasonic examination of her breasts as part of a routine health check-up. She was entirely asymptomatic clinically. Wild and Reid detected a tiny lesion in the areolar area, the existence and malignancy of which was later confirmed by biopsy.[136]

Wild's ultrasonic technique did have certain limitations. Breasts differ greatly in tissue density, so the equipment had to be carefully calibrated for each individual. This meant that one patient could not be compared with another. The precise calibration was, as Wild acknowledged, something of a craft skill, which required considerable experience to perfect. Moreover, given that one breast was used as the benchmark for the other, no reliable diagnosis was possible if both breasts were affected by disease. Nevertheless, by the end of 1953, Wild and Reid described a series of forty-one comparisons between echographic and histological diagnosis of solid lesions, with agreement in thirty-eight cases.[137]

In 1953, Wild and Reid successfully diagnosed a breast cyst for the first time.

> All the while we worked with scanners, the nagging question was, would we ever see a cystic lesion? We had been talking about what a cyst would look like in both A- and B-mode machines for some time, but had never seen a characteristic pattern. Wild was afraid that we had been missing cysts, and that there was something wrong with the machine. I insisted that the cysts should have hollow centers and even drew on a piece of paper what I thought a cyst would look like. One day . . . I looked up from adjusting the knobs and saw on the scanner the picture we had predicted. "Look, John, a cyst!" I said, forgetting that the patient would be unnecessarily worried by such talk between us. But Wild was overjoyed. It was, indeed, a hollow cyst. In fact, she had several of them and they all showed up beautifully. We explained these were a non-malignant growth and the patient was equally happy. For the following week, we seemed to see nothing but cystic patients, one after another had cysts. Until Wild again became worried that something was wrong with the machine. This was not an unusual pattern, however, since the doctor seems to blame the machine and the engineer is certain that he has made some new medical discovery.[138]

Cysts, which are filled with transonic liquid, return very few echoes from their interior, and appeared as blank "holes" on the Echograph screen.

Wild's report to the NCI in July 1953 was a confident summary of a remarkable period of sustained, creative research. As well as the successful breast investigations, he and Neal had built a prototype Echo-endoscope, with which they hoped to undertake two-dimensional echography of the rectum and lower bowel. They also described a prototype of a transvaginal scanner to examine the cervix and adjacent pelvic organs. Wild also indicated how his breast scanner might be modified to allow routine mass screening for breast cancer.

By 1956, Wild reported that 117 palpable breast abnormalities had been examined ultrasonically, with an accuracy of diagnosis as to whether malignant or benign of more than 90 percent. Using his skill in navigating the gastrointestinal tract, Wild had also obtained endoscopic ultrasound images from the sigmoid colon. But technical difficulties and problems in the interpretation of complicated echo patterns had delayed the clinical application of both the rectal and vaginal scanners. These were not Wild's only problems. His relationship with Wangensteen and with the Department of Surgery had continued to deteriorate. Nor was the situation at St. Barnabas wholly satisfactory. Bioengineering was a relatively new area of medical inquiry, and many clinical staff had difficulty accepting the presence of an engineer in their midst. Wild and Reid were also facing problems with the dissemination of their ideas, as Reid later described.

> Imaging in medicine was done with X-rays and people did not know what to do with us . . . We had difficulties getting papers accepted for publication because the only available reviewers were apt to be radiologists who knew nothing about what we were trying to do, or physicists who knew too much about low frequency sound waves . . . [We] found ourselves treated as misguided or demented investigators at most of the scientific meetings.
>
> The whole concept of transcutaneous diagnosis using human beings was very difficult to get across. Most cancer scientists in those days assumed that we were working on animals or surgical specimens. We could not seem to get it through their head what we were actually doing . . . We were involved in controversy almost from the beginning, with Wild being a character who rather seemed to enjoy this sort of thing, and who could go out and bring it upon himself in case things were getting a little bit dull. It was an exciting life.[139]

The NCI, moreover, had for some time not been happy with the way Wild spent its money. In the 1950s, the principles governing the funding program of the NIH enshrined the absolute priority of laboratory over clinical inquiry. It was assumed that extensive basic research should always precede any clinical application. Wild, by contrast, was applying his new equipment directly to human subjects without preliminary animal studies. This made the directors of the NCI uneasy. In 1953, it was made a condition of the renewal of their funding that Wild and Reid should establish the ultrasound distinction between benign and malignant tumors through a series of animal trials. Wild calmly continued his work on clinical material and "thumbing his nose at the NCI," as Koch puts it, entitled his next research report "Clinical Results of Echographic Diagnosis of Living Intact Lesions of the Breast of Primate, *Homo sapiens* (Female)."[140] Wild's disputatious spirit was provoked, and he vigorously defended the principle of purely clinical research against the precepts of the NCI.

By the mid-1950s, the NCI had another problem with its funding of ultrasound research. The institute was now also generously supporting the work of Howry and his colleagues in Denver. The NCI's research directors were understandably concerned with the possibility of duplication of effort. Accordingly, a special review of the merits of the two ultrasound research projects was commissioned. Two of the leading members of the review committee were

Theodor Hueter, lately of MIT, and William Fry, Head of the Acoustics Laboratory, University of Illinois. Both men were physicists and, as Koch documents, both strongly supported the policy that methodical testing in the laboratory should precede clinical application.[141] This opinion led the review committee to favor Howry's approach over Wild's. There was also concern that Wild's method was overdependent on his subjective craft skill at manipulating the controls of the Echograph, and his work on tissue characterization had not been independently confirmed—which was hardly surprising, given that no one else was working with 15 MHz ultrasound. Lower frequencies could not achieve the fine definition required to detect significant differences in reflectivity at the cellular level.

Remarkably, the review panel chose to minimize, indeed virtually to ignore, the differences between the research aims and practices of the two groups of workers. Despite Howry being interested primarily in producing better pictures and Wild in characterizing tissue, despite Howry's transducers operating at 2.5 MHz and Wild's at 15 MHz, and despite Howry's work using a probe in a large water bath and Wild's using hand-held scanners or endoscopes, the two research projects were represented as essentially identical in character and purpose. Wild's equipment, however, was deemed technically inferior, and the review panel recommended that he be given funds to buy a machine from Howry with which to continue his diagnostic work.

If Wild had accepted this advice, he would have had to radically change the direction of his research. As it was, he continued plowing his own furrow and supplemented the support he received from the NCI with grants from local sources in Minnesota. His relationship with St. Barnabas was souring, however. The senior members of the hospital staff were eager to see Wild contribute to the routine detection of breast cancer and were impatient with his insistence on pushing forward with experimental developments. They had, or so they believed, been promised in 1953 that clinical deployment was imminent. Wild's style of work, moreover, was not always easy on his colleagues. In his view, a good researcher "kicks and shoves and pushes people . . . Creativity must come from struggle."[142] Holmes described Wild as a "rugged individualist," which would seem to be something of an understatement.[143] In 1957, Wild's key collaborator, John Reid, left to undertake graduate study at the University of Pennsylvania, and Wild's relationship with Reid's successors was always problematic.

In the early 1960s, under pressure from Congress, the funding policy of the NIH changed. Projects with direct clinical relevance were now favored. In

1962, Wild received a substantial grant to develop his ultrasound research. He recruited new staff and reequipped his laboratory. However, before this new influx of funding could bear fruit, his long-running dispute with Wangensteen reached a crisis point. In 1964, under a court order, Wild's equipment was seized and his laboratory closed. He was to spend the next fourteen years engaged in a legal battle for redress.[144] During this time, he could do very little scientific work. Meanwhile, his claims that benign and malignant tumors could be distinguished on the basis of their ultrasonic characteristics remained unconfirmed by other workers, none of whom chose to work with 15 MHz transducers.[145]

Wild would have to wait many years for recognition by the scientific community of his pioneering efforts.[146] In 1978, he received the Pioneer Award of the American Institute of Ultrasound in Medicine, and in 1991, the prestigious Japan Prize. In 1998, he was named a Columbus Scholar and received the Frank Annunzio Award. He was nominated for a Nobel Prize. However, neither his transcutaneous nor his endoscopic instruments were accepted into the routine clinical repertoire. In this respect, his contribution to ultrasound scanning was, like Howry's, and indeed like Hueter's and Dussik's, a failed innovation.

CHAPTER THREE

Ian Donald before Ultrasound I

St. Thomas's Hospital and the Royal Air Force

Ian Donald, Regius Professor of Midwifery at the University of Glasgow, was the leading clinician involved in the introduction of obstetric ultrasound. In this chapter, we explore his early life and career with a view to understanding how and why he developed his distinctive practice of obstetrics and his interests in medical technology. Donald was not solely a clinical and technological innovator. Rather, his involvement in diagnostic ultrasound was one expression of a holistic conception of the nature and scope of obstetrics and gynecology. An investigation of his medical and moral education reveals the background to his characteristic concern with combining the clinical, research, and social roles of the obstetrician, a concern that was to be formative in his deployment of the ultrasound scanner. We also explore his first venture into technological innovation: his invention of a device to support neonates with breathing difficulties.

Ian Donald was born on December 27, 1910, in Liskeard, Cornwall, where his father was a general practitioner.[1] Despite his place of birth, his arrival might be said to have added a new member to a family of Scottish doctors. Ian Donald's paternal grandfather, James Turner Donald, was a general practitioner and medical officer of health in Paisley in the late nineteenth century.[2] James's son, John, graduated in medicine from the University of Glasgow in 1898. He contracted tuberculosis as a young man and never fully recovered his health. To escape the British winters, he regularly accepted engagements as a ship's doctor. It was on one of these trips that he met his future wife, Helen Barrow Wilson.

Miss Wilson was the daughter of a wealthy shipowner from Liverpool. She was an accomplished musician, and if her elevated social position had not precluded her working for a living, she might have been a concert pianist. She asserted her independence by traveling, with a chaperone, in the Far East.

While staying in Government House in Penang, Malaya, she was invited to play the piano after an official dinner. Dr. John Donald was one of the dinner guests.

Shortly afterward, Helen Wilson and John Donald sailed back to England together, already engaged to be married—an arrangement that shocked her conventional, upper-middle-class family. Nor did Mr. Wilson think that a general practitioner had sufficient social status to be welcomed as a prospective spouse for his daughter. Dr. Donald, for his part, delighted in shocking his fiancée's family with forthright expressions of his egalitarian views, on occasion describing himself as a Bolshevik. Despite her father's continued opposition, the couple married in 1908, and John Donald, previously a Presbyterian, adopted his wife's Anglicanism.

Ian Donald was the eldest of the four children of Dr. and Mrs. John Donald who survived infancy.[3] He had two sisters, Margaret (b. 1912) and Alison (b. 1914), and a brother, Malcolm (b. 1915). Ian was educated first at Warriston Preparatory School in Moffat in southern Scotland and then at Fettes College, Edinburgh (which he detested).[4] His father placed great emphasis on the importance of a broad education, conversing in French at the dinner table and encouraging his children to memorize passages from Shakespeare and the Bible.[5] Dr. Donald also set his children a personal example of charitable sympathy and compassion for those less fortunate, often inviting needy patients into his house for food and warmth.

In 1925, the Donalds moved to South Africa, with the hope that a warmer climate might improve Dr. Donald's health. The family settled in Kenilworth, near Cape Town, and Ian attended Diocesan College, in Rondebosch, on the outskirts of Cape Town. Diocesan College, perhaps South Africa's leading public school, was an Anglican foundation. Ian enjoyed the school's religious ethos and the quality of the teaching of literature, music, and classics.[6]

In South Africa, Ian developed new leisure interests. His father, whose physical condition was worsening, began to feel that he was not playing a sufficiently active part in his son's life. He employed a Mr. Hawkshurst to teach Ian woodwork and had a workshop built at the rear of their house. Hawkshurst also taught Ian some elementary electronics, enabling him to build, among other devices, a "cat's whisker" radio set. The boy developed a fascination with mechanical contrivances and inventions of all sorts. He began to attend exhibitions of engineering and manufacturing equipment. He also learned to sail, becoming a skilled and enthusiastic yachtsman.

Eighteen months after the Donalds arrived in South Africa, when Ian was just sixteen years old, tragedy struck. All the members of the family except Dr. Donald and Alison became seriously ill with what was diagnosed as diphtheria. But there can be little doubt that they had contracted a streptococcal infection and were suffering from rheumatic fever.[7] Mrs. Donald died of heart failure. Ian and Margaret recovered, but both were later to develop serious valvular disease of the heart.

John Donald, overcome with grief, outlived his wife by only three months. In his will, he named their housekeeper, Maud Grant, as his children's guardian. As Mrs. Grant had been in the post for only two months at the time of Dr. Donald's death, this was a somewhat unconventional, not to say risky, arrangement. Nevertheless, it seems to have worked quite successfully. The Donald children were able to continue living together, which had been their father's principal intention, and Mrs. Grant stayed with them for many years. They were supported financially by a trust fund set up under the terms of Mrs. Donald's will. Whereas Dr. and Mrs. Donald had been broad-church Anglicans, Mrs. Grant was an ardent Anglo-Catholic. The children followed her lead in religion, which had a lasting effect on Ian.

Before his illness, Ian had been an enthusiastic football player, but now he had difficulty keeping up with play. On one occasion, his games master caned him on the playing field for "lack of effort." This injustice soured Ian's attitude toward Diocesan College and perhaps helped encourage the development of his formidable independence of mind.[8]

In 1927, still only sixteen, Ian Donald enrolled at the University of Cape Town. He studied music, classics, and French, graduating with first class honors in 1930. Shortly after his graduation, all the Donald siblings moved to London to continue their education. Ian had finally resolved to fulfill his parents' wish that he enter the medical profession. The accidental discovery of his father's box of surgical instruments, which impressed upon him that medicine could be a practical as well as an intellectual activity, seems to have been influential in his change of heart.[9] In October 1930, he enrolled at St. Thomas's Hospital Medical School.

(((((Situated on the banks of the Thames, across the river from the Houses of Parliament, St. Thomas's Hospital, founded in 1552, was—as it is today—one of the great London teaching hospitals.[10] In the 1930s, like the other London schools, St. Thomas's Medical School was effectively self-governing and only loosely linked to the University of London.[11] Its principal activity was clinical instruction, and it did not wholly participate in the wider academic culture of the university.[12] Donald's time at St. Thomas's as student and junior doctor undoubtedly exerted a considerable influence on his later professional activities, so the type of education and training he received at St. Thomas's Hospital and Medical School is worth investigating. We pay particular attention to how the institutional ethos of St. Thomas's was expressed in the teaching of obstetrics and gynecology and the professional identity of its practitioners.

Donald had entered an establishment with a distinctive character. The senior members of the clinical staff, together with their peers in the other major London voluntary hospitals, constituted an elite and exclusive stratum of Metropolitan medicine.[13] The London "greats," as they were called, generally maintained extensive private practices, with consulting rooms in Harley Street or Wimpole Street. The patrician style and grand manner of the London consultants during the Edwardian and interwar periods found expression in a characteristic set of attitudes to medical practice, which Christopher Lawrence terms "clinical holism."[14] Lawrence argues that the leading consultants of Guy's, St. Bartholomew's, and St. Thomas's embodied a distinctive set of professional and social attitudes. The London greats especially valued breadth of experience in medicine, and they celebrated diagnostic skill at the bedside. They gave only conditional approval to laboratory tests and other nonclinical sources of information. Beyond medicine, they valued broad cultural attainment and humanistic learning. From their point of view, the better sort of doctor was necessarily not merely a technical healer but rather a discerning and civilized gentleman. They presented themselves not only as authoritative arbiters on medical matters but also as custodians of moral values and proper social conduct.

Lawrence identifies Lord Horder, of St. Bartholomew's Hospital, as one of the most influential of the greats in the period between the wars. Sir Maurice Cassidy, consulting physician at St. Thomas's during the 1930s, might be another example. As a young man, Cassidy had turned down the offer of a Cambridge fellowship and an academic career to pursue socially exclusive private practice. He had risen in the ranks of London consulting physicians and acquired the patronage, and indeed the personal friendship, of King George VI. Because of his reputation as an outstanding clinician and his elevated social position, Cassidy exerted considerable influence throughout St. Thomas's. As was typical, he published relatively little. Many of the other physicians and surgeons at St. Thomas's in the interwar period—Sir Henry Tidy, for instance—broadly shared Cassidy's professional and social aspirations.[15]

Emphasizing as they did the importance of breadth of clinical expertise, the greats particularly denigrated organ-specific specialization. "The essential vice of specialism," as Robert Hutchison, physician at the London Hospital and president of the Royal College of Physicians, put it, is "that it tends to concentrate attention on the parts and ignore the whole."[16] Thus, while Cassidy was famous for his interest in diseases of the heart, he insisted that his teaching clinic at St. Thomas's should be a general one, including patients with a wide range of conditions. Tidy scorned the electrocardiograph and defined the "clinical approach" as the study of "the patient and his problem . . . as a whole," a sentiment expressed in similar terms by several of his colleagues.[17] Men like Cassidy and Tidy prided themselves on their ability to comprehend each patient as a unique individual, a skill they believed to be the basis of their superior clinical acumen. Such an understanding related not merely to a patient's physical condition but also to his or her psychological state. The accomplished clinician was able to achieve, it was asserted, a finely tuned personal discrimination that the routine procedures of laboratory diagnosis could not emulate.

Lawrence stresses that the greats did not wholly disdain laboratory methods of diagnosis. Their concern was, rather, that the devolution of diagnostics to laboratory staff would undermine the basis of the clinician's personal interaction with his patient. Laboratory tests were regarded as potentially valuable but secondary and subservient to clinical judgment. Likewise, innovation in medical instrumentation and technology was usually accorded only a guarded and cautious welcome. It is telling that Cassidy was eulogized by his peers as "a general physician who had not been carried away by the mechanism of modern medicine."[18]

Many of Donald's teachers at St. Thomas's would have agreed with Hutchison that whatever the significance of the latest scientific developments, elite clinicians were the heirs of an older and prouder medical tradition. "One cannot help being impressed by the signs of a return towards the Hippocratic outlook," Hutchison wrote. "This revival . . . is called by its adherents by various names . . . the 'science of the individual' . . . but it may perhaps be conveniently described as 'neo-Hippocratism.' It lays great stress . . . on the fundamental unity of the living body, and on the interdependence or integration of its parts."[19]

To London's patrician clinicians, the key medical sciences were morbid anatomy and clinical pathology.[20] It was no coincidence that St. Thomas's had one of the most prestigious departments of pathology in Britain.[21] It is also revealing that, at St. Thomas's, even the pathologists were imbued with the clinical holism that characterized their medical and surgical colleagues. Joseph Bamforth, for example, who served as pathologist from 1922 to 1954 and taught Donald in the 1930s, was praised thus by a clinical colleague for his style of diagnostic inquiry: "The patient as distinct from his illness always took first place, and such ancillaries as test-tubes, manometers, and similar apparatus were relegated to their proper positions." According to another colleague, Bamforth "saw the patient as a whole" and was a good pathologist because he was also a "sound clinician."[22] In many respects, Bamforth was following the example of his illustrious predecessor at St. Thomas's, Professor Stanley Dudgeon, dean of St. Thomas's throughout Donald's student years. Dudgeon insisted on visiting the wards to collect specimens from patients in person and to confer with the patient's clinician.[23] Likewise, the clinicians at St. Thomas's visited the Pathology Department daily for postmortem conferences. The barrier between pathology and clinical practice at the hospital was a very permeable one.

A certain amount of fundamental clinical and scientific research was undertaken at St. Thomas's during the interwar period. For instance, the physiologist Arthur Huggett developed innovative techniques to measure blood-gas tensions in the placenta and fetus of the goat. But the Physiology Department, like most of the preclinical departments, was understaffed and inadequately equipped for high-quality research.[24]

(((((Ian Donald received his MBChB from St. Thomas's in 1937. Shortly afterward, he married Alix Mathilde de Chazal Richards, whom he had known in South Africa. Dr. and Mrs. Ian Donald were married for forty-nine years, until his death in 1987.[25]

Donald remained at St. Thomas's, becoming a house physician in the Department of Obstetrics and Gynaecology and subsequently, in February 1939, a resident.[26] It is fair to say that, in the 1930s, the best graduates were not regularly attracted to obstetrics and gynecology. Obstetrics remained the "Cinderella of the medical curriculum."[27] At St. Thomas's, however, Donald was introduced to the subject by very influential teachers—John Shields Fairbairn, John Prescott Hedley, James Montagu Wyatt, and Arthur Joseph (Joe)

Wrigley. Fairbairn, Hedley, and Wyatt were senior staff in the 1930s, and their teaching and practice exerted considerable influence on Donald at the start of his professional involvement in obstetrics. We discuss Wrigley's impact on Donald later in the chapter.

Fairbairn graduated from St. Thomas's Medical School in 1895.[28] He was appointed to the staff as assistant obstetrics physician in 1902 and retired in 1936. It is salutary to recall that when Fairbairn was an undergraduate, the compulsory teaching of obstetrics was not yet ten years old. Until passage of the Medical Act Amendment Act of 1886, there had been no legal requirement that medical undergraduates be instructed or examined in midwifery. Many students graduated from English medical schools, including St. Thomas's, without even a rudimentary knowledge of the proper management of childbirth. Indeed, disparagement and neglect of obstetrics was characteristic of the discourse of patrician medicine. As Irvine Loudon puts it, "the elite physicians and surgeons of the medical schools . . . saw obstetrics as a messy and unscientific activity divided between ignorant, illiterate, unskilled, untrained midwives and the lowest level of medical men, the general practitioners."[29] Active opposition by senior hospital consultants long prevented the formation of departments of obstetrics and gynecology in several of London's teaching hospitals.[30]

In 1888, in response to the provisions of the new Medical Act, St. Thomas's appointed Charles Cullingworth as obstetric physician and lecturer on midwifery.[31] He had previously been professor of obstetrics and gynecology in Manchester. Although Cullingworth instigated a course of undergraduate lectures on obstetrics, St. Thomas's Hospital had only very limited facilities for the practical teaching of midwifery. Students gained most of their practical training in the management of childbirth "on the district," in the homes of the poor, where they were supposed to be under the supervision of a house officer but frequently were not supervised at all.[32]

On Cullingworth's retirement in 1904, Fairbairn became the senior obstetrician at St. Thomas's and its principal teacher of obstetrics and gynecology. Like his predecessor, Fairbairn vigorously endeavored to improve the teaching of obstetrics. The important difference was that Fairbairn was an insider, a product of St. Thomas's, who wholeheartedly embraced the patrician, holistic ideology of London elite medicine and sought to deploy those values to improve the status of his subject. To Fairbairn, clinical pathology was the fundamental medical science. He had worked as a pathologist at the Chelsea Hospital for Women and regarded his experience there as central to his development as a clinician.[33] Back at St. Thomas's, Fairbairn worked very closely with Joseph Bamforth, as much of the content of Fairbairn's influential textbook *Gynaecology with Obstetrics* exemplifies.[34]

In 1910, Fairbairn presided over establishment of a new maternity facility, the Mary Ward, to improve the provision of clinical instruction in midwifery.[35] This initiative was taken by St. Thomas's in response to recommendations made by the General Medical Council, following the critical report of the Williams Committee in 1906.[36] Fairbairn claimed that the new ward, which had twenty-one lying-in beds, gave St. Thomas's the best facilities for undergraduate training in obstetrics of any general teaching hospital in England. This expansion of services required the engagement of new staff. Hedley and Wyatt, both alumni of St. Thomas's, were appointed.

A prolific writer, Fairbairn was the author of several influential textbooks and was for many years the editor of *Journal of Obstetrics and Gynaecology of the British Empire*. He was one of the principal movers behind the setting up in 1929 of the College of Obstetricians and Gynaecologists, and in 1932 he was elected the college's second president. Thus he was a figure of major significance within British obstetrics in the early decades of the twentieth century. Hedley and Wyatt, likewise, exercised considerable influence on the development of British obstetrics in the interwar years, Hedley taking over as head of department at St. Thomas's in 1928.[37]

In 1925, St. Thomas's introduced, on Fairbairn's initiative, a new scheme under which each student had to devote six months full-time to the combined study of obstetrics, gynecology, and pediatrics.[38] This arrangement remained substantially in place during Ian Donald's time as an undergraduate. The obstetrics component of the course required two months' residence in the hospital, during which Donald would have attended not only the maternity ward but also antenatal and "well baby" clinics. In his second month, he would also have attended district midwifery cases. The next two months were occupied with clerking and dressing in the gynecological department. The final two months were spent in the clinics for sick children and in attendance at gynecological outpatient sessions. Sir John Crofton, also a student at St. Thomas's in the 1930s, remembers with appreciation the breadth and interest of this part of the curriculum and the value of the teaching of obstetrics, gynecology, and pediatrics being combined. He also recalls that Hedley and his colleagues in the Department of Obstetrics, unlike most of the consultants in other departments, encouraged undergraduates to ask questions and discuss clinical matters with senior staff.[39]

A. J. Wrigley wrote appreciatively of Fairbairn as follows:

> After trudging stolidly through the first three years of the preclinical curriculum . . . I arrived eventually before Fairbairn. For many of us for the first time we found the teacher we had always sought, and for that matter had expected to find at the onset of our clinical studies. Here was a man who . . . lived for his work, who understood his subject and to whom patients were patients, not individuals who might (or might not) present interesting symptoms and signs. Here we were made to understand the importance of the background to each case and here we received our initiation into what is now called social medicine.[40]

Fairbairn, Hedley, and Wyatt are central to our understanding of Donald's background as a clinician, not only because they were charismatic teachers at the forefront of a sustained effort to improve the professional status of British obstetrics. They are important also because all three closely identified themselves, socially and professionally, with St. Thomas's Hospital and its patrician culture. They practiced obstetrics and gynecology in a way that expressed the values of that culture. In his writings, Fairbairn articulated a form of obstetric discourse that was harmonious with the ethos of Metropolitan elite medicine and was calculated to emancipate obstetrics from the disregard and denigration it routinely suffered at the hands of London's physicians and surgeons. Study of Fairbairn's texts enables us to see how Metropolitan clinical holism structured obstetrics and gynecology, as taught to Donald.[41] As we shall see in later chapters, certain of the concerns most characteristic of Fairbairn continued to resonate within Donald's own writing and teaching throughout his career.

Fairbairn explicitly identified the clinical holism of patrician culture with the proper practice of obstetrics and gynecology. In November 1931, he gave the Bradshaw Lecture to the Royal College of Physicians. Fairbairn emphasized the close similarity of his position to that of Robert Hutchison, who had given the Harveian Oration only a fortnight earlier. "The terms I have used are not those of the Harveian orator," Fairbairn said, "but I, in another way, have been pleading for the stronger infusion into gynaecology of what he describes as 'neo-Hippocratism' and the restoration of the idea of constitutions, and for the same individualistic study of the patient that he has advocated."[42]

A recurring motif in Fairbairn's writing is that obstetrics and gynecology should not be regarded as a distinct specialty or specialties but rather that they together constituted a branch of general medicine. Specialization, as we have noted, was particularly abhorred by the London elite. Fairbairn's quarrel with the gynecological surgical specialist was that he had too limited a conception of his patient: "My contention is that those professing it [gynecology] should be much more than surgeons with a special flair for the female pelvic organs. Their insight into womankind should surely be more than that disclosed by their inspections of the varying anatomical and pathological appearances met with in the reproductive apparatus." Dismissing the case for specialization, Fairbairn urged that, on the contrary, obstetricians and gynecologists should aspire toward a greater generalism. This involved giving due weight to precisely those issues that were held by Hutchison and Horder to lie at the heart of patrician medicine. "In spite of increased knowledge of morbid anatomy and skill in the craft of surgery," Fairbairn wrote, "the work of the gynaecologist will still be open to criticism if the personal factors in all his patients are not taken fully into account." He argued eloquently that many of his colleagues did not properly recognize the importance of the psychological dimension in both gynecology and obstetrics.[43]

Fairbairn pointed to several other ways in which the obstetrician could broaden his range of professional activities. Appropriate obstetric care should not, in his view, be focused solely on parturition and the perinatal period. It should also encompass the welfare of the woman throughout her pregnancy and of the child in the months and, indeed, years following birth. As we have seen, under his direction, the teaching of obstetrics and gynecology was closely integrated with pediatrics.[44] As a historian of St. Thomas's puts it, Fairbairn saw "maternity and child welfare as an indivisible whole."[45] He was instrumental in the establishment of a baby clinic in 1914, and shortly afterward a similar facility for toddlers was set up. In 1921, he and Hedley founded the first antenatal clinic to be established in an English voluntary hospital. Fairbairn argued explicitly that, besides providing a service for his patients, involvement in antenatal care protected the obstetrician-gynecologist against the dangers of specialization, bringing him "into closer contact with general medicine."[46] Fairbairn was remarkable among obstetricians and gynecologists of his era in urging a professional focus not merely on individual women and children but on society itself. He emphasized that social background directly affected maternal and child health and affected women's attitudes to labor, breast-feeding, and child care. Hence the obstetrician needed to be interested in social medicine and sensitive to welfare issues. He should aim to work closely with the medical almoner.[47] Such a wide range of professional concerns was the badge of the generalist obstetrician-gynecologist as opposed to the narrow surgical specialist.

To Fairbairn, the obstetrician-gynecologist should also exercise moral leadership. He was forthright in his opposition to widening the criteria under which termination of pregnancy was permitted. While acknowledging the need, on occasion, to resort to abortion for medical reasons, Fairbairn saw the trend toward allowing termination on social grounds as a product of a "slackening of moral standards," which the obstetrician should vigorously resist.[48]

In the 1930s, Fairbairn and his colleagues at the College of Obstetricians and Gynaecologists were striving to raise the status and standards of obstetrics. There was much work for them to do. At the time, there was an acute crisis of public confidence in the quality of obstetric care.[49] Donald had entered a branch of medicine that, in the opinion of many contemporaries, both lay and medical, was lagging far behind other fields.

In 1926, Francis Browne, the first full-time professor of obstetric medicine at University College Hospital, critically surveyed the state of his subject thus:

> It is a striking fact that while most rapid advances have been made in the science and art of surgery since the introduction of Listerian methods, the mortality and morbidity rate in child-bed and the puerperium are almost as high as they were in the pre-antiseptic days. I believe . . . in this country alone about 3000 women lose their lives every year as a result of one or other of the diseases and injuries incident upon parturition. In addition to this, about 40,000 infants are annually either born dead or do not survive the first months of life, largely as a result of preventable injuries and diseases. When we add to this, the thousands of women who survive but are more or less permanently injured . . . we are face-to-face with a condition that calls aloud for remedy. There is little doubt that this appalling mortality and morbidity is due largely to the fact that the medical practitioner has hitherto been insufficiently skilled in the practice of midwifery.[50]

Despite similar calls to action by several commentators, however, the situation was deteriorating. In the decade between 1925 and 1934, the annual maternal mortality rate in England and Wales averaged 2.7 per 1,000 live births.[51] This was worse than in any decade since 1875. A woman was more likely to die in labor in the early 1930s than in 1880, even though overall mortality rates had fallen sharply over the intervening period. Serious long-term morbidity among women resulting from childbirth injuries continued to be a major problem.

Irvine Loudon, in his magisterial survey *Death in Childbirth*, unreservedly lays the blame for this disgraceful situation at the door of the leaders of the medical profession. The efforts of Fairbairn and other obstetricians to assimilate their subject into the culture of London medicine had only limited success. Far into the twentieth century, the men who dominated the London Royal Colleges and determined the curricula of the Metropolitan medical schools continued to regard the practice of obstetrics with, at best, condescension, and at worst, contempt. While asserting their traditional right to oversee all branches of medicine and surgery, the Royal Colleges declined to concern themselves with raising standards of training in midwifery. Obstetricians were underrepresented on the General Medical Council, a result of active exclusion by their medical and surgical colleagues. In the medical schools, instruction in "midder" was often presented to undergraduates as a tiresome formality that the student should get through as soon as possible to allow him to move on to more interesting and important clinical matters.[52] For all these reasons, the standard of obstetric education in most English medical schools in the 1920s and 1930s was very poor indeed.

The twenty-one beds of the Mary Ward at St. Thomas's may well have been, as Fairbairn claimed, the best facility for the teaching of midwifery in an English voluntary hospital, but it was, nevertheless, wholly inadequate for the numbers of students in the school. Lying-in wards, whether in voluntary or municipal hospitals, were often poorly resourced in terms of both staff and materials. Such circumstances were not conducive to the inculcation of best practice. As Sir John Crofton recollects:

> Part of our obstetrics, because of shortages at St. Thomas's, was at St. James's which was the LCC [London County Council] hospital and that was a revelation. I went and lived there for a month and was absolutely horrified. The patients were treated like cattle. The medical superintendent was the official clinician for the whole hospital and they had a number of junior people who were paid, I think, rather poorly . . . But patients weren't considered at all. The medical superintendent went to an ante-natal, he was rushing doing PV [per vaginam] examinations and the nurse is trying to keep up the screens for these poor,

embarrassed women having all these things more or less done in public . . . I was really quite horrified and this poor medical superintendent . . . did all the major operations . . . and it all had to be done in such a hurry.[53]

In the community, as we have noted, much obstetric work was undertaken by general practitioners, whose education in midwifery was seriously faulty. Even in the teaching hospitals, standards of training and practice were often deficient. Major obstetric surgery was often delegated to inadequately prepared staff, either general surgeons without special training in obstetrics or junior obstetricians with insufficient experience to work unsupervised.[54] Many obstetrics departments maintained standards of cleanliness and antisepsis significantly lower than those considered acceptable elsewhere. Into the 1930s, it was still commonplace for hospital maternity units to be closed for long periods owing to outbreaks of septic infection. The tardiness with which modern methods for the management of cardiac cases were taken up by obstetricians also caused widespread concern among general physicians and cardiologists.[55]

There can be no doubt whatsoever that this neglect of education, training, and innovation in obstetrics had serious implications for the quality of care received by pregnant and parturient women. The Ministry of Health's *Report of an Investigation into Maternal Mortality*, published in 1937, concluded that at least half of maternal deaths in childbirth were due to avoidable causes. The chief of these causes was medical mismanagement—notably, unwarranted or unskilled use of obstetric instruments.[56]

By the time Donald graduated in 1937, the maternal mortality rate in England remained a national scandal; the figures for Scotland and Wales were still worse. While the rest of medicine had advanced, obstetrics and gynecology had stagnated, or so it appeared to many observers. There was much for a new generation of obstetricians to accomplish in bringing their subject up to the standards being established in other clinical fields. Donald was soon doing what he could to raise standards. In July 1939, shortly after becoming a resident, he wrote to a general practitioner reprimanding him for reckless use of forceps on a patient whose cervix was only partially dilated. Admitted to St. Thomas's, the woman later died of "generalized peritonitis."[57]

Undoubtedly one of the reasons Donald was attracted to the then unfashionable and comparatively neglected subject of obstetrics and gynecology was the intellectually stimulating teaching he had received at St. Thomas's. As we have seen, for the students of Fairbairn and his colleagues, training in obstetrics and gynecology was not just a matter of acquiring clinical technique, important as that was. The student's sense of ethics and moral purpose was engaged, as was his awareness of social and welfare issues.[58] There was an invigorating campaigning character to Fairbairn, Hedley, and Wyatt's efforts to raise the standard of their discipline. Obstetrics also has several other intrinsic attractions, when approached with a positive attitude. For most undergraduates, obstetrics provides their first professional contact with well people rather than sick ones; there is great job satisfaction inherent in presenting happy mothers with healthy babies. And just as important to a man of Donald's interests and predilections, obstetrics was a field in which he could set out to cultivate a broad range of practical as well as intellectual skills. As an obstetrician, he was effectively training to be both surgeon and physician.

It was during his spell at St. Thomas's as a house physician that Donald first began to apply his interest in inventions and mechanical contrivances to medical problems. In the pre-antibiotic era, the clinical management of bladder infections was difficult, and such conditions could be very debilitating. For their treatment, Donald designed an "automatic bladder irrigator." The irrigator was a remarkable device, consisting of a large water tank atop a column, seven or eight feet high. An elaborate system of pipes and catheters produced a continuous flow of water in and out of the patient's bladder. This invention seems to have been well received by patients, but somewhat less so by the nursing staff. Alix Donald describes one incident: "One day there was an old, old man, I think he was a Bishop . . . and he said 'My dear, this is the wonderful young man who has changed my life,' and just then the whole thing overflowed and water poured over the poor old man and his wife and everything and the nurses had to clear it up, they were so cross."[59] Donald demonstrated a more refined version of his irrigator to the Section of Urology of the Royal Society of Medicine in February 1940.[60] It was not only the nursing staff who tended to look askance at Donald's innovations. Some of his senior medical colleagues regarded his creative attitude to established clinical procedures as presumptuous in a young doctor. We might also note that, in treating male patients while an obstetric houseman, Donald was emphasizing a commitment to general medicine worthy of a student of Fairbairn.

(((((In May 1942, Donald was called up for active service in the Royal Air Force as a general duties medical officer. While serving in the RAF, Donald gained considerable knowledge of radar. He received a personal introduction to the world of military echolocation through his sister Alison, by then Mrs. Munro. Early in 1942, Mrs. Munro had been appointed personal assistant to Sir Robert Watson-Watt, scientific adviser to the Air Ministry.[61] One of the major pioneers of radar, Watson-Watt had written the first scientific report outlining the possibility of detecting aircraft by radio waves.[62] He was also responsible for pioneering the application of the cathode-ray oscilloscope to measurement of the time taken for a radio pulse to travel to and from a target.[63] In the late 1930s, as superintendent of Bawdsey Research Station, Watson-Watt had led the team of physicists and engineers who designed and constructed the Chain Home system of radar stations. These stations constituted a major part of the air defenses of the eastern coastline of Britain and played a key role in the successful prosecution of the Battle of Britain.

Mrs. Munro, who had studied mathematics while an undergraduate at Oxford, found the company of Watson-Watt's scientific staff exhilarating. "All these brilliant physicists," she recalls, "and on a Sunday morning they would all meet for coffee and lunch just to talk and you would see these brains firing off ideas coming from them, it was a most wonderful experience . . . and new ideas and new thoughts of equipment, new things radar could do, would emerge from these . . . discussions."[64] One of Mrs. Munro's tasks was to write technical reports on the work of Watson-Watt's group for the chiefs of staff. She was well-informed about developments not only in radar but also in sonar, in particular with the ASDIC system for the detection of submarines. She introduced Donald to Watson-Watt, an encounter that the younger man found memorable.[65] As Dame Alison remembers, her brother "took a great interest in this Watson-Watt thing."[66] From his association with Watson-Watt, Donald learned that radar had gone through a sustained period of technical development from 1936 onward and had become an indispensable instrument of the Allied war effort.

In March 1943, Donald was posted to Benbecula in the Western Isles, as medical officer to 206 Squadron, one of Coastal Command's most illustrious units.[67] Here he quickly gained hands-on experience with the latest echolocation technology. Donald joined the squadron at the climax of the Battle of the Atlantic, the defense of Britain's maritime supply lines against German U-boats.[68] Prior to 1943, the impact of aircraft on the antisubmarine campaign in the Atlantic had been negligible. But early in that year, Coastal Command's effectiveness was enormously enhanced by the introduction of much improved radar equipment. The ASV III was a microwave system, made possible by a remarkable invention, the cavity magnetron, which generated high-frequency radio waves at great intensity.[69] This powerful system of echolocation became operational in Coastal Command's aircraft just in time for the peak of the U-boat assault on Allied shipping, in April and May 1943. Over two months, 206's B-17 Flying Fortresses sank at least six German submarines.[70] This unprecedented success rate in airborne antisubmarine combat was entirely due to the enhanced ability of aircrew to detect U-boats. In the assessment of one historian, air-to-surface radar was "electronic warfare's greatest influence on the course of the Second World War."[71]

There was a health concern, however. Nazi broadcast propaganda repeatedly asserted that the use of radar transmitters in aircraft caused erectile dysfunction in aircrew. Anxiety on this matter was widespread and was having deleterious effects on morale in the RAF generally and in 206 Squadron in particular.[72] The squadron's new medical officer was convinced that these fears were groundless and volunteered to fly several missions as a demonstration of the complete safety of the equipment. With his interest in ships and the sea, Donald thoroughly enjoyed his flights over the Atlantic. No adverse medical consequences were reported.

Despite such adventures, Donald, like most of the RAF medical officers in the Western Isles, was often conspicuously underemployed. So much so that Donald's commanding officer in Benbecula became concerned that the long periods of idleness experienced by the medical personnel were having a detrimental impact on the morale of the other officers.[73] Therefore, he encouraged the doctors to find useful activities to do around the base when their professional services were not required. Donald chose to involve himself with the radar station. Indeed, by his own private account, he seems to have acted as a supernumerary radar operator. It would have been typical of Donald if his participation in radar was considerably more intensive than official regulations allowed.

Working with wartime radar equipment would have been a demanding learning experience. Even in 1943, despite much improvement in the design of radar sets, their effective operation required some craft skill and a basic understanding of the underlying physical principles.[74] While stationed at Benbecula, Donald also followed developments in sonar as closely as he could. Thus, during his service in the RAF, Donald gained considerable familiarity with techniques of echolocation. Like many in the armed forces, he would have been impressed with the transforming potential of technological innovation, particularly in electronics.[75]

In October 1943, 206 Squadron moved to a new base at Lagans in the Azores. Lagans was a very difficult environment for the RAF medical staff.[76] A large number of British service personnel were stationed on the island, but the medical accommodation consisted largely of prefabricated huts and tents, which regularly blew down in the frequent gales. There was no reliable water supply. In 1944 there was an epidemic of polio, and typhoid and typhus were endemic in the local population. Great endeavor and perseverance were required from the medical staff to establish reasonable standards of sanitation, public health, and clinical care.[77] Donald worked with enormous energy under the difficult circumstances of the Azores posting and enjoyed a very successful tour of duty (fig. 3.1). In 1945, he was mentioned in dispatches for his bravery in helping several airmen escape from a crashed and burning aircraft. In 1946, he was awarded the military MBE.

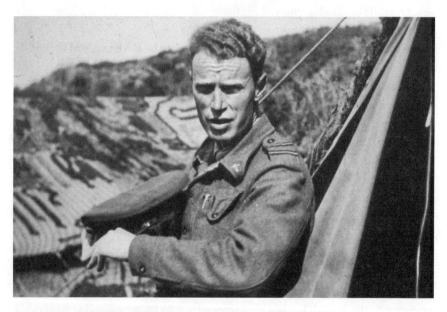

Figure 3.1. Ian Donald, while serving as an RAF medical officer in the Azores. During his service he became familiar with radar and sonar. *Reproduced with permission of the BMUS Historical Collection*

In May 1944, in preparation for D-Day, 206 Squadron returned to Britain, to St. Eval in Cornwall. Here, one of Donald's main tasks as medical officer was offering support to aircrew suffering from the stress and fatigue of long hours in the air and too many combat missions. These clinical responsibilities made a deep impression on him and rekindled an interest in psychiatry that he had developed in his student days. Toward the end of the war, Donald considered a change of career direction. Influenced by his close friend Denis Hill, he thought of becoming a psychiatrist. In Dame Alison's opinion, "becoming a gynaecologist was a second choice for him."[78] Later to become president of the Royal College of Psychiatrists, Hill was not a typical psychiatrist. Indeed, he and Donald had a lot in common. Like Donald, Hill had an avocational interest in mechanical and electrical gadgets. After graduating from St. Thomas's in 1936, Hill studied neurology at Maida Vale Hospital. There, he met Grey Walter, who was using the newly invented technique of electroencephalography (EEG) to investigate neurological disorders. Hill was fascinated by the technical aspects of the EEG machine and was impressed with Walter's early successes in the location of brain tumors. Later, Hill pioneered the application of EEG to psychiatric conditions. A man of broad general interests, in his writings, Hill encompassed philosophy as well as psychiatry and neurology.[79] His style of psychiatry, biologically focused and technologically sophisticated but not narrowly reductionist, would doubtless have appealed strongly to Donald.

In 1946, as his demobilization approached, Donald began to make plans for his future. He wrote to the distinguished psychiatrist Professor Aubrey Lewis (a close associate of Denis Hill), applying for a post at the Maudsley Hospital.

> The period I have spent in the RAF has at least taught me to take increasing notice of the psychological effects of illness, bad airmanship and delinquency and my desire to make a real study of psychiatry has . . . outgrown the wish to return to the somewhat mentally restricted field of midwifery and gynaecology in which I now realise the exercise of a certain manual dexterity affords the main interest.[80]

One might discern here Fairbairn's emphasis on the importance of psychological factors in medicine.

This plan for a change of career had to be abandoned, however. Under the terms of Government's Ex-Service Specialist Scheme, Donald was eligible for employment, and a substantial supplement to his salary, only if he went back to the specialty in which he had already trained.[81] Joseph Wrigley, now Head of the Department of Obstetrics at St. Thomas's, also exerted himself to persuade Donald that his best prospects lay in returning to his old department.[82] Accordingly, Donald applied for the post of obstetrics registrar at St. Thomas's and on July 8, 1946, was duly appointed.

(((((In the reform of medical education that followed the recommendations of the Goodenough Report, the London medical schools ceased to be independent institutions and were fully integrated into the University of London.[83] After the war, the policy of both the University of London and the Ministry of Health was to encourage the development of a research culture in the hospital schools, partly by establishing closer links with other university personnel.[84] The ministry therefore insisted on university representatives sitting on the appointment committees set up to select staff under the Ex-Service Specialist Scheme, with the understanding that preference should be given to candidates with an interest in research. Donald's scientific credentials were indeed meager at this stage in his career. However, he must have impressed his interviewers with a commitment to developing research interests, since not only was he given a post in 1946, but his appointment to St. Thomas's was renewed in June 1947.[85]

Donald was later to recall the immediate postwar years as a period of profound crisis in his life: "I returned from the war to a job with a salary of £225 a year, without a single publication and without any senior qualifications. The . . . situation was sufficiently obvious to me then to make me drastically reorganise my life . . . with considerable concentration of effort." War service had been less advantageous to obstetricians than many other doctors, since few of them had been able to practice their specialty while on active service. Donald was thirty-six years old and had a wife and two children to support. Rebuilding his career meant "terribly hard and apparently unrewarding work."[86] "I set out to make myself indispensable," he later wrote. "Every foul and boring clinic was thrown at me and I got to pulling my Chief's irons out of the fire and doing as many as three operating lists in a day until they soon found that they could not do without me. Exams too."[87]

Donald's mentor during this period at St. Thomas's Hospital was Joseph Wrigley. In later years, Donald frequently acknowledged that Wrigley had exercised a major influence on the ethos of his own clinical practice. Following in Fairbairn's footsteps, Wrigley was a pillar of St. Thomas's. He had graduated from the Medical School in 1925 and remained attached to its Department of Obstetrics and Gynaecology throughout his career, assuming the headship of the department in 1946, the year Donald returned from the RAF.

Like his predecessors, Wrigley had a considerable reputation within obstetrics and gynecology that was based on his standing as a clinician and a clinical teacher. He published little, and mostly on clinical or related matters.[88] In the manner of Fairbairn, Wrigley cultivated a conservative, expectant attitude to the management of pregnancy and labor. He was deeply suspicious of the encroachment of diagnostic technology at the bedside. "I have a poor opinion of unnecessary or routine investigations," he wrote to Donald, "and an unbounded admiration for strong clinical knowledge." He was content, as noted in his obituary, to be "essentially a clinician," to rely "on his senses for information, diagnosis and decision."[89]

It is ironic, given Wrigley's generally negative attitude to medical technology, that he is most widely remembered for the design of obstetric forceps bearing his name.[90] The Wrigley forceps, however, may be characterized as a conservative rather than a radical technological innovation. Their design embodies the inventor's cautious attitude to instrumental intervention in labor.

> The history of the "Wrigley" forceps is simple. When I acquired a position of responsibility at STH [St. Thomas's Hospital], I got fed up with (a) Residents who rang up every time they wished to use the long curved blunderbuss instrument that alone was available at the time or (b) others who misused said instrument and killed the baby and sometimes the mother. So I took a short straight forceps of Smellie to Allen and Hanbury's [instrument makers] and asked them to copy it with the addition of a slight pelvic curve in the shank. After a few modifications the final result was delivered.[91]

The shortness of the blades of Wrigley's forceps prevented them from being clamped around the fetal head prematurely. The design of the handles made it difficult to exert traction on the head excessively or with an undue turning movement. Overall, the Wrigley forceps were cleverly designed to minimize the damage an inexperienced or overenthusiastic operator might do to the woman or the fetus. The forceps have been credited with preventing much perinatal injury.

Under Wrigley's guidance, Donald's career development quickly began to recover from the hiatus of the war. In 1947, he gained the Membership of the Royal College of Obstetricians and Gynaecologists and successfully submitted his MD thesis. In a display of cultural versatility worthy of a London great, his dissertation was a medico-literary essay: "A Collection of Quotations about Medical London."[92]

In 1949, Donald accepted the newly created post of tutor in Obstetrics and Gynaecology at St. Thomas's. This appointment was of historical significance in the development of obstetrics and gynecology as an academic subject in Britain. In 1944, the Goodenough Committee had noted that there were only two chairs of obstetrics and gynecology in the whole of London—at University College and the Postgraduate School of Medicine, Hammersmith. The committee's report strongly recommended that to improve undergraduate education in the subject, the other London medical schools should found academic departments. St. Thomas's did not move quickly on this matter, however. Having not yet fully absorbed the values of research, the clinicians, as Philip Rhodes puts it, "found it difficult to know what an academic department would do that was not already being done by them."[93] Donald's tutorship was thus the first academic post in obstetrics to be created at St. Thomas's. He was chosen for this position because he had already established a reputation as a "superb teacher of students and those in their early graduate years."[94]

It was also in the late 1940s that Donald began to collect the case histories that were to form the basis of his very successful textbook, *Practical Obstetric Problems*. In 1951, he was promoted to a readership, a post he held together with a chief assistantship at the Chelsea Hospital for Women. (In British universities, a readership is an academic post, above senior lecturer and below professor.) While at the Chelsea, Donald undertook a study of the etiology of vaginal discharge, which provided the material for his first substantial research publication. Though the subject matter of this paper does not relate directly to any of the major projects he was later to conduct, it is nevertheless noteworthy for the light it sheds on how the training Donald received at St. Thomas's was expressed in his clinical and research practice.[95]

Donald's paper on vaginal discharge was wholly clinical in character, essentially a contribution to the natural history of gynecological disease. Similarities in structure to Wrigley's earlier papers on puerperal infection are apparent.[96] Donald provided carefully observed accounts of cases, complemented, where appropriate, with the results of microbiological tests and some rudimentary statistics. Refusing to delegate diagnostic matters wholly to support staff, he undertook many of the microscopic investigations himself: "The importance of

examining the fresh set specimen immediately in the clinic and without relying exclusively on subsequent laboratory diagnosis is emphasised." Throughout the paper, Donald speaks not with the descriptive neutrality of the natural
scientist but with the prescriptive authority of the head of a clinic. Much of the
discussion relates to the proper conduct of a gynecological clinic rather than
specifically to the research topic being discussed. Equally, the cases are not reduced to the pathological phenomena of tissues or microbes. A strong sense of
the patient's individual, psychological concerns is retained. "Vaginal discharge
is a common symptom," Donald writes, "and is often accompanied by fears that
may be more distressing than the complaint itself . . . while feelings of guilt or
uncleanness are reinforced by the patient's own repeated observations . . . To
prescribe treatment . . . without a convincing examination is to ignore a large
part of the patient's real need."[97] The tenor of the paper also retains the moral
overtones with respect to sexual behavior that characterized the writings of
his teachers. Donald's 1952 paper is a virtuoso performance, very much in the
St. Thomas's mold.

In the years following the Second World War, however, St. Thomas's Hospital and Medical School were changing.[98] A new emphasis was being placed
on research, and a research culture was gradually developing. The number of
scientific staff greatly increased as existing preclinical departments were expanded. New professorial appointments were made with a view to enhancing
leadership in research. Henry Barcroft was appointed to the Chair in Physiology, and Peter Sharpey-Schafer was attracted from the Postgraduate Medical
School to take up the Chair in Medicine.

With incorporation into the National Health Service (NHS) in 1948,
St. Thomas's no longer needed to spend its investment income on patient
care.[99] Much of this money was now allocated to the improvement of its laboratories and related facilities. A School Endowment Fund was set up to provide
financial support for staff research projects. Having obtained a grant to cover
engineering costs, Donald began a major investigation into the management
of neonatal breathing difficulties and, in particular, of atelectasis neonatorum,
failure of the lung to expand completely after birth.[100]

The nature of Donald's new research interest is an indication that obstetrics
was also changing in the postwar years. In the late 1930s, the maternal mortality rate had finally begun to improve.[101] By 1950, in most of England and Wales,
the incidence of death in childbirth had fallen dramatically and was continuing

to decline. Overall, maternal mortality was down to about 20 percent of what it had been in 1935. While there was still much to be done, standards of obstetric education and practice had considerably improved, and obstetricians had new tools for the secure management of complicated labor, such as ergometrine to stimulate uterine contractions postpartum, a reliable blood transfusion service, and improved anesthesia.[102] The sulfonamides and, later, antibiotics greatly diminished the dangers of puerperal infections. As confidence grew in the safety of the mother, obstetricians were able to accord greater attention to the well-being of the baby, during and immediately after birth.

Here also there was much to do. Infant mortality (deaths in the first year of life) had declined steadily in Britain since the beginning of the twentieth century. But the rate of neonatal mortality (deaths in the first four weeks of life) had fallen far less quickly. Long-term morbidity and impairment due to perinatal injury were also serious problems. Indeed, neonatal health had become, in the 1940s and 1950s, a matter of considerable concern in both professional and lay circles.[103] Thus, in beginning his work on the breathing difficulties of neonates, Donald was riding the new wave of research in obstetric medicine.

A baby that does not breathe easily in the first hours of life presents a very pressing clinical challenge. In the course of work with these cases, Donald became concerned that the available neonatal respirators were often ineffective.[104] Sometimes the machine imposed a breathing rhythm that conflicted with that of the baby, causing the little patient to waste energy "fighting" the respirator. Moreover, if gases were pumped into the newborn when its diaphragm was not contracting, they might flow into the esophagus rather than the trachea. Forced hyperventilation could produce respiratory alkalosis (disturbance of acid-base balance) with consequent tetany (disordered nervous and muscular activity). Donald sought to address these problems. For assistance, he turned to Maureen Young.

That Miss Young (later Dr. and, subsequently, Professor Young) was available at St. Thomas's to assist Donald was remarkably fortunate. Donald had stumbled across someone with a state-of-the-art training in fetal and neonatal physiology. Young joined St. Thomas's in 1947. She had graduated in physiology from Bedford College, London, and later returned as a member of staff. During the war, Bedford College was evacuated to Cambridge. There, Young worked under the tutelage of perhaps the most famous respiratory physiologist in the world, Sir Joseph Barcroft. After a distinguished career during which he had illuminated many aspects of adult respiration, Barcroft had, in his sixties, turned his attention to the little explored area of fetal and perinatal physiology. He and his team conducted a brilliant series of experimental investigations, elucidating such matters as birth reflexes and development of the circulation. Barcroft's book *Researches on Prenatal Life*, published in 1946, established the subject as a major branch of physiology.[105] Young had assisted Barcroft on several aspects of his fetal work, providing the elderly scientist with, as he put it, "accurate eyes and accurate hands."[106] Barcroft sought to understand how the fetus responded to the challenges of adapting to independent life.[107] He demonstrated that, contrary to contemporary orthodoxy, the physiological and structural changes undergone by the fetus in the transition from placental to pulmonary respiration occurred very quickly, within a few minutes of birth. These findings greatly interested obstetricians who were beginning to pay more attention to laboratory research.

Central to Donald's project was his idea for an improved design of negative-pressure respirator, one that, by means of a simple yet clever innovation, would follow the intrinsic cadence of the baby's breathing. Donald's respirator had two chambers, one for the head and one for the rest of the body. Air was delivered to the baby through a face mask. A mirror was attached to the flap of the valve that allowed air into the mask, and a beam of light was shone on the mirror. The movement of the flap as the baby began a breath caused the returning light beam to be deflected from a photoelectric cell. This triggered the respirator, creating negative pressure in the body chamber and thus inflating the lungs. Thus, mechanical assistance was given only to breaths that had already been initiated. A key feature of the design was the absence of a bellows, which kept the inertia of the system very low. Response to the initiation of a breath was correspondingly rapid. The pressures used in the system were determined both by observations on newborn infants and by a series of experiments that Young conducted on cats. In these latter investigations, Donald was wholly dependent on his physiologist colleague, since he did not hold, nor would he ever hold, a Home Office animal license.

Donald and Young also addressed another shortcoming in the design of negative-pressure neonatal respirators. The baby was pushed and pulled up and down in the chamber. Donald's solution to this "pistoning" was twofold. First, the effect was minimized by keeping the pressure changes in the body chamber as small as possible. Second, the opening between the head chamber and the body chamber was sealed using a quick-setting alginate compound. However, as Young recalls, "the sealing material sometimes solidified and sometimes did not!"[108]

Donald's "automatic respiratory amplifier" was quite a complicated piece of medical equipment for its time. He received considerable technical assistance from Commander Patrick Slater, an electrical engineer in the Fleet Air Arm. Acknowledging Slater's input, Donald wrote, "I did not even know what an electro-magnetic relay was when I first met him and he has taught me much."[109] The functioning of breathing equipment is, of course, a major concern in aviation engineering and medicine. Donald's debt to airplane technology was apparent: "The negative and positive pressures employed are pre-set on aircraft contacting altimeters which, being connected with the system of relays . . . cut out at these pressures as soon as they are reached, prevent their being exceeded and immediately initiate the next phase of the respiratory cycle as appropriate." In January 1952, Donald and Young demonstrated the new respirator at a meeting of the Physiological Society at the Royal Free Hospital.[110] The apparatus arrived in pieces and, with no technicians available, Donald demonstrated his understanding of its workings by putting it back together again. Young recalls that the demonstration created considerable interest, if partly for the loud clanging of the solenoid-operated valves.

Young greatly enjoyed collaborating with Donald. Both workers relished the manual, dexterous aspects of scientific research. It is evident that Donald benefited greatly from this collaboration. Although less senior than Donald, Young was a much more experienced scientist. Donald learned a great deal from her about physiological methods—how to measure blood oxygen tensions, for instance. But there was also a more intangible debt. The papers Donald published before he started his respirator project can fairly be characterized as those of a clinician dabbling in research.[111] His later publications were, by contrast, those of a fully fledged clinician-scientist. Much of this improvement was doubtless due to their author's greater maturity, but a close collaborative association with an experienced research physiologist can only have aided Donald's development as a scientist.

In 1952, Donald left St. Thomas's to take up a readership at the Institute of Obstetrics and Gynaecology at the Royal Postgraduate Medical School.[112] The senior staff at St. Thomas's were disappointed to see him go. As the minutes of the School Council record:

Tribute was paid . . . to the distinguished work he had done here, and special reference was made to his Respiratory Machine . . . as an excellent example of good team work between the Departments of Obstetrics, Physiology and Diseases of Children . . . Mr Howard enquired if the Hospital could in any way have helped in retaining his services, but the Dean said that only reconstruction could have realised this by overcoming the lack of space and dispersal of the Department over various hospitals.[113]

This last sentence is ironic, given the circumstances under which Donald was to work during his first few years in Glasgow.

CHAPTER FOUR

Ian Donald before Ultrasound II

Hammersmith and Glasgow

In the years before he began his work on diagnostic ultrasound, Ian Donald developed a characteristic approach to clinical work, and to the professional and social role of the obstetrician, that would be formative in his relationship to the new technology. In this chapter, we explore his maturing as a clinician and a researcher, with particular attention to his first innovative use of diagnostic imaging and his enthusiasm for applying technology to clinical concerns. It was his prior commitment to the clinico-anatomical method, acquired at St. Thomas's, that provided the focus for his earliest imaging research. We also explore the background to his appointment to the Regius Chair of Midwifery at the University of Glasgow and describe the medical environment he encountered on taking up this post.

The character of the Royal Postgraduate Medical School at the Hammersmith Hospital, where Donald began his readership in 1952, was distinctly different from that of the Medical School at St. Thomas's Hospital. Far from being a venerable voluntary foundation, the Hammersmith Hospital had opened in 1905 as a Poor Law infirmary. It was taken over as a municipal hospital by London County Council in 1930, then incorporated into the National Health Service in 1948. The Postgraduate Medical School was established in 1935, in response to concerns about the quality of postgraduate medical education in London. The aim of its founders was that the school should be a "university centre with whole-time academic staffing and with research opportunities for the staff."[1]

The first professor of medicine at the Postgraduate School was Francis Fraser. Since 1921, Fraser had been professor of medicine at St. Bartholomew's Hospital. But Barts, like St. Thomas's, was not a congenial environment for the scientifically minded physician, and Fraser eagerly grasped the opportunity for a fresh start at the Hammersmith. He set about recruiting like-minded colleagues and cultivating a strong institutional commitment to research. In 1938, John McMichael joined Fraser's department, quickly securing an international reputation in cardiovascular physiology. McMichael's style of investigation, which employed the controversial technique of atrial catheterization, was interventionist and technically sophisticated—as was that of his colleague Sheila Sherlock, who developed liver biopsy techniques that helped elucidate the pathology of hepatitis.[2]

In the years following the war, the Postgraduate School made a large number of new appointments. In 1947, Ian Aird was recruited from Edinburgh to become professor of surgery, and John McClure Browne became professor of obstetrics and gynecology. McClure Browne developed techniques for studying placental function and localization, while Aird emerged as one of the most innovative surgeons in Britain.[3] In the Department of Medicine, Guy Scadding, Peter Sharpey-Schaffer, and John Crofton undertook original and important work in respiratory and cardiovascular medicine. Thus, by 1952, when Donald joined the staff, the Postgraduate School had established its preeminence within British clinical research.

Nevertheless, it must have required a degree of moral courage for Donald to leave his post at St. Thomas's, where he certainly had career prospects, to move to the Hammersmith. Despite the growing international reputation of the Postgraduate School, a prejudice remained among the elite circles of London medicine against the school's style of work. As John Crofton, who moved from St. Thomas's to the Hammersmith in 1947, recalled, "At the stage I went to the Postgraduate School, the teaching hospital thought it was terrible. These were places where they put needles in the liver and catheters in the heart! You don't go to a place like that. There was a sort of ambivalence, which of course gradually changed as such distinguished work came out."[4]

Donald must have been aware, however, that to reach the heights of his profession in the changing climate of British medicine after the Second World War, he would need to consolidate his reputation as a researcher. At St. Thomas's in the 1950s, an active involvement in research was still rare among senior clinicians. By contrast, every member of staff at the Postgraduate School had his or her own research project.[5] Moreover, given that Donald's major interest at St. Thomas's had been neonatal respiratory problems, the attractions of the Hammersmith, which was now a major center for applied respiratory physiology and related clinical research, must have been considerable. In the 1950s, the Postgraduate School was also one of the few academic centers within British medicine with an active research interest in bioengineering and technology. Its laboratory facilities were excellent, by contemporary standards. There was a well-equipped technical workshop, able to build experimental apparatus to order. In 1949, the school took the pioneering step of establishing a Department of Biophysics.[6] Thus the Hammersmith offered many attractions for an ambitious clinical researcher interested in working at the interface between medicine and technology.

(((((Shortly before Donald arrived at the Postgraduate School, a major project had got underway. Aird had become convinced of the possibilities of open-heart surgery but recognized the need for an oxygenation pump to maintain the patient's respiration and circulation while the heart was stopped.[7] A colleague, Denis Melrose, began work on techniques of keeping isolated organs functioning by fluid perfusion. This research eventually culminated in the development of a prototype heart-lung machine. Donald, always eager to be involved with the latest technological innovations, followed this work closely. In 1954, another Hammersmith colleague, William Cleland, used Melrose's heart-lung machine to support the circulation of a patient undergoing cardiac surgery.[8] Donald was a member of the team that undertook this pioneering operation, his job being to monitor the oxygen saturation of the patient's blood—a task for which his research on respiratory problems in neonates had prepared him well.[9]

The 1950s were an exciting time to study respiratory physiology. Barcroft's classic experiments had stimulated much further work in the laboratory and the clinic. To obstetricians and pediatricians, improving their understanding of oxygen exchange was far from a matter of merely academic interest. In 1952, in England and Wales, the death rate in the first four weeks of life remained above 18 per 1,000 births.[10] Nearly one-half of these approximately twelve thousand fatalities were attributed to respiratory conditions, and atelectasis neonatorum remained a major medical problem.[11] There was, however, a great increase in activity within pediatric medicine following the setting-up of the NHS.

At the Postgraduate School, Donald continued his investigations into the breathing difficulties of neonates. The Hammersmith Hospital had a modern, well-staffed Premature Baby Unit.[12] However, the school did not, at this time, have a separate department of pediatrics. The Premature Baby Unit was under the aegis of the Department of Obstetrics, with the senior pediatrician, Professor Alan Moncrieff, visiting once a week from Great Ormond Street Hospital. Under these institutional circumstances, the obstetricians worked closely with their pediatric colleagues. McClure Browne was very supportive of Donald's work, being keen to improve the research profile of his department.[13]

Initially, Donald focused on improving the performance of the "Servo patient-cycled respirator," as Donald and Young's respiratory amplifier came to be called. Working with Josephine Lord, neonatal registrar in the Premature Baby Unit, Donald also developed a new piece of equipment, the Trip spirometer. Its purpose was to measure the volume of air inspired with each breath and thus provide an assessment of a baby's respiratory efficiency.[14] Donald presented his invention as an aid to the diagnosis of primary atelectasis. It could be used to help decide whether treatment with the Servo respirator was indicated and to monitor the effectiveness of such treatment. Donald described an occasion when, with only a single respirator available, the staff of the Premature Baby Unit were faced with triplets, two of whom were in respiratory distress. The spirometer was used to identify which baby was in the greater need of mechanical assistance with its breathing.

The Trip spirometer was not used solely as a diagnostic instrument. Donald and Lord also used the device on healthy babies to measure the parameters of normal respiration, their ultimate goal being to elucidate the physiology and pathology of neonatal pulmonary disease. In 1953, a leading article in the *Lancet* gave a warm endorsement to Donald and Lord's endeavor to base "rational treatment" of atelectasis on the quantitative determination of both normal and impaired respiration. However, Dr. Donough O'Brien, at Harvard Medical School, soon voiced strong criticisms of Donald and Lord's lack of precision in measurement and absence of a benchmark calibration against "basal conditions." Donald's reply was robust and indicative of the general thrust of his research.

> Basal conditions are not applicable in the face of respiratory distress, and maximal respiratory capacity is more indicative of the child's ability to survive. It would be wanton to forgo any contributory information . . . in making a clinical assessment; and Dr. O'Brien's objections ignore the practical needs of the case. Let us not widen the existing gap between scientific experiment and clinical reality.[15]

In other words, to the hard-pressed clinician, a partially calibrated measurement was preferable to no measurement at all.

In 1953, Donald published a review of best practice in the resuscitation of the newborn.[16] He stressed that the ultimate objective of neonatal care could not be merely the restoration of physiological function. The long-term good of the patient, in particular his or her quality of life, had to be kept in mind. Noting the strong association between perinatal asphyxia and mental deficiency, he concluded: "This is a sobering thought. In resuscitating the newborn one is not only, for the time being, a trustee for the child's life but also for its intellectual future."[17]

While at the Postgraduate School, Donald also began developing a third device, a positive-pressure respirator. Neonatal respiratory distress often presented as an emergency, and Donald was aware that the negative-pressure respirator that he had developed at St. Thomas's was not of great utility under such circumstances. The machine was complicated, it needed to be carefully set up, and its operation required the presence of more than one fully trained member of staff. The Servo respirator was better suited to the prolonged treatment of babies with established respiratory difficulties. In a crisis, immediate positive-pressure ventilation seemed to be preferable. However, existing positive-pressure respirators were designed to deliver oxygen through an endotracheal tube, since positive pressure applied to the face tended to force gas into the esophagus rather than the lung. But intubation of small, sick babies could be a fraught business. As Donald put it, "We clearly needed a respirator which could be operated at once via a mask with the child still in its cot or incubator."[18] He set about devising such a piece of equipment, his "positive-pressure patient cycled respirator," known in the Hammersmith Hospital as the Puffer.[19] The Puffer conveyed an oxygen mixture, at positive pressure, to the baby's face. Like the Servo respirator, its activity was controlled by a photoelectric trigger mechanism. In the case of a sudden cyanotic attack, the Puffer could be applied to the ailing baby in under a minute.

Donald's colleagues in the Departments of Medicine and Surgery took a keen interest in his work on resuscitation. He was encouraged to adapt the Puffer for use on adults. Having done so, he was shortly asked to treat one of Aird's patients, a woman who had failed to reestablish spontaneous respiration following a cholecystectomy. After five minutes with the Puffer, "an adequate depth of respiration" was achieved, and the patient went on to make a full recovery. On another occasion, Donald was asked to treat a baby at University College Hospital. Again, there was a successful outcome. These achievements prompted interest from the British Oxygen Company, which made a copy of Donald's prototype with a view to commercial development.[20]

Meanwhile, Melrose and Cleland were having problems with funding. Despite an impressive run of early successes, they were unable to secure the support of the Medical Research Council for continued investment in the heart-lung machine.[21] The initiative in further development of cardiopulmonary bypass equipment passed to surgeons and engineers in the United States. Likewise, nothing substantial came of the British Oxygen Company's interest in the Puffer. At the Hammersmith, therefore, Donald gained experience both of the excitement and fulfillment to be found in successful technological innovation in clinical medicine and of the difficulties, financial as well as technical, in moving from invention to wider implementation and commercial development.

The research ethos of the Royal Postgraduate Medical School extended, as Calnan emphasizes, to its nonclinical departments.[22] In his investigations of neonatal respiratory distress, Donald worked closely with Albert Claireaux, a pathologist who took a special interest in perinatal mortality. Breathing difficulty in the newborn is frequently associated with hyaline membrane disease, in which the pulmonary alveoli become lined with a layer of dense material. Claireaux's histological studies of hyaline membrane did much to clarify the cellular pathology of the disease.[23]

Claireaux undertook postmortem examination of all of Donald's respiratory patients who died during treatment. In true St. Thomas's fashion, Donald attended nearly every one of those autopsies. In the early 1950s, the presence of hyaline membrane could not be confirmed until autopsy. Yet, as Donald was painfully aware, the efficacy of any treatment for hyaline membrane disease could not be rationally assessed without confidence in the pretreatment diagnosis. The various causes of neonatal respiratory distress—hyaline membrane, primary atelectasis, cerebral hemorrhage, even infectious disorders—were difficult to distinguish from one another. What had those few babies who recovered following treatment with the respirator really been suffering from? Was hyaline membrane disease an irreversible condition, for which no therapy could be effective?

Donald wondered whether it might be possible to use radiography to address these questions, and this led to his first foray into medical imaging for research purposes—thus his deployment of imaging technology sprang initially from his commitment to the value of the postmortem examination. Because of his training in pathology, Donald was accustomed to trying to understand disease in terms of structural lesions. Claireaux's work clarified for him the pathological changes in the lungs of neonates suffering from hyaline membrane disease. Donald then sought to identify these same lesions in clinical subjects. In his hands, medical imaging was indeed the "anatomization of the living," an extension of the clinico-anatomical method.[24]

Donald approached Dr. (later, Professor) Robert Steiner of the Department of Radiology with his idea. Steiner was one of the cohort of research-oriented staff recruited by the Postgraduate School in the 1950s.[25] He was keen on collaborative research with clinicians and responded enthusiastically to Donald's suggestion. For the remainder of Donald's time at the Hammersmith, he and Steiner worked together on the radiological investigation of neonatal respiratory distress. They undertook several series of examinations of neonates in respiratory difficulty; in most cases, infants were X-rayed several times as the disease progressed. These inquiries were driven by Donald's usual energy and enthusiasm, one baby being X-rayed when only thirteen minutes old. The recent institution of a twenty-four-hour radiography service at the Hammersmith facilitated this research, as did the availability of mobile X-ray machines that could be taken into the Premature Baby Unit or even the labor ward.[26]

Donald's determined use of radiography was a radical departure from normal clinical practice in cases of prematurity. Accepted protocol was to handle ill neonates as little as possible, since disturbance was thought to irritate and weaken them. Donald was not insensitive to this consideration—he frequently emphasized that care of the sick baby should be based on "warmth, oxygen and minimal handling."[27] Nevertheless, he felt that the positive potential of radiographic imaging, both in aiding diagnosis and in assessing the progress of therapy, outweighed any deleterious effect. Steiner's considered opinion was that the disturbance to the baby was relatively small: "We brought the machine right over the incubator, lifted the lid, slipped a film behind the body . . . It was a matter of survival. They were so ill and the dose was minute. So we were helping them, trying to make a diagnosis."[28] Nevertheless, X-raying neonates in their incubators was a bold initiative by contemporary standards. But as Steiner later put it, "when you work at Hammersmith you have the moral courage to do many things."[29] An institution that had seen Sherlock stick needles in the liver and McMichael catheterize the heart was evidently one into which Donald readily fitted.

By 1953, Donald and Steiner were able to publish a study of twenty-eight cases of hyaline membrane disease.[30] They outlined the radiological features of what they believed were three distinct stages in development of the membrane. The initial phase was characterized by a "diffuse miliary mottling." This feature of the radiographic appearance of the premature lung had been described previously but was considered to be physiological.[31] Donald and Steiner regarded it as both pathological and pathognomonic. There were some false positives but no false negatives in their series; no baby without mottling on radiography was subsequently found, at necropsy, to have hyaline membrane. The finer the granularity of the mottling, they argued, the earlier the stage of development of hyaline membrane. In the second stage, the lesions gradually became "coarser and more confluent" until, finally, the signs of lobar consolidation and collapse were observed.

Donald and Steiner's conclusion was that radiographic imaging did indeed have much to offer in the elucidation of neonatal respiratory distress.[32] In particular, they asserted that the diagnosis of hyaline membrane disease could now be arrived at with confidence while the patient was still alive. Donald and Steiner cautiously suggested that the condition could be, on occasion at least, reversible. Sometimes, as a baby began to breathe more easily, its lungs lost the radiographic signs suggestive of the membrane.

> When you then watched the hyaline membrane progressing from hour two, three, or four after birth and for the next eight or ten hours, and you suddenly realised, very occasionally, that the snowstorm [miliary mottling] disappeared. We saw the snowstorm disappear and the child improved and the child survived. That was very exciting. The baby survived. Now when that happened the effort on the paediatric side became much stronger to do something about treating this disorder.[33]

Donald's growing salience as clinician and researcher led to an invitation to give the Blair-Bell Lecture to the Royal College of Obstetricians and Gynaecologists in May 1954. Predictably, he chose to speak on his major research interest, atelectasis neonatorum.[34] In an address liberally sprinkled with literary allusion, Donald broadly surveyed both the scientific and the clinical aspects of neonatal respiratory distress. He emphasized the potential of his respirators for improving the management of atelectasis. Enthusiast for clinical innovation though he was, Donald's focus as an obstetrician was never narrowly technological. On the contrary, he stressed that the best remedy for the problems of prematurity did not lie with mechanical ventilation or even in the Premature Baby Unit.

> The surest defence against dying from atelectasis is vaginal delivery at term and clearly, the prevention of premature labour, which is very much the obstetrician's concern, would be the ideal solution. Baird (1945) has shown that the prematurity rate is more or less inversely proportional to the social status of the patient and a rising standard of living amongst the poorer classes would progressively reduce it.[35]

Thus, to Donald, obstetrics remained the essentially social medicine it had been to Fairbairn.

This broad perspective is also evident in the other major product of Donald's time at the Hammersmith, his textbook *Practical Obstetric Problems*.[36] With the benefit of an awareness of Donald's later research interests, it is interesting to note the several passages in which he voices frustration at the difficulty of understanding what is going on, as he puts it, "behind the iron curtain of the maternal abdominal wall."[37] He discusses, for instance, the uncertainty surrounding the diagnosis of twin pregnancies and looks "forward to the day when a safe and certain method of diagnosing placenta praevia is possible without local examination and disturbance."[38] The potential of the imaging techniques he had explored with Steiner had evidently stimulated his imagination.

(((((While Donald was hard at work at the Hammersmith, the University of Glasgow was looking for a professor of obstetrics and gynecology. Leading the search was University Principal Sir Hector Hetherington. From the beginning of his tenure in 1936, Hetherington had sought to modernize the university's Medical Faculty. His aim was, as Hull puts it, to "academicize" Glasgow medicine.[39] In the 1930s, all the university's clinical chairs had been held part-time. The professors devoted much of their energies to their private practices and, with some outstanding exceptions, did little research. Hetherington felt that if Glasgow University were to maintain its status as a leading medical school, the clinical chairs would have to be made full-time, with the professors becoming the leaders of research teams.

Obstetrics and gynecology was an area of direct personal interest to Hetherington.[40] However, midwifery, as it was still called in Scotland, presented his modernizing project with particular difficulties. Glasgow's Medical School was unusual in having two chairs of midwifery, the Regius and the Muirhead, each with its own academic department and clinical unit. This situation pertained partly because the city had two large teaching hospitals, the Western Infirmary, beside the university at Gilmorehill, and the Royal Infirmary, on the High Street, the old center of Glasgow.[41] The Regius Professor had gynecological wards in the Western Infirmary, whereas the Muirhead Professor had gynecological wards in the Royal Infirmary. Both professors had their obstetrics beds in the Glasgow Royal Maternity Hospital, situated on Rottenrow, near the Royal Infirmary.

The Royal Maternity Hospital, commonly known as Rottenrow, was one of the largest maternity hospitals in the United Kingdom.[42] As well as its two professorial clinical units, it housed a third, nonprofessorial unit and a training school for midwives. Obstetrics in Rottenrow had a distinguished history. The Regius Chair was held from 1894 to 1927 by Murdoch Cameron, pioneer of the cesarean operation,[43] and from 1927 to 1934 by his most famous pupil, John Munro Kerr. Munro Kerr's improvements to Cameron's operation were central to the international acceptance of cesarean section as a justifiable procedure.[44] Acknowledged as one of Britain's leading obstetricians, Munro Kerr was a pioneer of postnatal care and the author of the influential textbooks *Operative Midwifery* and *Clinical and Operative Gynaecology*.[45]

It is fair to say, however, that following Munro Kerr's retirement, the reputation of the Royal Maternity Hospital had declined. The retirement of Robert Lennie from the Regius Chair in 1954 presented Hetherington with a golden opportunity for reform. He sent letters to several leading figures in British medicine to elicit their opinions on how to fill the midwifery vacancy. "The Professor will . . . have more ample research facilities than have been enjoyed by his predecessors," he wrote. "We hope therefore for a considerable development in the post-graduate teaching and research of the Department . . . this is an extremely important appointment."[46] As one correspondent reminded him, a difficult balance had to be sought.

I believe that in Glasgow of all places a professor could not possibly succeed in inspiring the necessary loyalty and enthusiasm unless he was already a fully trained clinician, fit to take his place on terms of complete equality with your very able non-professorial teachers. Clinical ability and academic leadership do not often go hand in hand.[47]

The consensus among Hetherington's correspondents was that the best candidate was Thomas MacGregor, senior lecturer at the University of Edinburgh.[48]

Several correspondents thought Ian Donald not yet quite mature enough as a clinician.[49] One writer, while recommending MacGregor as first choice, gave the following assessment of Donald: "As a research worker, and as a source of original ideas for research, Dr Donald should take first place, but his clinical attainments are hardly up to Glasgow standards. In addition, his splendid enthusiasm has about it a fiery impatient quality which is not without its dangers."[50] Hetherington was sufficiently intrigued by this comment to mark it in red in the margin of the letter.

Only one of Hetherington's correspondents came down unequivocally in favor of Donald as first choice, and he was not an obstetrician. Henry Dible, professor of pathology at the Postgraduate Medical School, wrote:

> I can . . . tell you something about Donald. In the first place, he is regarded as absolutely first-class in his clinical work, both in obstetrics and gynaecology. Secondly, his research work is of a high order. He has a physiological approach to problems and is well-versed in all the modern techniques of investigation. I understand that his work upon . . . failure of respiration, in the new born is extremely good. He is a man of outstanding energy and drive . . . It may be said that he is a little impatient in the face of obstruction, but this I personally regard as a virtue. I gather . . . that there is a need in Glasgow of a vigorous personality who will bring the status of the Department of Obstetrics and Gynaecology to something much better than it is now and, if this is so, I am sure that you would get what you want from Donald . . . I have confirmed my opinion of Donald by talking to Professor Browne and John McMichael.[51]

In the 1950s, if one wanted to find a prospective professor inculcated in the culture of academic research medicine, the Royal Postgraduate Medical School was the obvious place to look. Accordingly, Hetherington must have considered Dible's recommendation carefully.

Hetherington was evidently faced with a choice between settling for the safe option—MacGregor was undoubtedly a reliable clinician and would be wholly acceptable to the Glasgow medical establishment—or gambling on a more exciting, if risky, alternative, a candidate who might ruffle a few feathers, who might yet have something to learn, but who might also provide the dynamic research leadership that the specialty required in Glasgow. A university principal with a less clear vision for the Medical Faculty might have opted for caution. Hetherington, however, remained true to his reforming mission and determined to appoint Donald.

Now forty-four years old and an ambitious academic clinician, Donald was seeking a professorial appointment as his next career move. He knew the Glasgow Maternity Hospital, both by repute and through personal contacts. His father had done his obstetric training in Rottenrow. However, after applying for the chair, Donald visited the hospital and was unimpressed by what he encountered. When invited for an informal chat with Hetherington at the principal's London club, Donald "treated the matter with a certain amount of indifference," because he "had seen the department in Glasgow and was aware of its glaring defects."[52] Hetherington, however, took great pains to persuade Donald to reconsider, assuring him that a "new hospital with the most modern accommodation would be provided within five years" and that the new professor would be allowed a major role in its design. With these incentives, Hetherington secured Donald's services for Glasgow University. Donald later confided to a friend that another important factor in convincing him to come to Glasgow was the prospect of the excellent sailing available off the west coast of Scotland.[53]

Between his acceptance of the appointment to the Glasgow chair and taking up the post at the end of September 1954, Donald had a chance encounter with John Wild. As described in chapter 2, Wild had successfully used pulse-echo ultrasound to visualize lesions in the human breast. Invited to give the University of London's University Lecture in Medicine, Wild arrived in Britain several weeks before he was due to speak. In August 1954, he attended the British Association for the Advancement of Science meeting at Oxford, where he met the distinguished obstetrician John Chassar Moir. They spoke about Wild's ultrasonic research, and Moir, intrigued, raised the possibility that Wild's technique might be applied to localization of the placenta.[54] Moir also suggested that Wild visit Professor Valentine Mayneord at the Royal Marsden Hospital, which he duly did. Mayneord was experimenting with ultrasound to locate the midline of the brain, and he expressed great interest in Wild's images of breast lesions. Wild was also eager to meet Ian Aird at the Postgraduate Medical School. Before Wild had left for Minnesota, Aird had expressed skepticism about his plans to develop a device to facilitate intestinal intubation, and Wild wanted to show the famous surgeon that he had been wrong. During Wild's visit to the Hammersmith, a still skeptical Aird, eager to be rid of his vexatious visitor, introduced him to Ian Donald.[55]

Donald had read Wild's 1951 *Lancet* paper and took the opportunity to have a long conversation with him about ultrasonic imaging and its possible application to obstetrics. Wild showed Donald the slides of breast lesions, including cysts, which he had prepared for the University Lecture, and discussed the "cystic" nature of the gravid uterus.[56] Wild also pointed out that the equipment he was using in Minneapolis would not be suitable for uterine investigations. Imaging of deep structure through the abdominal wall would require a probe with a frequency considerably lower than 15 MHz.[57] Wild suggested, however, that the frequencies employed by industrial flaw detectors, such as that used by Mayneord, might be more suitable.

Donald was not able to attend Wild's lecture, having departed for Glasgow. If he had done so, he would have heard Wild give a brief account of his scanning apparatus, outlining his earliest investigations of postmortem specimens.[58] Wild then discussed the issue of safety, concluding that a "cautious but positive approach" was justified, given the absence of evidence of tissue damage at the intensities of ultrasound used for imaging. The greater part of the lecture was taken up with a description of the visualization of breast tumors and cysts. Wild concluded with an account of how the ultrasonic method might be applied to examination of the lower bowel. He must have discussed most of these issues in his conversation with Donald, and Donald also got a second-hand account of the lecture from Mayneord—who described Wild as "outrageously provocative."[59] Donald thus arrived in Glasgow with the impression fresh in his mind that ultrasound could be diagnostically useful. He was intrigued, but far from convinced.[60]

(((((Donald took up his duties in Glasgow in September 1954. Initially, his research effort continued to focus on the respiratory difficulties of the newborn. He secured financial support from the Scottish Hospitals Endowments Trust and forged collaborative links with the Western Hospital Board's Regional Department of Medical Physics. Cordial relations with the director of the department, Dr. (later, Professor) John Lenihan, were established, and Donald began a fruitful partnership with Lenihan's colleague, the physicist and engineer Dr. John Ronald (Ron) Greer. Donald and Greer built an adult version of the Servo respirator, which Donald used to treat some of his gynecological patients in the Western Infirmary.[61] Further improvements were also made to the neonatal version of the Servo respirator—it was, for example, modified for use with an endotracheal tube. Greer also designed two new tools to aid the precision of Donald's research: a novel type of optical electromanometer and a more accurate "integrating" spirometer.

Donald particularly wished to record the pressure changes associated with the initial inflation of the lungs. He sought to do this by insertion of a catheter into the esophagus of a baby being delivered by cesarean section as soon as the head was clear, even before the shoulders were delivered. Owing to many clinical and practical exigencies, this technique failed more often than it succeeded. Nevertheless, Donald managed to secure more than twenty records of respiratory pressure changes in the thorax during the first breath. This pathfinding research indicated that the respiratory effort of a healthy newborn is considerably greater than had been suspected, and it confirmed animal work suggesting that, normally, the lungs fully inflate quickly after the first breath.[62]

In Rottenrow, Donald also continued his radiological investigations of neonates with hyaline membrane disease. He was able to persuade the hospital's Board of Management to buy a new "rotating anode" X-ray machine, which he considered more suitable than standard radiological equipment for this class of patient. Using this equipment, Donald achieved the remarkable feat of X-raying a healthy neonate only one minute and fifty-five seconds after birth.[63] In 1956, however, doubts were expressed about the justifiability of this type of investigation. Alice Stewart and her colleagues detected a significant correlation between exposure to diagnostic radiation in utero and the occurrence of leukemia in childhood.[64] Donald was one of a number of obstetricians and pediatricians who remained, initially, skeptical of the statistical conclusions of Stewart's study. In later editions of *Practical Obstetric Problems*, he cited two further investigations, those of Court Brown et al. and Lewis, both of which found no greater incidence of leukemia among children born to irradiated mothers than in a control group.[65] He remained convinced, for instance, of the value of X-ray pelvimetry in cases of apparent disproportion. Nevertheless, Donald could not and did not deny the wisdom of minimizing, for all patients, the exposure to ionizing radiation. The hardening of medical attitudes to the use of radiography in pregnancy could not be ignored by those working with pregnant women or, indeed, with very young babies. The intensive use of X-radiology for research purposes became difficult to justify, and thus the attraction of an alternative form of imaging was enhanced.

Overall, despite the considerable refinement of his ventilation apparatus by Greer, Donald's research into the treatment of atelectasis neonatorum was, by the mid-1950s, making slow process. Neonatal respiratory distress was proving an intractable problem. The "disappointment-rate," as he put it, was "very high."[66] With the benefit of hindsight, we can see where the difficulties lay. In the 1960s, it was discovered that the lungs of premature babies are deficient in surfactant, a substance that normally lines the alveoli, reducing surface tension and maintaining the integrity of the alveolar mucosa.[67] The absence of surfactant causes hyaline membrane, and without replacement, artificial ventilation of the neonate's lung is likely to be futile.

Donald also became aware that even apparent success with intensive ventilation treatment might be equivocal. On one occasion, he made heroic efforts to maintain respiration in a tiny baby of twenty-seven weeks' gestation and achieved adequate aeration.

> Thereafter progress was satisfactory until the sixteenth day when the infant suddenly collapsed and died. At necropsy it was found to have had a severe intraventricular haemorrhage whose existence we had not expected . . . It is chastening to reflect that this child came very near to surviving, thanks to our meddlesome interference and zeal, and it is as well to pause to consider how far this sort of work is worth while. Our failures have been numerous enough to provide us with plenty of food for thought.[68]

The child's cerebral pathology was incompatible with normal mental development.

The intensive care of very sick and dying babies is one of the most emotionally demanding areas of clinical medicine. It is a field in which "disappointments" are particularly hard to bear. However, given Hetherington's expectations, not to mention Donald's energy and ambition, it was unthinkable that Donald should not establish himself in Glasgow as the leader of a successful research team. Thus, toward the end of 1954, Donald began to look for a new project.

As we noted at the end of chapter 2, neither Howry nor Wild achieved unequivocal success with their innovations in ultrasonic diagnosis, if we define success as incorporation of their instruments into routine clinical procedure. The same might be said of Donald's excursions into medical technology at this stage in his career. The reasons for this relative failure are of interest. Donald's first invention, the bladder irrigator, was awkward to use in a ward, occasionally failed in a spectacular fashion, and was not received enthusiastically by the nursing staff. He was a very junior member of the medical profession at that time and did not have the authority to enforce the use of his appliance against such opposition. Moreover, the introduction of antibiotic therapies made bladder infections less of a persistent clinical problem by the 1950s.

Likewise, none of Donald's respiratory inventions secured a long-term place in the treatment of neonatal breathing difficulties, for several reasons. One is that nothing came of the interest initially expressed by commercial companies in developing the devices. Changes in the professional structure of medicine also worked against him. When Donald became involved in respiratory medicine, he was riding a wave of innovative research. However, as McAdams describes, by the 1950s, research into the treatment of neonatal breathing difficulties had become the property of a dedicated and highly trained cadre of researchers who had extensive experience in laboratory physiology and identified themselves, not with obstetrics, but with the rising specialty of pediatrics and, in particular, the subspecialty of neonatology.[69] The time when an obstetrician, working in the clinic, could provide leadership in the treatment of sick babies was rapidly passing. Moreover, the consensus among neonatologists was in favor of positive-pressure ventilators, rather than the negative-pressure devices that Donald had largely concentrated on. But perhaps the most important reason for the relative failure of Donald's innovations in the area of neonatal respiratory distress was that the biology of the human body did not cooperate. Without the missing factor of surfactant, mere ventilation of the infant lungs, whether by positive or negative pressure, could not achieve consistently satisfactory results. Indeed, Donald's sole unequivocal success in the field of medical technology at this stage, the imaging of hyaline membrane that he undertook with Steiner, showed how rare and problematic such successes were. Hence, Donald could not, for any of his early inventions, put together the heterogeneous nexus of technical, biological, social, and commercial factors that would have gained these devices the status of a successful clinical innovation. As we shall see, his luck, in this respect, would change dramatically.

CHAPTER FIVE

A-Scope Investigations in Glasgow

By 1955, Ian Donald was established in his post as Regius Professor of Midwifery and had already begun working on a new research project. In this chapter, we investigate his earliest attempts to apply ultrasound technology to clinical problems. In the course of our investigations, we employed an unorthodox historical method: a reenactment of Donald's first applications of the industrial flaw detector to biological materials. Later in his career, Donald was to represent these early experiments as an unequivocal success. However, our reconstruction revealed that he had been both fortunate in the results he obtained and naive in his interpretation of them. He did not wholly understand—indeed, could not have wholly understood—the nature of the modality he was working with. The contingent and emergent characteristics of scientific research are thus tellingly revealed. We also follow another fortuitous turn of events that was to have a crucial role in the development of Donald's research program: his meeting with Thomas Brown, who became his principal engineering collaborator.

Given Donald's institutional and vocational commitments, any new research project had to combine scientific interest with clinical potential. It seems to have been in October 1954 that Donald seriously resolved to investigate the medical possibilities of ultrasound.[1] He had been intrigued by his conversation with John Wild, during Wild's visit to the Hammersmith Hospital, and afterward, began to study Benson Carlin's *Ultrasonics*, a standard textbook on the physics of ultrasound.[2] Donald now knew of the industrial flaw detector and thought he had some understanding of how it worked.

Early in 1955, he managed to borrow, from a local engineering company, a powerful ultrasonic generator. This machine, which came with a tank of carbon tetrachloride, was probably used for the ultrasonic cleaning of industrial components. When the transducer was activated, considerable turbulence was produced in the tank. The energy levels generated were clearly far too large for the machine to be safely employed in diagnostic investigation, and Donald used the equipment to explore the biological effects of high-power ultrasound. He exposed vials of blood to the ultrasound beam for varying lengths of time, and by counting the numbers of intact cells remaining, he was able to measure the degree of hemolysis caused by the exposure. He concluded that the destructive effect on blood cells was in direct proportion to the heat generated by ultrasound.[3] Donald never published these results, but they seem to have convinced him that, at the levels likely to be useful diagnostically, ultrasound would not be harmful, as no significant heating of tissue should occur.

In the spring of 1955, one of Donald's patients, grateful for the successful outcome of an operation, introduced him to her husband, who happened to be a director of Babcock and Wilcox, an industrial fabrication company.[4] This was a stroke of good fortune. Babcock and Wilcox was a major user of industrial ultrasound. The company manufactured boilers for ships and for the nuclear power industry, employing ultrasonic flaw detectors to check welds and steel plate for cracks and other defects. Donald duly secured an invitation to the factory in Renfrew, near Glasgow. After lunch with the directors, he visited the fabrication yard and was introduced to Mr. Bernard (Benny) Donnelly, a technician in the nondestructive testing department. Donnelly was asked to demonstrate the ultrasonic flaw detector to Donald—he was using a Kelvin and Hughes Mk IV instrument (see fig. 5.1B) at this time.

Confident and voluble to the point of garrulousness, Donnelly was later to become well known in Glasgow as a businessman. Although only in his mid-twenties when he met Donald, Donnelly was sufficiently self-assured not to be cowed by the distinguished visitor. Indeed, he had not been intimidated by visitors even more awe-inspiring than the tall, red-haired professor. A colleague described the meeting thus:

> Benny was a very assertive shop steward, and after a threat to call a strike of the plate testers, he was given a week's notice to quit. However a visit of the Queen and Prince of Edinburgh to Babbies [Babcock and Wilcox] was due midweek and the route through the Drum shop carefully painted in and personnel detailed as to their conduct. Benny, as a known Communist, was positioned well back from the pathway . . . but the Prince, seeing Benny, and the flickering [screen] of the [flaw detector] set left the party and asked him what he was doing. The Duke was so intrigued by Benny's explanation that he called the Queen over, to the

consternation of the security, and had Benny explain again. After a demonstration, Benny asked the Queen if young Prince Charlie, at school in Australia, was writing regularly home. On being told by an *aide de camp* that he could not address the Queen directly, he told him to get stuffed, and the Queen, amused, told Benny that Charlie was doing well. Photographs were taken and the Press, when the party moved on, insisted on [hearing about] Benny's conversation. When Benny said that the conversation was personal, they went to the Drum Shop manager . . . and demanded the story. When he tried to persuade Benny, he was promptly reminded that Benny's sacking would be part of the story. He withdrew the notice [of dismissal] and Benny [re]told the conversation on condition that he got a large photo in return.[5]

Donnelly's character is noteworthy because the success of the meeting with Donald must be seen in the context of the class relations prevailing in British industry. In the 1950s there was a considerable social distance between employees and their bosses. Donnelly was a blue-collar shop-floor worker; he spoke with a broad Glaswegian accent. Donald was a well-spoken, high-status professional, who had just emerged from lunch in the boardroom. The commanding presence of the Regius Professor tended to overawe even those who were his social equals. Interaction between the two men could easily have been polite but strained and superficial. Donnelly had shown other visitors around the yard on those terms. But, unexpectedly, his exchanges with Donald turned out to be engaging and stimulating for both parties.

Donald and Donnelly most likely recognized each other as fellow enthusiasts. Within Babcock's, there was a competitive tension between the ultrasound technicians and those who undertook more traditional means of nondestructive testing, such as industrial radiography. A committed and articulate advocate for ultrasound, Donnelly was well practiced in the exposition of its virtues and industrial potential. Donald, ever intellectually curious, was keen to learn about the technology from a skilled exponent.

Watching Donnelly's demonstrations of flaw detection, Donald noticed that ultrasound technicians were in the habit of testing their equipment by bouncing the beam off the bone in their thumbs.[6] If an echo spike of approximately the right size appeared in the right place on their oscilloscope screens, they could be confident that the sensitivity and time-base settings were adjusted appropriately. Obtaining a strong echo from the thumb requires some expertise; the bone is small and round, presenting only a narrow target.

Donnelly located his thumb bone with a facility that was the product of constant practice. A wet thumb may have been a rough-and-ready method of calibration, but to an experienced craftsman, it was good enough for most engineering purposes.[7] A technician could quickly check his equipment in this way several times a day, as he moved from task to task or changed his probe. Thus, during Donald's first encounter with the flaw detector, he saw it being effectively applied to biological material, albeit to a limited extent.

Donnelly was aware, moreover, that the trace obtained from the thumb indicated something more than merely the presence of a strongly reflective surface. What appeared on the screen was not a simple spike, but what Donnelly termed an *envelope*—a spike with a broad base and more than one peak. Donnelly knew that the appearance of the envelope was different from the signal received from a flaw in a steel plate and that this difference must relate to the nature of the reflective surfaces within his thumb. In effect, Donnelly tacitly demonstrated to Donald that the trace contained some biological information about the tissues around the bone. Furthermore, Donnelly showed that if the probe was pressed harder against the thumb, the echo from the bone moved along the oscilloscope display nearer to the transmission spike. Donald also learned that Babcock's technicians sometimes bounced the beam off the bones in their shins, where similar phenomena could be observed. Donnelly demonstrated that different echoes were obtained if the beam was directed through the calf muscle rather than toward the bone and remarked that the technicians were themselves curious about which structures within the limb produced the complex envelope spike. Donald was "very very interested in this sort of thing."[8]

Donald was sufficiently intrigued by what he saw in Babcock's yard to arrange a further visit. On July 21, 1955, he and his colleague, the surgeon Wallace Barr, loaded up their car trunks with pathological specimens—uterine fibroids and a large ovarian cyst—all removed from patients in the operating room that morning. Babcock's provided "an enormous lump of steak by way of a control material."[9] Donald wanted to know whether the echoes obtainable with the flaw detector could differentiate between a solid tumor such as a fibroid and a fluid-filled, cystic structure.

There then followed a series of fascinating experiments behind closed doors in their [Babcock's] research department. We applied their ultrasonic probes directly to the various tissues and noted the type of echoes which appeared on their cathode ray screens. There were no facilities for photography and the factory artist was called in to sketch the results. All I wanted to know . . . was whether a metal flaw detector could show me on A-scan . . . the difference between a cyst and a myoma . . . To my surprise and delight the differences were exactly as my reading had led me to expect, the cyst showing clear margins without intervening echoes because of its fluid content and the fibroid progressively attenuating the returning echoes.[10]

Using the unmodified industrial equipment (fig. 5.1B), Donald was able to readily distinguish between the two sorts of pathological specimen.

Barr recalls that, on their return to the Western Infirmary, Donald was elated. For Donald, the afternoon had been an unequivocal success. In later decades he was to retell the story of their visit to Babcock's many times, always emphasizing that what had inspired him to further investigation was that the image they obtained from a solid tumor was clearly and unequivocally different from that obtained from a cyst.[11] Donald never published any of these early images, however, and none of the sketches made by Babcock's "factory artist" seem to have survived.[12]

To assist our understanding of these events, we organized a reconstruction of Donald's earliest investigations. We were fortunate in having the cooperation of Wallace Barr and Benny Donnelly in staging the reenactment (fig. 5.2), which both were able to attend. Mr. Donnelly lent us a working example of the instrument he had demonstrated to Donald. Dr. Barr advised us on the characteristics of the specimens they had taken to Babcock's. Our purpose was to achieve a better understanding of the events of July 21, 1955, and to gain an impression of what Donald's first ultrasound images might have looked like.[13]

Staging the reenactment proved a fascinating and rewarding exercise. We realized that it was fortunate for Donald that the difference between a fibroid and an ovarian cyst turned out to be quite as clear-cut as it apparently had. In the passage quoted above, Donald alludes to the twin-spiked echo pattern (fig. 5.3A), which was later recognized as characteristic of cystic, as opposed to solid, tumors. When an A-scope image is obtained from a fluid-filled structure in situ in the abdomen, a sharp echo is obtained from the far wall.[14] If the cyst is a simple one (without internal divisions), the fluid-filled space between the two walls returns, at most, only a few weak echoes and appears as virtually a flat line on the oscilloscope trace. A strong echo is also received from the near wall, although this may be obscured by echoes and reverberations

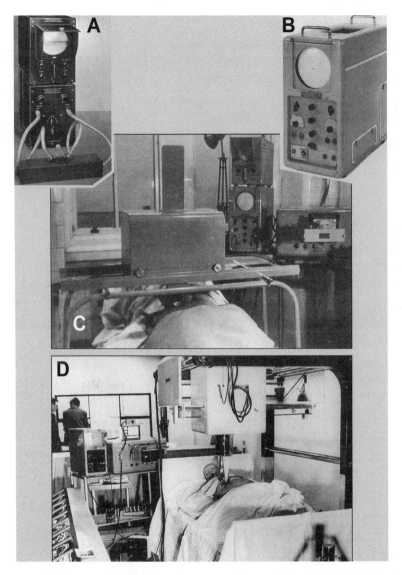

Figure 5.1. Prototype instruments, 1956 to the 1960s. *A*, Henry Hughes Mk IIb Supersonic Flaw Detector used by Ian Donald before the involvement of Tom Brown. *B*, Kelvin Hughes Mk IV Supersonic Flaw Detector (A-scan), as demonstrated to Ian Donald on his first visit to the Babcock and Wilcox factory, ca. June 1955, and used for the experiments there on July 21, 1955. A similar instrument was obtained by Brown for the early work by Donald and MacVicar. (A Mk IV was borrowed from Mr. B. Donnelly, Axiom NDT Ltd., for our reenactment in 1996.) *C*, Bed-table Scanner in the Western Infirmary, Glasgow, ca. 1957 (Brown acting as patient). *D*, Automatic Scanner in exhibition at Third International Conference on Medical Electronics, Olympia, London, July 1960. In the background, Tom Brown (*left*) and Brian Fraser. *Reproduced with permission of the BMUS Historical Collection*

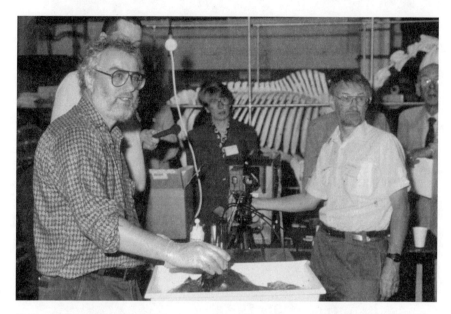

Figure 5.2. Reenactment, in July 1996, of Donald's first experiments on July 21, 1955. Nicolson is manipulating the transducer, Fleming adjusting the video camera that is viewing the flaw detector, partly hidden by his arm. The A-scan trace is displayed on a screen on the wall behind the photographer. Also pictured: Dr. Ian H. Spencer (with microphone) and Drs. Margaret B. McNay, Wallace Barr (behind Fleming), and James Willocks. The reenactment was conducted in the Department of Veterinary Anatomy, Glasgow University. *Photograph from the authors' files*

from structures lying between the cyst and the skin surface (fig. 5.3A); compare the trace of a solid tumor, the far wall of which gives only a few weak echoes (fig. 5.3B).

The unambiguous distinction between the ultrasonic characteristics of a simple cyst and a solid tumor, however, is crucially dependent on the sensitivity setting of the apparatus. Too high a setting will make fluid-filled objects appear solid, by picking up echoes from turbulence and small particles within the fluid. A very low sensitivity setting, by contrast, can give a solid tumor an ultrasonic appearance somewhat like that of a cyst, because the echoes from the internal structures of the tumor are not picked up. Indeed, when A-scope ultrasound was first used clinically, this feature was often exploited to aid in distinguishing cysts from solid tumors. The question then posed by Donald and his colleagues was often, how high does the sensitivity setting have to be

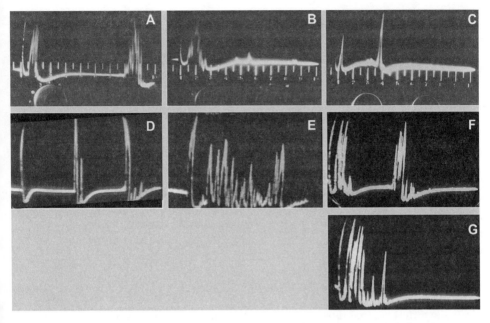

Figure 5.3. A-scans recorded by Donald, MacVicar, and Brown, ca. 1956: *A*, "ovarian cyst, abdominal swelling 30/52 size" (i.e., as expected at 30th week of pregnancy), "looking down through the cyst"; *B*, fibroid to the level of the umbilicus, "looking obliquely through the mass"; *C*, "full bladder." A-scans recorded during reenactment, July 1996: *D*, water-filled bovine bladder; *E*, piece of beef; *F* and *G*, human bladder (Fleming), in vivo, full and empty. *A, B, and C reproduced with permission of the BMUS Historical Collection; legends as on original slides, with minimal editing; D, E, F, and G from the authors' files*

to reveal information about the internal structure of the object? If the answer was "quite high," then the presence of a cyst was suspected.

But, of course, Donald did not know this in July 1955. Donnelly was not involved in Donald's second visit to Babcock's and it is unclear whether Donald had any technical assistance, on this occasion, from a competent user of the flaw detector. Somewhat patrician in manner, Donald was concerned both with the prerogatives of the medical profession and with protecting the sensitivities of laypeople, so he undertook the examination of the pathological material himself. Barr recollects that Donald initially had difficulty achieving acoustic coupling between the specimens and the probe—a problem that an ultrasound technician would have quickly solved.[15] The sensitivity of the Mk

IV flaw detector can be adjusted, and this function was sometimes used in the technical examination of steel plate. But for Donald, there must have been an element of good fortune in the fact that the sensitivity of the machine he used was set so as to provide him with a two-peaked trace for a cyst and a more complicated echo for a solid structure.

Donald must also have been fortunate in the nature of the pathological specimens he had brought with him. Mature fibroids may develop cavities due to degeneration, and they then display ultrasonic characteristics that are more cystlike. On the other hand, an ovarian cyst may display an A-scope appearance more like that of a solid tumor, if it has many internal divisions or its cavities contain a large amount of cellular debris, or both. Donald was lucky, therefore, that the fibroids he and Barr had harvested that morning were solid and that the ovarian cyst was simple, thus maximizing the ultrasonic distinction between the two types of tumor.

It should be noted that the results of the ultrasonic examination of a cystic structure removed from the body and placed on, say, a metal tray are somewhat different from those from the same structure in vivo. The A-scope trace of the extirpated specimen consists of two spikes with an anechoic gap between them, as does the trace from a cyst in place in the abdomen. But the origins of the spikes are not the same. This difference can be seen by comparing figures 5.3A and 5.3D. The first shows an ovarian cyst in vivo. At the left-hand end of the trace is a sharp, needlelike deflection indicating the transmission pulse. Then, after a gap of half a division, is the echo from the near wall of the cyst. After a gap of six full divisions, the echo from the far wall of the cyst is seen. Compare this with figure 5.3D, which was recorded during the reenactment. It is from a bovine bladder, used to simulate a cyst, resting on a metal tray, with the probe pressed against its upper surface. There are two very clear echoes, one in the center and another close to the right-hand end of the trace. These could easily be taken as the near and far walls of the bladder, but the right-hand spike is an artifact produced by reverberation. The central spike is the echo generated when the ultrasonic pulse reached the far wall of the specimen (and the metal tray). When that echo reached the face of the probe, some of its energy was again reflected and repeated the journey, thus producing a second echo. The near-wall echo is in fact the spike at the left-hand end of the trace; it has merged with the transmission pulse.

That a significant echo is not received from an interface in immediate contact with the probe of a Kelvin and Hughes Mk IV flaw detector is partly due to the characteristics of the probes used in industrial applications. In the non-destructive testing of steel plate, the operator is not interested in the characteristics of the surface, which may be inspected visually. Therefore, probes designed to detect deeper defects are used.[16] In the Mk IV, the transmitting and receiving transducer elements were placed side by side, usually at a small angle to one another. This produced a V-shaped sound path in the test material. The area immediately in front of the probe, inside the V, was not in the direct track of the beam, and thus the system had a low sensitivity at, and close to, the probe face.[17] The Mk IV also had a relatively long pulse length, again rendering it insensitive to echoes generated close to the transducer. When ultrasound is reflected from an object nearer to the probe than half the pulse length, the receiver begins to receive the pulse before the transmitter has finished transmitting it. Echolocation cannot work under these circumstances.

The difference between in vivo and in vitro A-scans of cystic structures had been deduced long before Donald published his account of his first experiments, "Medical Sonar—The First 25 Years," quoted from above, in 1980, but he seems not to have fully appreciated its significance. (Alternatively, perhaps he did not want to spoil a good story.) One may certainly conclude that, in 1955, Donald did not quite understand what he was seeing. Barr's recollection is that Donald was indeed convinced that the twin-spiked A-scan meant that he had detected echoes from both walls of the cyst.[18] This interpretation was strengthened, in Donald's mind, by his observation that if he moved the probe to a thinner part of the cyst, the two spikes came closer together on the oscilloscope screen. But, of course, the path length of the secondary reflection would also shorten.

The precise distance between the reflective surfaces and the probe could have been determined by interposing a test object at a known position or by reading the x-axis of the oscilloscope screen. Such refinements, however, were beyond Donald at this stage—he was content simply to see a trace that looked something like what his reading had led him to expect. It may be acknowledged that neither test would have been entirely straightforward to apply. First, interposing a test object requires the use of a water tank. Second, the x-axis of a flaw detector screen consists of a graticule, marked in arbitrary units representing echo times of between 4 and 1,200 microseconds, depending on the settings of the instrument. The scale would not have meant much to Donald. Moreover, given that the velocity of sound in tissue is only a quarter of that in steel, even an experienced industrial user of the flaw detector, unfamiliar with the acoustic properties of biological objects, might have been confused. It would have been a brave technician, and one confident of his ground, who dared contradict Donald in one of his moments of intense enthusiasm.[19]

In July 1955, despite extensive reading and his experience of radar, Donald was evidently still a naive user of ultrasound. It is revealing that, later, he recalled that the steak "gave confusing and intermediate results which was rather a waste, especially since nobody would accept it to take home for cooking!"[20] This is puzzling, since one would expect steak to have ultrasonic characteristics similar to those of a solid tumor—which was the result obtained in our reconstruction (fig. 5.3E). Thus it was fortuitous that the image Donald saw on the screen when he applied the flaw detector to an ovarian cyst corresponded with his intuitive idea of what the echo pattern from a fluid-filled object should be—two spikes with a gap in the middle. Donald's earliest experiments with ultrasound were certainly successful. But, like many an experimenter before him, he did not wholly know, and indeed could not have wholly known, exactly how he had produced these results.[21]

Donald was applying the flaw detector to a task quite different from that for which it was designed. Flaw detectors are used to find hairline cracks, or voids, within a solid, homogeneous medium—metal. Donald, by contrast, was attempting to characterize structures within a more or less fluid, far from homogeneous medium—tissue. He may have achieved what he regarded as the right results for the wrong reasons, but he had stumbled upon an application of ultrasound for which the material characteristics of the target object happened to be very favorable. We noted in chapter 2 how attempts at ultrasonic visualization of brain pathology were unsuccessful owing to distortion of the signal by the bones of the skull.[22] Abdominal cysts and fibroids proved to be comparatively amenable to ultrasonic investigation. Thus, part of Donald's good fortune as a pioneer of the biological application of ultrasound lay simply in his being a gynecologist.

(((((One might point to two further lessons that Donald learned during his visits to Babcock and Wilcox's yard, although neither was deliberately taught. One was the possibility of contact scanning. Earlier researchers had interposed a water column between the probe and the target. This procedure had certain advantages. Water transmits ultrasound readily and provides acoustic coupling. Also, by distancing the probe from the specimen, the water column eliminates the masking effect of paralysis produced in the amplifier by the transmission signal. In the industrial context, water baths were sometimes used in the examination of small components. Water baths also have some disadvantages, the most significant being secondary reflections within the tank. Moreover, an immersion technique was impractical for testing the welds of a large structure, such as a ship's boiler. Under these circumstances, the technicians at Babcock's applied their probes directly to the surface of the test object, relying on the generous application of a coupling agent, such as oil, to ensure acoustic coupling. With practice, reasonably precise detection of cracks could be achieved. Thus the investigative technique that Donnelly demonstrated to Donald was uncomplicated by quantities of water and would have seemed, in principle, compatible with diagnostic procedures. If the transfer of ultrasound to the clinic had appeared, from the outset, to entail putting patients in water baths, Donald would probably have been less excited about its potential. It may also be relevant that Carlin's *Ultrasonics* contains a more detailed account of contact scanning than was typical of textbooks on nondestructive testing in the 1950s.[23] The utility of contact scanning was a lesson that Donald learned only imperfectly, however, and would later have to be retaught.

Second, during his conversations with the personnel at Babcock's, Donald would have been aware of their presumption that ultrasound, at the power levels used in flaw detection, was not a health hazard. The technicians were happy to direct the beams from their transducers onto their thumbs or legs. Indeed, the fundamental rationale behind the deployment of ultrasound by Babcock's was that it was a safe alternative to the standard method of testing welds, X-radiography. In its main yard, Babcock and Wilcox had X-ray machines of enormous power that could "turn bottles blue."[24] When a test was being carried out, the shop-floor workers were supposed to retreat behind twenty-ton lead-lined doors. But stopping production and evacuating the floor for every test was inconvenient for both the management and the workforce, most of whom were being paid piecework. Some men chose merely to take shelter wherever it was available. With machines of that power, in a very reflective environment, considerable scattering of the radiation was inevitable, with consequent exposure of personnel not in the direct line of fire. Moreover, it was difficult, on a busy shop floor, to uphold the best standards of safe practice in the operation and maintenance of powerful X-ray machines.

The dangers associated with X-ray testing were, understandably, of increasing concern to what was a highly unionized, politically well-educated workforce. For a number of reasons, therefore, Babcock's head of engineering,

Dr. H. Harris, had sought to minimize the use of X-rays on the shop floor and so was keen to explore the possibilities of ultrasonic testing, which promised to be both less of a danger to personnel and less disruptive of production.

In the mid-1950s, as noted in chapter 4, the medical profession in general, and the specialty of obstetrics and gynecology in particular, were also becoming increasingly concerned with the dangers of X-radiation, following the careful statistical work of Alice Stewart and her colleagues.[25] Despite the initial skepticism of a number of clinicians, including Donald, her claims received widespread acceptance. Routine X-ray pelvimetry of pregnant women was abandoned in Britain and the United States, and X-ray imaging of the fetus was henceforth resorted to only for pressing clinical reasons. It was undoubtedly significant, therefore, that Donald's earliest experiments with ultrasound took place in a context in which it was regarded as essentially benign. With obstetric opinion hardening against X-radiography, the presumed safety of ultrasound would have increased its appeal as an alternative means of obtaining information from within the abdomen—even if, at this stage, Donald was envisaging the initial applications to be in gynecology rather than obstetrics.

(((((As we have seen, Donald wished to explore whether ultrasound could be employed to distinguish fibroids from ovarian cysts. This was an important diagnostic problem within Donald's clinical practice as a gynecologist in the 1950s. The setting-up of the National Health Service in 1948 had made health care available, free of charge to all, at the point of delivery. A hitherto unsuspected abundance of morbidity among the populace was revealed as patients took advantage of the new service. But, especially among working-class women, consultation with the doctor still tended to be delayed until their condition was relatively advanced. Thus, even in the mid-1950s, the hospital gynecologist was regularly confronted by women with gross, sometimes asymptomatic, distensions of the abdomen. Clinical history and physical examination were often unreliable guides to the underlying pathology, whether solid tumor, ovarian cyst, ascites, some other abdominal disorder, or even simple obesity. This clinical problem was not, of course, confined to the West of Scotland, but Donald believed it to be particularly prominent there, owing to the high prevalence of both gynecological morbidity and obesity among the Glaswegian working class.[26]

The NHS had responded to the unexpectedly high level of demand for treatment by effectively imposing rationing, accomplished then, as now, by means of waiting lists. But whereas a patient with a large fibroid could be safely left for several months until a convenient opportunity for intervention arose, ovarian cysts demanded more urgent investigation. Their underlying cause might be a malignant tumor.[27] Furthermore, bleeding from or rupture of a large cyst, even one of benign origin, could cause acute illness. Gynecologists were, understandably, reluctant to subject their patients to exploratory laparotomy (surgical opening of the abdomen)—hence the pressing need, within postwar Glaswegian gynecological practice, to find a reliable and minimally interventionist means of distinguishing between the two conditions. Donald, not surprisingly, responded to the apparently clear-cut distinction between the echo pattern of a solid tumor and that of a cystic structure with the conviction that further investigations into the diagnostic potential of ultrasound would be worthwhile.

Shortly after his visit to Babcock's, Donald contacted Professor Mayneord, at the Royal Cancer Hospital (the Marsden) in London, of whose work with diagnostic ultrasound he was already aware. He was also introduced, around this time, to Dr. Douglas Gordon, radiologist to the Willesden General Hospital.[28] Like Mayneord, Gordon was attempting to use A-scope equipment to detect shifts in the midline of the brain, in the hope of being able to locate brain tumors and subdural hematomas.[29] Donald visited the Marsden, where Mayneord and his colleagues received him very courteously. Donald found that they had encountered great difficulties in getting consistent echo patterns from within the skull and had become discouraged. Gordon, by contrast, was still very optimistic about the long-term potential of diagnostic ultrasound, and at his instigation, Mayneord lent Donald a flaw detector, which was duly transported to Glasgow. This was an old model, a Mk IIb (fig. 5.1A), rather than the more advanced Mk IV that Donnelly had demonstrated to Donald at Babcock's. Moreover, the loan instrument was the set that had been inappropriately modified by Turner to operate with a single probe, as described in chapter 2.

To help in his investigations, Donald enlisted the aid of Glasgow's Department of Clinical Physics, and in particular of Ron Greer, who was already assisting his respirator work. Together they set out to recreate the success achieved at Babcock's in distinguishing between cysts and solid tumors in vitro, and to begin investigating the intact abdomen.

(((((Donald's first trials with the flaw detector in Babcock and Wilcox's yard had been remarkably successful. In the Western Infirmary, however, he and

Greer were unable to reliably reproduce the earlier results. It was soon determined that the machine Donald had acquired had a long paralysis time. No echoes were discernible from targets nearer to the probe than eight centimeters. It was impossible to gather useful information from within the abdomen under these circumstances. The obvious solution was to interpose a water column, at least eight centimeters long, between the probe and the patient's skin. Donald experimented with large Perspex tubes, covered at one end with a flexible rubber membrane. The rubber was coated with grease and applied to the patient's abdomen. The tube was then filled with water, into which the ultrasonic probe was "gingerly dipped."[30] Wet beds and soaked patients were, more often than not, the result.

The decision was made to try to contain the water column within a flexible membrane. The obvious device was a water-filled rubber condom. In the 1950s, however, contraceptive sheaths were not commodities that a respectable medical gentleman found easy to buy in his home town.

> Being rather well-known, by sight if not by repute, in a city like Glasgow, I was naturally a little reticent in those days about being seen entering one of those shops for surgical rubber goods . . . My friend the late Professor James Louw from Cape Town was visiting me at the time and . . . offer[ed] to buy them for me. On being asked . . . whether he wanted teat-ended or plain, he astonished her [the shop assistant] by saying that he would go out to the car and enquire.[31]

This story quickly gained wide circulation in Glasgow medical circles and beyond.

The association of Donald's clinical investigations with objects as unspeakable as condoms did not endear him to the prim and proper nursing staff of the Western Infirmary. The nurses might have been less inconvenienced by wet beds, but they were far from enthusiastic about the latest disturbance to the decorum and good order of their wards. Donald soon reverted to Perspex or glass cylinders. It seems to have been around this time that the Regius Professor was first dubbed "Mad Donald." The sobriquet encapsulated the character of the initial response of the local medical establishment to his eccentric technological enthusiasms and unconventional behavior.

Sometime in 1956, Donald enlisted Dr. John MacVicar, registrar in the Department of Midwifery, to help with this research. But, despite the extra assistance, little or no progress was being made. Donald and MacVicar were unable to get consistent echo patterns from within the abdomen. What limited echoes they were able to discern, they could not reliably interpret. More-over, the only means of recording their results was by making sketches of the rapidly flickering oscilloscope traces. Even given Donald's considerable artis-tic skill, this method was clearly limited and scientifically unsatisfactory, as well as time-consuming and thus inconvenient to both doctor and patient—on whose abdomen the heavy tube of water had to be precariously balanced until the sketch was completed.

One evening in late 1956, Donald received a phone call that was to transform his project's chances of success. It was from Thomas (Tom) Brown, twenty-three years old, an engineer with Kelvin and Hughes Ltd. at their Hillington factory, in Glasgow. Brown was to be a major force in the development of diag-nostic ultrasound, and we now consider his earlier career in some detail.

(((((Like Donald, Brown had been interested in electronic and mechanical devices from an early age.

> I had been a hobbyist, brought up during the war in fairly isolated circumstances and got into crystal sets and valve radios and what have you . . . I was in the Air Training Corps and I had a chance of going to the RAF camps . . . I got myself a wee bit of a reputation because I came back from one of the RAF camps with a complete gyroscopic compass system out of a Stirling Bomber and I took it to bits and found out how it worked, put it back together again and got it all work-ing as a demonstration.[32]

Brown attended Allan Glen's School in Glasgow, which had a science-based curriculum and a good reputation as a feeder school for the science and engi-neering faculties of the Scottish universities. He gained sufficient qualifica-tions for university entry but did not wish to continue formal full-time educa-tion. "I had had enough of schooling for my tastes, but didn't really know what I wanted to do with my life," he recalls. A teacher "arranged for me to visit Kelvin & Hughes after school one afternoon, to meet Mr. Peter Turner, the Chief Engineer. It was like wandering into a kind of intellectual 'Aladdin's Cave,' and within half an hour I had made up my mind that this was for me, and in April 1951 I joined as a 'Technical Apprentice.'"[33] While an apprentice with Kelvin and Hughes, and studying part-time for professional qualifications, Brown gained experience of many aspects of electronic and instrumentation engi-neering. Furthermore, he acquired an appreciation of the work of the crafts-men who built instruments or used them in the industrial setting.

As we described in chapter 2, Kelvin and Hughes manufactured marine radar apparatus and underwater echo sounders. They also made "Supersonic Flaw Detectors" for the nondestructive testing of industrial materials. Brown was initially attached to the company's marine products division, where he worked on some radar applications and "big sonar systems for catching whales."[34] Then, in 1953, he was assigned to assist Alexander Rankin, head of Applications Engineering. Rankin was a metallurgist by training and an enthusiast, by vocation, for the industrial application of ultrasound.[35] Kelvin and Hughes's main ultrasound research and development department was located in its factory in Barkingside, near London, but Rankin had been sent up to Glasgow to be nearer the major industrial customers on the Clyde. He had established a small "applications research" unit in an old air-raid shelter within the grounds of the Hillington factory. His remit was to develop the market for ultrasonic flaw detectors by designing special transducers and other hardware to meet the specific needs of individual clients.

One of Kelvin and Hughes's most important customers for ultrasound equipment was Babcock and Wilcox's Renfrew factory. The head of engineering at Babcock's, Dr. Harris, had posed Rankin a particularly difficult technical problem. As we have seen, Harris sought to minimize the use of X-ray testing on the shop floor and to replace it as far as possible with ultrasonic flaw detection. There was a problem, however. To obtain insurance coverage for the welded pressure vessels they manufactured, Babcock and Wilcox was required to supply the insurance companies with documentary evidence of the integrity of every weld. X-radiography could produce an acceptable record, on a photographic plate; ultrasonography, as then practiced, could not. Recordings taken from the oscilloscope screen of a flaw detector were not acceptable for insurance purposes, since the position of the ultrasound probe at the time any image was taken could not be precisely specified. Moreover, the conditions under which each trace was obtained were difficult to define exactly, since the identification of weld defects with a flaw detector depended on the craft skill of the individual operator.

Rankin came to the conclusion that only a fully automated system could produce a record of the ultrasonic inspection that was sufficiently standardized to satisfy the insurance companies. "There were formidable practical problems involved," Brown recalls, "and even today such techniques are only feasible in strictly limited circumstances, but of course we did not know then just how difficult it would be."[36] Rankin felt that this project was not getting the support it merited from Kelvin and Hughes's main ultrasound department at Barkingside. So he welcomed the addition to his small staff of an evidently bright and promising young engineer who already had a noteworthy track record within the company.

> With all the benefits of youthful inexperience and enthusiasm, I plunged in, and ran into all sorts of practical problems. These were mainly associated with the hostile electrical environment in a welding shop, and the unpredictable acoustic contact between transducers and the rough surfaces of the vessels. I ended up developing quite an ambitious system, which would select for recording only echoes from particular regions of the test piece, by means of electronic time "gating." I also found it necessary to stabilise the overall sensitivity of the system by selecting a reference echo from the test piece boundary, and using it indirectly to control the overall sensitivity. It sounds simple, but in practice it was quite difficult. I did get a system working, really quite well, and the company applied for patents.[37]

In building his prototype, Brown was greatly assisted by the handbooks published by the Radiation Laboratory at the Massachusetts Institute of Technology and by the greater availability and reliability of electronic components that had followed the development of radar.[38] Thus, like many other innovations at this time, Brown's flaw detection instrument was made possible by the transformation of electronics technology that had resulted from wartime investments in echolocation in Britain and the United States.

Although proud of how well his prototype worked, Brown was a little diffident about the quality of the design and was not displeased when it was proposed that the project be taken over for further development by the main research group at Barkingside. Impressed with the performance of Brown's prototype, Rankin went ahead and took a number of advance orders, unknowingly building up a legacy of trouble for the company and for Brown.

Brown's seniors at Kelvin and Hughes's Glasgow branch were very pleased with his performance as an apprentice and proposed that he should undertake further academic study.

> I got a pat on the head and [they] said "You ought to go to university, young man, we'll pay," and they said, "What would you like to do?" and I said, "Medicine." And they said "Get lost." So . . . I said, "What about Applied Physics because that is what I am doing, acoustics and so on?" "All right, Applied Physics."[39]

Brown enrolled in a course of applied physics at the Royal College for Science and Technology (now the University of Strathclyde). But there was a bureaucratic difficulty. He had not yet done his National Service, and his period of educational deferment could not be extended indefinitely. Accordingly, he negotiated an arrangement with the college whereby, in the light of his existing qualifications in engineering, he would go straight into the second year of the course, simultaneously taking extra evening classes in the subjects in which he was weakest.

> Now maths had never been my strong suit and there was more maths and heavier maths in the second year of the applied physics course than there would have been in the whole of the electrical engineering course, had I taken electrical engineering. I couldn't hack the maths. I learned a lot in the course of the year . . . but not enough to pass the exams, certainly not in maths or physics. So I did the sort of thing young men in those circumstances do, I saw too much of my girlfriend, a nurse in the Western Infirmary, and played too much snooker, and resat the exams to no avail, and eventually I had to go back to Kelvin Hughes, cap in hand, and say, "Can I have my job back?"

No longer quite the golden boy, Brown was put to work on a more mundane project: designing a smoke detector for factory chimneys.

(((((Kelvin and Hughes also made lamps for operating rooms. Edward Smith, a senior salesman, was responsible for marketing this equipment. Smith and Ian Donald happened to be acquaintances, having met while Donald was in London, through their common interest in sailing. When Kelvin and Hughes came up with a new design of shadowless lamp, Smith arranged that Donald should undertake a field trial in the Western Infirmary. A squad of men from the Hillington factory arrived in Donald's department to make the installation, one of whom noticed Donald's ultrasound equipment and later happened to mention to Tom Brown that "the doctor" was using a flaw detector "on people."

Brown had retained his interest in ultrasound, despite his fall from grace, and was intrigued. "Not knowing any better," he recalls, "I looked Donald up in the book, and telephoned him that evening. He was friendly and very courteous, but told me that he had all the technical help he needed from Dr Lenihan's Department of Clinical Physics . . . However I was welcome to come and see what he was doing." When Brown visited the Western Infirmary, he found Donald still using the equipment lent by the Marsden. It was an "ancient . . .

very much the worse-for-wear, black-crackle painted, Kelvin & Hughes Mk IIb Supersonic Flaw Detector," together with a "comical arrangement of glass tubes and water jugs and jars of petroleum jelly."

> The apparatus . . . hadn't even been made by Kelvin and Hughes, it had been made to Kelvin and Hughes's designs by some other company under a Ministry of Supply manufacturing contract, the sort of thing that happened towards the end of the war. One of the things that was noticeable about it was the front panel had a gaping hole in it where somebody had been at it with a hacksaw. Also sitting on the trolley was a big jar of Vaseline and a glass cylinder about 10 inches long and about 2½ or 3 inches diameter . . . and a large jug of water and plenty of towels. So the patient was wheeled in and the Professor, in his best bedside manner, pulled back the covers exposing this large abdomen. He picks up the glass cylinder and smears one end with Vaseline and sort of brings it on to the abdomen, picks up the jug of water, fills the cylinder up with water and then picks up the probe and sticks it in the end.

The transmitter of a Mk IIb flaw detector produced a pulse of approximately 1,500 V. The amplifier, however, could not process signals above 20 mV, orders of magnitude less than the transmission pulse. Accordingly, several features had been incorporated into its design to protect the amplifier, as far as was feasible, from the transmission pulse. The principal feature was two separate probes, one for transmission and one for receiving. To facilitate its application to the skull, the machine Donald was using had been modified to circumvent this. Brown recalls:

> During its journey to the Royal Marsden Hospital, somebody had thought "This is no damn good, we want one probe to do both jobs." So they connected the two together. Now this amplifier wasn't capable of handling that, so it got belted with fourteen hundred volts, went into paralysis and only very gradually came out of paralysis and was able to start amplifying signals again. So Donald's expedient was to use the glass cylinder with the patient, to allow the amplifier to recover from its paralysis. So, you got a paralysis with nothing at all and then a few little echoes at the end, which were from inside the patient. It was a travesty of the technology of the day, but they didn't know any better then. He [Donald] was doing his best with it. So the real fun started when he tried to get the water back out of the cylinder and into the jug, which is why there were plenty of towels.

However, it was clear to Brown that even under these unfavorable conditions, some potentially useful information was being obtained from within the body.

Brown telephoned Rankin, who was back in Barkingside trying to sort out the problems created by his overenthusiastic selling of products based on Brown's mechanized flaw detector. Rankin was receptive to the news of the Glasgow trials, partly because of his commitment to finding novel uses for ultrasound and partly because it was not his first encounter with medical application. Rankin had supplied equipment and advice to Lars Leksell in Sweden, who had undertaken experiments in the ultrasonic detection of the cerebrum's midline. He had also had some contact with Douglas Gordon.[40] Only a few days after receiving Brown's phone call, Rankin dispatched to Glasgow a brand-new Mk IV flaw detector, retail price £600.[41]

> [It] arrived at Glasgow Central Station, without any paperwork marked "To Be Called For by Mr Tom Brown." I didn't drive then, but got that brute of an instrument out of the station and into a taxi, and up to the Western Infirmary, then on to a patient cart, and up to . . . Donald's Gynaecology Unit. The Mk IV was also a double-transducer machine, but when used with a decent double-transducer probe, the results were strikingly better than anything Donald had seen before, I was "in" . . . and Dr. Lenihan's Department took a bit of a back seat.[42]

Donald and MacVicar were immediately impressed with the new apparatus and were fascinated by the extra information it enabled them to gather.

It is a telling illustration of the state of Donald's knowledge of ultrasound at this time that he was unaware of the deficiencies of the machine inherited from Mayneord. Even if it had been working properly in its unmodified form, the Mk IIb flaw detector was, in terms of technological development, about five years behind the instrument Donald had used at Babcock's. Its electronics were markedly inferior to the Mk IV. Moreover, Donald's advisors in the Department of Clinical Physics seem to have neither understood the inherent deficiencies of the Mk IIb nor appreciated that the machine they were using had been modified in a deleterious manner. At a stroke, Brown sorted these problems out. Donald now had state-of-the-art equipment and authoritative advice. The improvement in the performance of the apparatus was very evident. The success of Brown's intervention was embarrassing to Greer and to his head of department, Dr. Lenihan, whose doctoral research had been on the physics of sound. Brown's star quickly rose, and relations between Donald and

Lenihan cooled significantly. The arrival of the Mk IV flaw detector effectively brought Donald's collaboration with Greer to an end.

Brown also managed to acquire for Donald a Cossor oscilloscope camera that could record the A-scan traces on rolls of 35 mm film. Both Brown and MacVicar recall that Donald regarded the arrival of the camera as a significant addition to the project.[43] Not only was photography more convenient and accurate than making drawings of the oscilloscope trace by hand, but reproducible and objective images were essential if the results of their ultrasound investigations were to be disseminated effectively within the academic community.

By far the most important addition to Donald's project at this time, however, was Brown himself. The dynamic and innovative clinical professor, fascinated by technology, had met his ideal foil: the brilliant young engineer intrigued by medicine. Brown was admirably equipped to assist Donald in his pioneering research. As well as possessing a creative technical intelligence, Brown had a broad background in instrumentation and had worked on virtually every aspect of industrial ultrasound technology. Grappling with the difficult, in some respects intractable, problems of his pioneering mechanized flaw detector had provided him with excellent training for further innovative endeavors with pulse-echo ultrasound. He had developed a depth of understanding of the electronic and mechanical intricacies of the technology that can have been rivaled by few of his contemporaries. Brown was, moreover, eager to restore his reputation within Kelvin and Hughes. "Shame was the spur," as he later put it.[44]

Brown's involvement with Donald's ultrasound research was initially on a purely informal, unpaid basis. He would go to the Western Infirmary in the evenings, after his day's work at Hillington, and work with MacVicar, developing and analyzing the film from that day's clinical examinations and performing maintenance, if required. Brown and MacVicar also experimented with applying the flaw detector to their own bodies to gain experience with biological materials.

Brown designed a Perspex water tank, which had on one side a circular window covered by a rubber membrane, against which an ultrasound probe could be placed.[45] It may seem odd that, with the acquisition of the Mk IV flaw detector, and having abolished the water column from their clinical investigations, the team should now introduce a water bath into their laboratory experiments. The principal purpose of this apparatus, however, was to mimic the circumstances of in vivo examination. The tank was, in effect, an experimental model of the abdomen, with the rubber membrane functioning as the patient's skin and abdominal wall. The hope was to explore the ultrasonic characteristics of tissue by scanning patients preoperatively and then examining excised specimens of tumors and cysts postoperatively in the water tank. The team made 165 or so A-scope records of this sort. But it gradually became clear that the ultrasonic characteristics of excised tissue were significantly different from those of living tissue in situ, largely due to the lack of blood flow. It was also difficult to replicate exactly the angle at which the tumor had been addressed while in the abdomen. Nevertheless, in the course of this work, MacVicar and Brown gained considerable experience in the relation between frequency and attenuation. They decided that, for the examination of large abdominal masses, a transducer vibrating at 2.5 MHz was generally the most suitable, providing a reasonable compromise between penetration and resolution.

MacVicar and Brown also tried to make model preparations that would simulate the ultrasonic appearances of other bodily structures. They experimented, for example, with filling condoms with water stained with meconium, to mimic the appearance of the amniotic sac. But, again, the results were disappointing.[46] Whatever study materials were used, these tank experiments were complicated by the recurring problem of secondary reflections from the walls of the tank and the water surface. Donald, moreover, had little interest in a sustained series of laboratory investigations.[47] The tank experiments were soon abandoned and their results were never published.[48]

Donald's real passion was always for clinical application. He was later to represent the termination of the team's in vitro experiments as an essential step toward the realization of ultrasound's diagnostic potential: "We . . . threw our tanks onto the top of the most inaccessible cupboards. As soon as we got rid of the backroom attitude and brought our apparatus fully into the department with an inexhaustible supply of living patients with fascinating clinical problems we were able to get ahead really fast."[49]

MacVicar and Brown carried an enormous workload at this time. Much of the work had to be done in the evenings, after Brown had finished his day's work at Hillington and MacVicar had finished his normal clinical duties. At this time, too, patients were available for nonroutine investigations. Also, it was often in the evenings that they discussed the clinical significance of the images with Donald. The professor, by now fired with enthusiasm, was driving his team hard. His impatience with any delay imposed heavy burdens on his colleagues, particularly on Brown, who had the responsibility of keeping the flaw detector working optimally. It was fortunate that a mutually supportive relationship grew between Brown and MacVicar. MacVicar, whose background was clinical and who had little experience of research, had become convinced that diagnostic ultrasound would eventually have a significant impact in obstetrics and gynecology. He therefore saw his collaboration with Brown and Donald as a major opportunity to further his career in academic medicine. He was aware, moreover, that the success of the project depended crucially on Donald's drive and vision and on Brown's technical brilliance. He was thus prepared to undertake many of the more routine tasks in support of his two colleagues. He was later to describe himself, with an undue degree of humorous self-effacement, as the "dogsbody" of the team.[50]

Donald's desire to make rapid progress was not merely another expression of his customary energy and motivation. He had a pressing, if personal, reason to be impatient—intimations of mortality. Donald was now aware that one of the valves of his heart had been seriously affected by the rheumatic fever he had suffered in his youth. His cardiac function was progressively deteriorating: he anticipated having to submit to major surgery in the not too distant future. The prospect of a heart valve operation was, in those days, a grave one indeed, and Donald approached his ordeal with even more than usual trepidation. His sister Margaret had also suffered damage to her heart as a teenager and had had to give up her medical studies at the Royal Free Hospital as a result. She had married and returned to southern Africa, but her condition had continued to deteriorate. Early in 1957, Donald arranged for her to travel to Scotland, to be admitted to Glasgow Royal Infirmary for surgery. Tragically, she died in the course of the operation. Grief-stricken, Donald was also increasingly apprehensive that he might suffer a similar fate. Thus, in relentlessly spurring Brown and MacVicar on, Donald was a sick man in a hurry.

(((((Gradually, Donald, MacVicar, and Brown began to gain confidence in their ability to interpret the information their equipment allowed them to obtain. They learned not only how to distinguish cysts from fibroids but also to recognize the ultrasonic characteristics of different types of cysts. The team received considerable encouragement from the first occasion on which the ultrasonic findings significantly improved upon clinical opinion. A woman was admitted to Donald's gynecological department with lower abdominal pain and purulent vaginal discharge. On examination, a midline swelling was palpable, from within the pelvis to well above the symphysis pubis. The patient was deemed to be suffering from pyometra, accumulation of pus in the cavity of the uterus. However, the echoes obtained with the flaw detector were suggestive of the presence of an ovarian cyst. Laparotomy confirmed the ultrasonic indications, revealing a cyst of the right ovary, which had twisted downward to lie on the anterior surface of the uterus.[51]

On other occasions, contradictions between the clinical and ultrasonic diagnoses were not resolved in the technology's favor. In one case, a patient presented with intermittent vaginal bleeding. Abdominal palpation revealed a firm swelling, extending from within the pelvis nearly to the umbilicus. On vaginal examination, a diagnosis of uterine fibromyoma was arrived at. However, when the flaw detector was applied to the woman's abdomen, one set of echoes was obtained from the anterior wall of the swelling and another set from a greater depth. There seemed to be no echoes originating from within the structure itself. Accordingly, a diagnosis of cyst was offered. At laparotomy, however, the swelling proved to be a highly vascular fibroid. The quantity of blood in the tumor had misled the ultrasound investigators, who had not previously encountered this sort of fibroid.[52]

This misdiagnosis is indicative of the difficulties that Donald, MacVicar, and Brown faced in trying to make sense of the A-scope traces they were obtaining. Their interpretative challenge was completely novel. There was no model for them to build on. Experience in the interpretation of ultrasonic echoes was slowly and painfully accumulated. Reflecting on their problem with the vascular fibroid, MacVicar later commented, perhaps more in hope than assurance, that they would not have made the same mistake twice.[53] This case also vividly revealed the limitations of in vitro ultrasonic experimentation. An attempt to recreate the in vivo A-scope trace by examining the fibroid in the water tank failed, illustrating the role of blood flow in producing the distinctive characteristics of the tumor.

One diagnostic coup was particularly noteworthy.[54] Donald was invited to demonstrate his new apparatus to colleagues in the Department of Medicine. A sixty-four-year-old woman with a grossly distended abdomen was chosen as the subject for the demonstration. She was vomiting regularly, was anemic from hematemesis, and was rapidly losing weight. Professor (later, Sir) Edward Wayne, Regius Professor of the Practice of Medicine, had diagnosed gastric cancer, a conclusion that radiological investigation, revealing a filling defect of the stomach wall, appeared to confirm. The abdominal swelling was attributed to ascites caused by secondary tumors in the liver. The patient's condition was deemed inoperable. She was receiving only nursing care, having effectively been abandoned to die.

Donald's physical examination supported the diagnosis of ascites, but while he was applying the probe to the abdomen, MacVicar looked over his shoulder at the oscilloscope screen and exclaimed, "Looks like an ovarian cyst!" In reward for venturing his opinion, MacVicar received a sharp kick underneath the bed screen from Donald. Brown, who was also present, supported MacVicar. Questioning a diagnostic pronouncement by the Regius Professor of Medicine was not a course of action to be embarked upon lightly. Wayne did not take offense, however, admitting that he was not certain in his diagnosis. The radiological evidence was equivocal, and no malignant cells had been found in fluid tapped from the woman's abdomen. Donald likewise conceded that the ultrasonic appearance of the swelling might be misleading and asked that the woman be admitted to his gynecological department for further investigation. Laparotomy duly confirmed the ultrasonic diagnosis, and a massive cyst was successfully removed. The patient made a complete recovery and lived healthily for decades thereafter.

It is an indication of the team's developing expertise in the interpretation of A-scans that MacVicar could instantly recognize the difference between the ultrasonic characteristics of ascites and those of a cyst. A simple cystic structure would show as an echoless space within the abdomen, bounded by echoes from the near and far walls. In ascites, the abdominal cavity fills with fluid, which, like the contents of a cyst, reflects few echoes. However, in most cases of ascites, the bowel floats free in the accumulated peritoneal fluid. The lumen of the bowel always contains gas, which is highly reflective of ultrasound. Thus, had the patient been ascitic, the echoless space produced by the fluid would have had dispersed within it a distinctive pattern of strong echoes from intestinal gas. The differential diagnosis of ascites and simple cyst was thus, like the discrimination between cyst and fibroid, a task well suited to A-scan investigation. The flaw detector's probes were, as an unintended consequence of being designed to find voids in a solid medium, effective in the detection of gas pockets within the bowel, the common feature between the two applications being strongly reflective interfaces. In other words, MacVicar benefited from the fact that Wayne's patient had a condition that, by lucky chance, was amenable to elucidation by ultrasound.

In later years, Donald repeatedly affirmed that saving this patient's life was a watershed in the development of his ultrasound research program. After such a dramatic success, there would be no turning back. That ultrasound had clinical potential in gynecology could no longer be doubted, and it would be unthinkable not to develop the technique as quickly as possible. It may be that such a view is a retrospective reconstruction, telescoping a gradual realization into a single moment of illumination. That certainly is Brown's view of events.[55] Yet it is undoubtedly the case that this and other diagnostic coups helped diminish the initial skepticism of Donald's colleagues in the Western Infirmary.

The members of the Department of Medicine evidently did not hold Donald's contradiction of their professor's opinion against him, for, sometime later, they again sought his advice.[56] A patient in the Western Infirmary who had been diagnosed with mitral stenosis was operated on for its relief. Having opened the chest, the surgeon palpated the heart and found a mass in the left atrium, which he concluded was a myxoma. A myxoma is a rare, benign tumor of the connective tissue of the heart that may, on occasion, produce symptoms confusingly similar to those of mitral valve disease. Its removal was within the repertoire of cardiac surgery by the late 1950s—the first successful operation was performed in 1954.[57] However, the procedure required cardiopulmonary bypass, for which preparations had not been made. Accordingly, the surgeon closed the chest with a view to proceeding on another day. The patient's physicians were annoyed; they were convinced that the palpable mass was a clot and that the operation to dilate the stenotic valve should have gone ahead. Donald was asked to use his new-fangled apparatus to adjudicate. He concluded that the physicians were correct in their suspicion of thrombus, an opinion confirmed when the chest was again opened. Unhappily, the patient did not survive the second operation.

In this case, Donald was again fortunate in the nature of the organ he was asked to look at. The heart has some of the characteristics of a cystic structure, consisting as it does of fluid-filled cavities containing solid structures. These are favorable circumstances for the application of A-scope ultrasound in diagnosis. Nevertheless, the ultrasonic differentiation of atrial myxoma from thrombus was challenging in the early years of echocardiography, and indeed remains so, at least on occasion, to the present day.[58]

Donald did not publish an account of this case. The first published description of ultrasonic diagnosis of atrial myxoma, by Effert and colleagues, appeared in the same year, 1957. Whether Donald or his physician colleagues knew of this German work before he attempted the differential diagnosis we have been unable to discover, although Donald did refer to Effert's paper in his first publication on ultrasound in 1958.[59] Later, echocardiography would become the technique of choice in diagnosing structural abnormalities of the heart.[60]

When Donald was asked to look at the patient with the supposed myxoma, his Mk IV flaw detector was in the Royal Maternity Hospital, and so the man was transported there to be examined. It is a measure of the physicians' determination to prove their diagnosis correct that they were prepared to transport an ill man across Glasgow. It also speaks of Donald's willingness to defy convention that he arranged for a bed to be prepared to receive a male patient in his antenatal ward. To some, his eccentricity was confirmed.

> It was at this point that I was delighted to see advancing upon the scene, like a ship under full sail, one of the senior nurses from another unit. Hitherto she had shown not the slightest interest in any of my research, but now she was all eager to behold with her own eyes the spectacle of a male, admittedly a sick male, in a bed in an antenatal ward of a maternity hospital. Her triumph was enormous. She came, she saw, she went away scandalized![61]

Donald rather relished such notoriety.

The location of Donald's flaw detector in the Royal Maternity Hospital indicates that, by late 1957, he had expanded his research interests from his initial concern with gynecological conditions toward encompassing the ultrasonic examination of pregnant women. That this development did not occur until the second year of the project can be attributed to a concern with safety. Donald's hemolysis experiments, together with the absence of damage associated with the use of continuous ultrasound for therapeutic purposes and the apparently sustained healthiness of the thumbs and lower limbs of the technicians at Babcock and Wilcox, gave him considerable confidence that ultrasound was not deleterious to human tissue at low intensities. This opinion was substantiated by the literature on the safety of ultrasound, which suggested that structural damage would be produced only at energy levels many times greater than those that Donald intended to use diagnostically. Wild, likewise, had concluded that his diagnostic apparatus produced no deleterious effects on the brains of experimental animals, while operating at an intensity roughly equivalent to an exposure, at the surface of the human body, of 1.3 W cm^{-2} (watts per square centimeter).[62] By contrast, Brown estimated the power output of the

Kelvin and Hughes Mk IV as less than 1.5 mW cm^{-2}, with only 0.7 cm^2 of the patient's skin irradiated at any one time.[63] Nevertheless, there was a significant ethical difference between, on the one hand, applying the flaw detector to a gravely ill adult patient in the hope of a potentially life-saving intervention and, on the other, exposing a developing fetus to ultrasound radiation. As the research team appreciated, moreover, the deleterious effects of X-radiation had not been recognized for some time after its clinical use began.

Convinced though he was that pulsed ultrasound at diagnostic intensity was harmless, Donald felt a need to demonstrate its safety more rigorously. At his instigation, Dr. P. Bacsich, of Glasgow University's Department of Anatomy, exposed the heads of a pair of two-day-old sibling kittens, under anesthesia, to the flaw detector for one hour. Two other kittens from the same litter were used as controls. One of the exposed kittens and one of the controls were sacrificed twenty-four hours later. The other pair were sacrificed after three weeks. Their brains were fixed and sectioned, and a detailed comparison was undertaken between the insonated kittens and the controls.

> In the microscopical examination of the brains of the 24-hour experimental kitten, signs of cavitation, coagulative necrosis, localised hyperaemia, haemorrhages, and chromatolysis were looked for; and the brain of the 3-week kitten was examined for any evidence of patchy cell destruction, neuroglial scarring, axonal degeneration and localised lack of myelination. All these tests were completely negative, and the brains of the experimental kittens and their respective controls were in every way comparable.[64]

On recovery from anesthesia, the exposed animals had exhibited completely normal behavior and, in the case of the kitten allowed to live for three weeks, normal development. The exposure of the kittens to thirty times the dose of ultrasound necessary for diagnostic use had caused no apparent neurological damage. Donald thus felt sufficiently confident of the safety of the modality to proceed cautiously with obstetric investigations.

Bacsich chose cats as his experimental subjects because kittens retain fetal-like structural characteristics in their brains for some time after birth.[65] By present-day standards, of course, a study involving only four animals, that focused solely on neurological effects, and that employed no fetal subjects, might seem hardly adequate.[66] However, Bacsich's investigation did compare favorably with other studies on the safety of ultrasound conducted in the 1950s.

Nevertheless, the main purpose of his investigation was, in effect, to put a cloak of scientific respectability around Donald's working assumption that the technique was safe. Donald now became fond of opining that being exposed to diagnostic ultrasound was "no more dangerous than listening to Beethoven's Fifth Symphony."[67]

Initially, Donald and his colleagues made uncertain progress with their application of ultrasound to obstetric cases. The only structure of the fetus that the team could identify with confidence was the skull. Indeed, it is ironic, given the future career of the technology, that obstetric scans were regarded as particularly difficult to interpret "because of the echoes from the fetal parts."[68] It was soon discovered, however, that A-scope ultrasound could reveal the presence of polyhydramnios, an excess of amniotic fluid relative to the size of the fetus; the gravid uterus is thus rendered more cystic than usual. Polyhydramnios may be associated with fetal abnormalities such as anencephaly, which could be confirmed by radiological investigation.

The first clear-cut demonstration of the utility of ultrasound in the monitoring of pregnancy was accomplished, not by Donald or MacVicar, but by one of the staff nurses of the Royal Maternity Hospital, Miss Marjorie Marr. Donald became intrigued by Marr's ability, whenever he did a staff round of her ward, to pronounce confidently on the position of the baby's head. Marr's predictions were impressively accurate, even in obese patients or other complicated cases. On interrogation by Donald, it emerged that she had been making surreptitious, early morning use of the flaw detector before the professor's arrival, and she had taught herself how to recognize the echoes of the fetal skull.[69]

By mid-1957, Donald was increasingly confident that he and his colleagues were making real progress toward establishing ultrasound as a clinically useful diagnostic modality. He and MacVicar had unexpectedly got their hands on an expensive and sophisticated electronic device. With this equipment, they could constructively address the problem that had first engaged Donald's attention as a potential application for ultrasound: the differentiation of cysts from solid tumors in the intact abdomen. It was evident that the flaw detector had other gynecological uses, such as in the diagnosis of ascites and in the monitoring of bladder function following surgery. Ultrasound was likely to prove a useful complement to established methods of diagnosis, particularly in cases in which abdominal palpation or vaginal examination was problematic.[70]

Its potential in obstetrics remained to be explored. But Donald was never one to confine himself rigidly to his own specialty, and he saw diagnostic possibilities in urology and cardiology. Thus Donald and MacVicar were understandably eager to continue developing diagnostic applications of A-scope. Brown, however, had another agenda, as we examine in the next chapter.

CHAPTER SIX

The First Contact Scanner

In the early months of 1957, Ian Donald, Tom Brown, and John MacVicar were hard at work in Glasgow's Western Infirmary, applying their Kelvin and Hughes Mk IV flaw detector to the abdomen of any patient who looked suitable and trying to understand the echoes they received. It was clear that a great deal of information was being obtained from within the body, but the display on the oscilloscope screen was often difficult, if not impossible, to interpret. Successful clinical application of the technique was still problematic in all but a few favorable cases.

From his experience of radar, Donald would have known that the one-dimensional A-scope display was not the only, or generally the best, means of visualizing the information obtained by echolocation. Early in the course of his experiments with pulsed ultrasound, he had tried to design a mechanical scanning device that would provide two-dimensional images.[1] Unfortunately, no evidence is available as to the nature of this apparatus. What is certain, however, is that Donald's attempts to build such a scanner were unsuccessful. He did not have the necessary expertise. He was, moreover, so excited by the vastly improved images that the Mk IV flaw detector produced that he became preoccupied with exploring the clinical potential of A-scope ultrasound and ceased to be interested in a more pictorial form of display.

Brown, however, looked at the problem from an engineering perspective. To him, the A-scope display did not seem well suited to the application to which it was being put. Industrial flaw detectors are designed to display stationary and fairly unambiguous signals coming from discrete defects in the study object. The human body, by contrast, contains a multitude of reflective surfaces. When Donald and his colleagues applied the flaw detector to the abdomen, they saw many echoes simultaneously, coming from a variety of depths. Moreover, the echoes moved about and fluctuated in intensity. Brown was certain that, within all this echoic activity, there was much information of clinical interest. The challenge was to develop a means of presentation that would make interpretation easier.

> It seemed plain, as the nose on one's face, that what was needed . . . was some kind of system which would display echoes in the position from which they were coming. Now I tried to explain this to Donald . . . I don't remember exactly what was said, but I do recall the recognition that it was heavy going. I could not really get over the thought that was in my head about finding some way of making a picture out of this information.[2]

The communication problem between the two men was compounded by an unwillingness on Brown's part to speak firmly to Donald on this matter. Brown's reticence sprang from his awareness of the differences in age, background, and status between himself and the Regius Professor. Donald was "a forceful personality" and was "not a good listener" when he had a fixed idea.[3] He evidently did not fully understand what Brown was proposing—a method of scanning both radically different from and considerably more sophisticated than any Donald had previously encountered. Indeed, for a time, Donald regarded Brown's commitment to an alternative means of display as a distraction from the main thrust of his clinical research.

(((((In his search for a means of providing a two-dimensional representation of ultrasonic echoes, Brown turned first to the technology of radar, a field in which Kelvin and Hughes Ltd. was an active innovator. A standard method of two-dimensional display for radar was plan position indicator, originally developed by the Air Ministry Research Establishment in 1939.[4] PPI had greatly simplified the work of the radar operator by providing a spatial representation of incoming information. In this system, the radar source is represented by a point at the center of a large oscilloscope screen. A narrow line, the time-base, which represents the beam of radio pulses transmitted by the antenna, extends radially from the central point to the edge of the screen. As the antenna rotates, the time-base line sweeps around the screen synchronously with it. An echo from an aircraft within the region scanned is represented by a bright spot on the line. Thus the bearing of the aircraft relative to the station may be read directly from the screen. Moreover, the position of the bright spot along the time-base line represents the distance of the aircraft from the radar source.

A map of the area surrounding the radar station is superimposed on the screen, enabling the operator to ascertain the precise location of the aircraft. In the modification of PPI known as sector scanning, rather than executing a full rotation, the antenna is swung forward and backward through an arc of 30 or 40 degrees.

Donald had acquired some experience of radar while serving with the Royal Air Force. Yet this prior knowledge may have impeded rather than assisted his comprehension of the innovation Brown was proposing. Donald certainly knew enough about military echolocation to appreciate that its display techniques were not immediately applicable to diagnostic imaging, the abdomen presenting a much more complex topography. Moreover, the applications of radar with which Donald was most familiar—locating a submarine on the surface of the sea or an aircraft encroaching on one's airspace—conveyed information about the position of a target but virtually nothing about its other characteristics.[5] In mid-1957, Donald's primary research focus was on the differential transonic qualities of tissue. As he and MacVicar then conceived it, the challenge facing the investigators was to exploit the ability of A-scope to distinguish between objects within the abdomen that strongly attenuated ultrasound, such as solid tumors, and those that did not, such as cysts. A considerable leap of the imagination was required to appreciate how two-dimensional visualization could contribute to this enterprise. It is understandable, therefore, that Donald was initially skeptical about the applicability to ultrasonic diagnosis of imaging techniques derived from radar.

Brown was able, however, to convince both his immediate boss, Peter Turner, chief engineer at Hillington, and, more importantly, William Slater, deputy managing director of Kelvin and Hughes and head of the Hillington factory, of the feasibility and potential of a two-dimensional display. A certain rapport had developed between Brown and Slater, who had been impressed with the younger man's track record within the company. Early in his career, Slater had himself been a significant technological innovator, pioneering an improved design of altimeter for commercial aircraft.[6] He also had experience of medical applications of industrial technology, having been involved in the development of ultraviolet light therapy. Slater had a sufficiently high estimation of his protégé to send Brown to Barkingside to discuss his ideas with William Halliday, Kelvin and Hughes's "chief scientist," in overall charge of all applied acoustics work. Halliday had worked in submarine echolocation for the Admiralty during the war. Brown recalls their meeting thus:

Halliday was an expert in acoustics, sonar, non-destructive testing . . . and he was deaf. One of those ironic situations, he had progressive nerve deafness and he got by for years with a boot lace and a shirt button. He would stick the button onto the end of the boot lace, stick it in his ear, stick the other end of the boot lace into his top pocket, and this was like a white stick, "I am deaf," people spoke up and that was all he needed. Anyway I found myself talking to Halliday and explaining what it was I wanted to do . . . So anyway he heard me through and just looked blank. So I started at the beginning again, but louder . . . I got about a third of the way through when he put up his hand and said "Stop, Brown, stop! I now appreciate the full enormity of what you are proposing." He is twinkling like mad and we get down to talking practicalities.[7]

Brown had been considering the possibilities of the marine "true motion" radar system, then in development at Kelvin and Hughes. On a true motion display, the transmitting ship appears to move relative to the surrounding seascape. This feature makes it easier to recognize the direction and speed of movement of one's own ship, relative to land and nearby vessels. Brown thought it might be possible to adapt true motion to medical use, "regarding the patient as [an] island, around which 'own ship' is travelling."[8] It quickly became clear, however, on talking to the radar engineers at Barkingside, that the working of the true motion system depended on a great deal of information being discarded in the process of constructing the image. Such a systematic and substantial loss of detail, Brown thought, would be unsatisfactory in medical application. Despite these difficulties, Brown was able to persuade Halliday that the idea of a two-dimensional representation was fundamentally sound. The chief scientist gave his blessing to the project, and Brown began work.

Meanwhile, Donald had sought, through his friend Edward Smith, an introduction to William Slater. Slater entertained Donald to lunch, and Donald showed the businessman the research with the flaw detector that was underway in the Western Infirmary. Slater was particularly impressed by the story of the woman whose life had been saved by the ultrasonic diagnosis of an ovarian cyst, as we described in chapter 5.[9] This vivid demonstration of the clinical potential of ultrasound seems to have played a major role in convincing Slater that it would be worthwhile to support Donald's project. For his part, Donald was eager to formalize Brown's connection with his department. Slater accordingly authorized Brown to spend one afternoon a week working on diagnostic ultrasound and allocated him a budget of £500 for his development expenses. As Brown was later to put it, "In the months to come, that £500 was to be a remarkably elastic sum of money, and if my other official duties got half a day per week from me it was unusual. But Slater was already weaving his protective screen around me and the project."[10] Slater's backing was a crucial factor in the success of the Glasgow-based research into medical ultrasound. For several years, he assiduously supported and defended the venture, to the extent of hiding its true cost from his colleagues on the board of Kelvin and Hughes.

Having gained the approval of his superiors, Brown began the process of building a working prototype. First, he retrieved what remained of his mechanized flaw detector system, then lying discarded in the Research and Development Department at Barkingside. This supplied him with some basic electronic components. With a relatively limited budget, Brown had to get hold of parts where and how he could. From the Barkingside factory, he obtained a second Mk IV flaw detector, rather older than the one he had acquired for Donald, which provided an amplifier and a high-voltage power supply. Since Brown envisaged some form of scanning arrangement in which the probe moved across the abdomen, he needed a means of detecting the position of the probe. The most crucial component he required was a sine/cosine potentiometer, a device that converts a mechanical rotation into two voltage outputs, one proportional to the sine and the other to the cosine of the angle of rotation. These potentiometers were used in radar systems to coordinate the sweep of the oscilloscope trace with the rotation of the antenna. Kelvin and Hughes manufactured sine/cosine potentiometers, but even at cost price, they were beyond Brown's means. He managed to find a defective one, which he was able to repair. Linear potentiometers, likewise a product of the radar industry, were readily available from government surplus stores. Brown used chains, sprockets, and so forth, from a Meccano set.[11] The mechanical part of the apparatus was built on the frame of a hospital bed-table, borrowed from the Western Infirmary (see fig. 6.2). Hence Brown's prototype became known as the bed-table scanner. The electronic units were assembled on a borrowed hospital equipment trolley (see fig. 5.1C).

Having concluded that true motion was not the answer to the problem he had set himself, Brown began to consider other forms of display. In A-scope, the pulse-echo signal is displayed in amplitude-modulated form, with the height of the spikes on the oscilloscope trace being proportional to the magnitude of the returning echoes. The same information may also be displayed in a brightness-modulated form. Here, the oscilloscope trace becomes a series of dots of light, the brightness of each dot depending on the strength of the incoming signal.[12] The distance of the dots along the time-base indicates the distance of the reflective surfaces from the transducer, as in A-scope.

Brightness-modulated displays can be used to create two-dimensional images. To achieve this, the changes in position and direction of the transducer must be followed by the trace on the oscilloscope screen. As the transducer is moved, the brightness-modulated trace forms a representation of the echo-producing surfaces within the target, if a long-persistence screen is used. This is an adaptation of the radar display known as B-scope, used when sector scanning with the target at one side of and some distance from the source. B-scope was the method of image generation used by John Wild and was, in effect, the starting point of Brown's own trajectory of innovation in ultrasound imaging.

Brown quickly concluded, however, that "radar-style 'sector-scanning' . . . did not appear to me to meet the case."[13] Ultrasound is reflected strongly only when the beam hits a reflective interface at or very close to 90 degrees. The topography of the deep structures of the abdominal cavity is complex, and many of its reflective surfaces are not aligned parallel to the surface of the body. Thus, at any particular angle of the beam, much of its energy is diverted away from the probe and hence lost to the receiving transducer. Brown realized that if each reflecting point within the abdominal cavity were exposed to the ultrasound beam from a range of angles, the likelihood of the beam hitting the surfaces at right angles and thus of a strong echo returning to the transducer would be greatly increased.[14] Achieving this consistently through the length of an abdominal scan, while keeping the probe in contact with the skin, was a complicated matter, however, both mechanically and electronically.

(((((Before examining how Brown overcame the limitations of B-mode imaging, we should consider the relationship of his endeavors to the work previously undertaken in the United States. As described in chapter 2, Wild and Howry had by this time built functioning two-dimensional imaging systems, but Brown proceeded independently of both these earlier developments. Donald had met Wild and discussed ultrasound imaging with him, but he seems not to have gained a wholly favorable impression of the quality of Wild's images. He did not show Brown any of Wild's published work.

The still photographs reproduced in Wild's publications do not fully convey the quality of the images his apparatus was capable of producing. Wild's breast images were created on an oscilloscope screen, in real time, as the probe was moved over the chest. They revealed their detail best if viewed on cine film.[15] Wild had not taken his films to Britain when he visited in 1956. When he lectured at the University of London, he made do with showing slides of the still pictures that appeared in his published papers.[16] Thus neither Donald nor anyone else in Britain had seen Wild's images under optimal conditions. It is likely, therefore, that Donald did not fully appreciate their significance—a conjecture corroborated by his remark that "other workers have made claims which . . . are more striking than substantial, judged by some of the illustrations offered."[17] From the context, it is clear that Donald is referring to Wild's publications.

There were probably several reasons for Donald being less than impressed with Wild's two-dimensional images. One is certainly that Donald, at this stage, did not have the skills necessary to interpret such images. Ultrasonic pictures, especially the early ones, are not easy to decipher. Indeed, in the 1950s, most observers would have had to take on trust Wild's reading of his breast echographs, and Wild himself could not make complete sense of the bowel images.[18] Also, Wild's eccentric manner, coupled with his boundless, even arrogant, confidence in his technique, could be off-putting. In particular, in common with most of his British colleagues, Donald was skeptical about Wild's claims that ultrasound could be used not merely to locate but to characterize the cytology of solid tumors.[19] Moreover, Wild's imaging system could not have been applied to Donald's clinical problems without considerable modification. The depth of penetration that Wild was able to achieve with his very-high-frequency probes would not have been adequate for gynecological work. Furthermore, the internal structure of the abdomen, normal and pathological, is much more complicated than that of the breast.

By 1957, Donald must also have known of the existence of Howry's Somascope, but again, he did not alert Brown to the developments in Denver.[20] When Brown began assembling his prototype, he was unaware of Howry's work, and he would remain so for some time. Brown attributes Donald's lack of communication on this matter partly to the awkward nature of his interaction with the Regius Professor at this time and partly to Donald not being fully in sympathy with the innovation Brown was proposing. Donald may not have seen the relevance of Howry's elaborate imaging technique to his own, more clinical, concerns.

Brown was working in an industrial rather than an academic environment. Among R&D engineers, it was not the custom to undertake comprehensive literature searches when initiating a project, as would be the norm in a university. Rather, they usually began with a feasibility study. Only when this had been successfully completed, and if a patent application was being considered, would a systematic survey of other relevant work be embarked upon. Commercial pressures ensured that feasibility studies were conducted expeditiously, and Brown felt time especially pressing, because he still expected to be called up, at relatively short notice, for his National Service.[21] Accordingly, he plunged enthusiastically into the practical process of invention, unaware of and unconcerned about similar work elsewhere. Working independently, Brown was free to construct an ultrasound scanner that was radically different from earlier instruments.

A distinctive feature of Brown's prototype was that the ultrasonic probe was in direct contact with the patient's body (see fig. 5.1C); it was not immersed in a bath of water. Interposing some fluid between transmitter and target is essential for adequate acoustic coupling between the probe and the surface of the study object. For this reason, Peter Turner tried to persuade Brown to experiment with water baths.[22] Brown, however, was convinced that close proximity between probe and skin, with acoustic coupling achieved by the application of oil, would be the preferable arrangement for clinical purposes. He resisted his boss's suggestion, and Turner did not pursue the matter. Turner, too, was unaware of Howry's work. But G. B. G. Potter, managing director of Kelvin and Hughes, knew of the Denver project and had obtained copies of Howry's publications. Potter was based in Head Office at Wembley, however, and Brown had no direct communication with him. Potter did eventually bring to Slater's attention the existence of Howry's Somascope, but not until Brown had successfully built his prototype contact scanner. In this crucial phase of the innovation process, Brown's ignorance of Howry's work was certainly fortuitous. Looking back on the episode years later, Brown expressed the conviction that, had he seen Howry's "quite extraordinary and beautiful pictures" before he was well advanced with his own design, he would not have been able to sustain his confidence in the direct contact method in the face of Turner's skepticism.[23]

There were several reasons underlying Brown's reluctance to use a water bath. From his experience of industrial ultrasound, he knew that reverberation of the signal from the walls of a tank, or between the probe and the target, caused spurious echoes. When metal objects were being examined, these artifacts did not necessarily pose a major problem. The velocity of sound being much greater in metal than in water, the geometry of the system could be arranged so that echoes from within the target arrived back at the probe well in advance of the reverberations. The speed of sound in tissue, however, is very similar to that in water, so the two sets of echoes would be more difficult to separate. Brown was also sensitive to the need for his scanner to be readily acceptable in a hospital environment and, in particular, within a department of gynecology. He was reluctant to suggest to Donald that his female patients, often elderly and seriously ill, should be subjected to the ordeal of sitting in a tank of water. Nor could these patients be reasonably expected to bear the weight of large bags of water on their abdomens. Brown was also aware of Donald's previous difficulties with spillage, wet beds, and irate nurses. He experimented briefly with a small water bag—in reality, a condom filled with an attenuating fluid—in the front of the probe to minimize distortion of the abdominal wall.[24] Reverberation of the signal within the bag immediately proved to be a problem, and Brown quickly returned to the direct contact method and did not again depart from it. His commitment to the contact principle was to be crucial to the further development of obstetric ultrasound.

A key element of Brown's scheme, as described above, was that each reflective interface in the target should be struck by the ultrasound beam from as wide a range of angles as possible. He referred to this technique as "compound B-scope."[25] To achieve this, Brown devised a mechanism whereby, as the probe was moved across the surface of the abdomen, it could be manually rocked backward and forward on a spindle (fig. 6.1). In effect this produced a series of mini sector scans, which could be combined either on a persistence oscilloscope screen or on photographic film. The integration of the sector scans had to be precisely calibrated so that echoes from the same reflective point appeared in exactly the same position on the screen, regardless of the angle from which that point had been scanned. Accordingly, Brown set out to build a hand-operated, electromechanical apparatus that would register the precise position and orientation of the probe (fig. 6.2).

To track the position of the probe, Brown chose to use an orthogonal measuring system. This was accurate and electronically relatively simple, if mechanically quite complicated. In his original design, the probe was built into a box, the "bread-bin," which ran on two parallel rails. On one rail, the box was mounted on two "kinematically correct vee-rollers" to ensure accurate tracking.[26] Longitudinal movement of the box along the rails was measured by a linear potentiometer, linked to it by a chain. Within the box, the probe was mounted on a narrow vertical shaft, the blade, by means of two vee-rollers

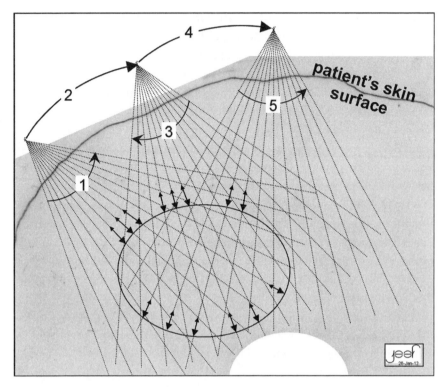

Figure 6.1. Compound sector scanning pattern, showing three overlapping sectors resulting from the sequence of movements of the transducer, or probe, indicated by 1 to 5. In practice, this was repeated at many points across the patient so that each tissue interface was scanned from many different angles. *Drawn by jeef*

along one side and one along the other, again to ensure accurate tracking. The probe could thus be moved vertically in a plane perpendicular to that of its longitudinal movement. A second linear potentiometer tracked its vertical displacement. As noted above, the probe could be rocked backward and forward as it was moved across the abdomen—but only in the plane of its vertical and horizontal movement. Its angle of rotation was measured by a sine/cosine potentiometer. By using the outputs from the three potentiometers, a time-base line was generated on the oscilloscope screen that precisely replicated the position and direction of the probe. Ultrasonic echoes returning to the probe were amplified and displayed on the screen, in brightness modulation, in their appropriate position along the time-base. This provided a cross-sectional image of the abdomen in a single plane.

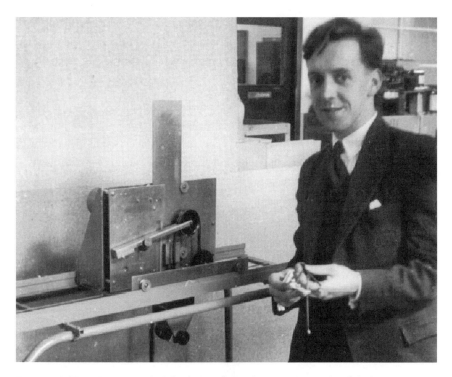

Figure 6.2. Tom Brown in the laboratories of Kelvin Hughes Ltd., with the scanning mechanism of the Bed-table Scanner, November 1956. *Reproduced courtesy of Mr. T. G. Brown*

Brown tested his system on an experimental model of the abdomen, the Perspex water tank that he had built for the team's in vitro trials of A-scope. While testing the B-scan instrument, the scanning mechanism was placed above the tank and a grapefruit, suspended on a wire, provided a mock internal organ.[27] But Brown found that, even using compound B-scope, the images remained unsatisfactory. The apparatus was less sensitive than he wished. Convinced that if ultrasound were to realize its potential as a clinical tool, it had to reveal as much information from within the body as possible, Brown set about designing a radically new form of signal processor. His objective was to allow the display of signals over an exceptionally wide dynamic range, ensuring that both very strong and very weak echoes registered on the oscilloscope screen. Ultimately, he managed to achieve a ratio of the order of 1,000 to 1 between the amplitudes of the maximum and minimum displayable signals, even when a weak echo was very closely preceded by a strong one. Brown was drawing here on his industrial experience—he had devised similar solutions to the problem of maximizing sensitivity and dynamic range while designing his mechanized flaw detection system.

> I had previous experience of this problem on the industrial job . . . the problem in weld testing was that the sensitivity of the technique would vary widely, depending on the surface roughness of the metal, on the thickness of the oil film between the transducer and the metal and on the mains supply voltage. And we were working in a boiler shop in which there were . . . great X-ray machines, there were welding machines going on and off and the mains voltage was jumping all over the place and the instruments we used with multistage valve amplifiers were quite sensitive to fluctuations in the mains voltage. So in order to do the sensitivity stabilisation trick I had to be able to observe echoes whose amplitude variation was very considerable so I was sort of familiar with that general area. So to an extent I was primed when it came to the medical thing.[28]

Many of the characteristics of the bed-table scanner were determined empirically. Brown settled on a transmission frequency of 2.5 MHz, partly because that was one of the standard frequencies for industrial instruments, and partly because he and MacVicar had found that 2.5 MHz gave a reasonable compromise between resolution and penetration. The transmitter had a pulse-repetition rate of 50 per second, again partly because that rate was available on the Mk IV flaw detector. Brown also considered that 50 pulses per second would be adequate in clinical application, given that the operator was unlikely to move the probe more than one beam width in 20 milliseconds. If the probe were moved too quickly relative to the pulse-repetition rate, returning echoes would be missed, causing gaps to appear in the resulting image.

Brown was well aware that increasing the pulse-repetition rate would improve the brightness of the resulting image. That he chose not to alter the rate is indicative that optimizing the sensitivity of the apparatus was not his sole objective. His thinking on scanner design was structured by another important consideration—namely, safety. Brown was convinced of the intrinsic harmlessness of ultrasound at the power levels that his prototype would use. Nevertheless, he wished to proceed with caution and sought to minimize the acoustic power output of the probe as far as possible. The lower the pulse-repetition rate, the lower the amount of ultrasound energy entering the abdomen. With the same end in view, Brown introduced a switched attenuator between the transmitter and the probe, by which the overall sensitivity of the system could be adjusted. He recommended that the operator begin scanning at the lowest power setting and then gradually increase the output to the minimum required to obtain a readable image. The receiver amplifier was set to the maximum gain compatible with a clear signal. In clinical use, the output of the bed-table scanner was less than 1.5 mW cm^{-2} of skin surface—much lower, as it turned out, than that of the machines built by Howry and Wild.[29]

Brown's first prototype had three oscilloscope screens—a dedicated A-scope monitor, a long-persistence B-scope display that allowed the operator to monitor the image as it was being composed, and a short-persistence B-scope display, in front of which was mounted an oscilloscope camera (see fig. 5.1C).[30] As well as providing a permanent record of the scan, the photographic film served to integrate the information displayed on the screen. Owing to the width of the sound beam, a point target would appear on the screen as a small arc. But if echoes were received from the same target many times, at a range of angles, the arcs would intersect at a single point, producing a bright spot on the photographic plate. In other words, an image would be built up that was the sum of the transient images on the short-persistence screen. Brown assumed that genuine echoes would tend to summate, whereas artifactual signals arising from reverberation and other causes would not repeat so regularly. Thus photographic integration would help reduce the number of artifacts in the final image.

(((((Eventually, Brown felt confident enough to transport his prototype to the Western Infirmary to demonstrate its capabilities to Donald. A patient with a suspected large ovarian cyst was chosen as the pioneer subject. A scan of her abdomen was undertaken by one of the clinicians, and a two-dimensional image was duly produced. Brown remembers being disappointed at how ill-defined and difficult to interpret the image was.[31] Nevertheless, he persevered. As they had done with the flaw detector, Brown and MacVicar experimented on themselves, taking scans of each other's thighs and abdomens. While Brown continued to make minor adjustments to the apparatus when necessary, the key, now, to improving the machine's performance was learning how to operate it in the clinical environment. Achieving acoustic coupling between the probe and the subject's skin was initially a problem, but this was solved by generous applications of olive oil (fig. 6.3).

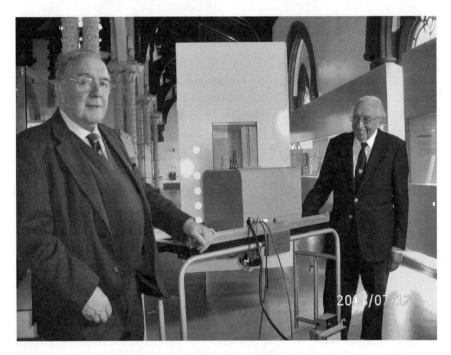

Figure 6.3. Tom Brown (*left*) and John MacVicar (1927–2011) with the Bed-table Scanner in the Hunterian Museum, Glasgow University, 2008. *Reproduced courtesy of Mr. T. G. Brown*

To produce a well-defined, compound B-mode image, the clinicians had to learn to maintain a smooth, consistent rocking motion of the probe as they moved it across the surface of the patient's body. This was not easy, partly because the ergonomics of the scanner were far from optimal. Brown's aim in constructing his prototype had been to demonstrate, as quickly as possible, the feasibility of two-dimensional abdominal ultrasonic imaging. Understandably, he had not given much attention to ease of use. To conduct a scan, the operator had to reach under the supporting frame to position the probe and move it across the abdomen, while simultaneously turning his head to view the oscilloscope screen. Inconsistent rocking of the probe or jerky lateral movement could leave blank spaces in the composite picture. Gradually, however, Donald and MacVicar gained confidence in their scanning ability. The quality of the images began to improve.

Despite his previous lack of interest, Donald was now convinced that two-dimensional imaging constituted a major advance toward realizing the diagnostic potential of ultrasound. The limitations of A-scope were obvious. If anything, his enthusiasm and commitment to the project redoubled. The burdens on his colleagues increased, and "hours of continuous work often late at night became usual," as MacVicar later described.

> Examination of countless patients and experiments with mechanical developments and picture display took up much of our time. Feelings of fatigue and frustration, despair and delusion, excitement and elation, became well known to us . . . we always considered Ian as the person who was heading the whole thing and driving it on and that Tom and I had to do our best to fulfil what he wanted to do and if we weren't able to do that then we were going to fall down in his expectations, because whatever else we felt we wanted to achieve this for him. And Ian was a very hard task-master . . . and he pushed quite a lot. And there is no doubt Tom and I worked hours which were crazy. We would start work probably when Tom finished at the factory at half-past four or five and I had finished doing the clinics and then work until eight or nine at night, because patients were available and we were available . . . [Donald] wanted to make progress and everything else and why wouldn't we try this and why wouldn't we try that and why wouldn't we try the other thing.[32]

The oscilloscope camera provided an invaluable record of each scan, but it was inconvenient to use. The camera back contained a thirty-foot roll of film. After every scanning session, Brown and MacVicar had to remove the cassette from the camera, extract the film from the cassette using a "portable darkroom" glove system, and seal it into a developing tank. Inevitably, accidents would occasionally occur, resulting in a ruined film and a whole series of scans having to be repeated.

The transfer of the bed-table scanner to the gynecological wards of the Western Infirmary and its application to clinical work did not bring Brown's technical development of the apparatus to an end. He occasionally transported his prototype back to the Hillington factory for maintenance and to refine aspects of its design. For instance, he replaced the original amplifier with a higher-performance model derived from a Mk V flaw detector. Another modification was prompted by clinical experience. Built on the frame of a bed-table, the prototype could scan across the abdomen only at right angles to the long axis of the body. But the clinicians soon realized that it would also be useful to perform scans in other orientations. Accordingly, Brown replaced the bed-table frame with a sheet metal construction, mounted on wheels, within which the scanner could be oriented transversally, longitudinally, or tilted in a non-vertical scan plane. To achieve this, he removed the mechanism of weights and pulleys that counterbalanced the vertical mounting of the probe and replaced it with a motor taken from a gramophone, which functioned as a constant tension spring.

By this time, MacVicar had decided to write his MD thesis on the use of ultrasound as a diagnostic aid.[33] He therefore sought to obtain scans of as wide a range of gynecological cases as possible. Emerging from his subordinate position in the team, MacVicar was beginning to take a leading role in the clinical investigations. However, the overwhelmingly pathological thrust of his research led to a degree of creative tension with Brown, who was equally concerned with improving the definition of the images and confirming the status of ultrasound as a reliable visualizing modality. For this purpose, Brown often preferred to scan normal structures, such as the body parts of the team members. On one occasion, for example, a neck scan was undertaken. Here the anatomy was known and the images obtained could be more directly compared with those in medical textbooks. Fortunately, the two research agendas, the normal and the pathological, effectively complemented one another, as Brown and MacVicar worked in a constructive collaboration to refine their skills in the production and interpretation of ultrasound images.

(((((Many of the clinical investigations undertaken with the bed-table scanner centered again on the problem of distinguishing cystic structures from solid tumors. Donald and his colleagues had already developed considerable expertise in achieving this discrimination with the flaw detector and its A-scope display. This prior experience undoubtedly assisted them in interpreting some of the earliest two-dimensional images of cysts and fibroids provided by the bed-table scanner. Where an A-scope trace of a cyst showed a gap between two spikes, there now appeared a dark space. In learning to distinguish cysts from fibroids using compound B-scope, the key point that had to be appreciated was that if the object were cystic, anatomical structure would be visualizable beyond the dark space. Owing to the transonic qualities of fluid, ultrasonic pulses passed through the cyst and were reflected from its far wall. Tissues lying behind the far wall, such as bowel, were often also revealed. Solid tumors, on the other hand, significantly attenuated the ultrasound waves, casting sonic shadows, which also appeared dark on the two-dimensional image. But the echoes received from beyond these darkened spaces were weaker, and less anatomical structure could be visualized. The crucial skill lay in being able to differentiate between those parts of the image that were dark because of the absence of reflective interfaces and those that were dark because the ultrasound beam had been prevented, partially or completely, from penetrating them. One might say that, in this context, enlightenment lay in learning to distinguish between two different forms of darkness.

The team also quickly learned to recognize the echoes that were characteristic of bowel.[34] In a normal abdomen, deep penetration of the beam cannot occur, owing to the strongly reflective interfaces between gas and fluid in the intestines. When bright loops of bowel could be identified as floating within a dark space, through which the ultrasound beam had penetrated more deeply than usual, ascites could be confidently diagnosed. The investigators later recognized that if, in ascites, loops of bowel adhered to neighboring structures rather than floating freely in the abdominal cavity, then a malignant causation should be strongly suspected.

The challenge posed by the interpretation of the early two-dimensional images can hardly be overstated. The pictures were technically quite crude, but also, and more importantly, they were radically novel. No one had ever looked at the female abdomen in this way before. Each gynecological image constituted a thin slice through the abdominal cavity, the position and angle of which was variable. The skills necessary to make sense of such images were quite different from those required to understand an X-ray shadowgraph, for example.[35] Direct visualization of the arrangement of the abdominal organs, during surgery or postmortem, was of considerable assistance but could not be unproblematically transferred to interpretation of the planar images obtained by ultrasound. Nor were anatomy textbooks wholly useful guides. Anatomical illustrations tend to portray normal rather than pathological structure. Moreover, in the 1950s, they rarely featured cross-sectional illustrations. Brown did manage to find one anatomical text devoted solely to transverse sections, which he studied carefully.[36] Even here, however, all the sections had been made at right angles to the long axis of the body. Furthermore, when interpreting an image in an anatomical textbook, one does not need to allow for sonic shadowing or the reflective indices of different tissue interfaces. Ability to interpret the images obtained by the bed-table scanner was gained slowly, by trial and error, helped by systematic correlation with structures revealed at laparotomy or autopsy. Images of earlier cases were frequently returned to in order to reassess earlier interpretations in the light of greater experience.

If it was not easy to interpret the images, it was still harder to explain them to outsiders. To convey the planar nature of the pictures, Donald devised a metaphor based on a sliced loaf of bread. The loaf represented the body of the patient. The ultrasound image was imagined to be constructed as if one lifted a single slice out of the loaf and looked perpendicularly at its cut surface. This was a useful pedagogic device. However, whereas a loaf is always sliced transversely, an ultrasound scanner could take images transversely, longitudinally, or obliquely. It is hardly surprising that many of Donald's Scottish colleagues were far from convinced of the value of the pictures.

Wallace Barr, for example, who had been present at Donald's experiments at Babcock's, had become doubtful of the professor's latest technological enthusiasm. He described the contact scanner as being of "use to a deaf and blind gynaecologist who had lost the use of his hands." Another Glaswegian consultant dismissed the ultrasound images as reminiscent merely of "a snow storm in Sauchiehall Street" (a street in the city center).[37] A jape circulated among Glasgow medical students that when attempting to distinguish between fibroids and cysts, the Regius Professor got it right 50 percent of the time.[38] Several members of the rival professorial unit in Rottenrow regarded Donald's experiments with ultrasound as bizarre, and his reputation for eccentricity was accordingly enhanced. Such attitudes continued for some years. In the early 1960s, a "distinguished colleague" from Edinburgh University visited the Western Infirmary and was shown an ultrasound examination. On his return, he announced, to the amusement of his audience of medical students, that in Glasgow obstetricians "were using a £10,000 machine to diagnose an ovarian cyst, which, in Edinburgh, was diagnosed using a tuppenny glove."[39]

Not everyone was skeptical. Donald received significant encouragement from key figures in Glasgow medicine, notably the two professors of surgery, Sir Charles Illingworth and William Arthur Mackey, who encouraged Donald to demonstrate the bed-table scanner at a meeting of the American College of Surgeons, held in Glasgow in the summer of 1958.[40] Donald was able to display diagnostic images of fibroids, ovarian cysts, and ascites. He was particularly proud of the ascites image, the ultrasonic appearance of which he considered to be virtually pathognomonic. Donald alluded to the cystic characteristics of the gravid uterus and asserted that pregnancy could be confirmed ultrasonically when the uterus had enlarged above the symphysis pubis. He also emphasized to his surgical audience that the utility of the visualizing technique was not confined to gynecology and obstetrics.

Around this time, the team received a considerable morale boost from an unexpected quarter. Donald's former teacher at St. Thomas's, Joe Wrigley, had been incredulous to the point of mockery about Donald's trials with the flaw detector. Wrigley was notoriously hostile to the intrusion of technology into medicine, preferring to emphasize the priority of clinical acumen. But, sometime in early 1958, he visited Glasgow as an external examiner. Donald showed him around his wards in the Western Infirmary and gave him a demonstration of the contact scanner. Wrigley was quickly convinced that two-dimensional ultrasound had genuine clinical potential in obstetrics and gynecology. On his return to London, he wrote an enthusiastic letter to Donald, urging him to press on with the development of the technique. Donald was profoundly gratified by his old chief's dramatic change of heart.[41]

(((((As with A-scope ultrasound, initially Donald and his colleagues obtained their best results by applying the contact scanner to cystic structures. In one early case, a fifty-five-year-old woman presented with lower abdominal swelling of four months' duration. It proved impossible to determine by clinical examination whether she was suffering from a fibroid or an ovarian cyst. Ultrasonic examination gave unequivocal indication that the swelling was cystic. The cyst appeared to be so big that its posterior wall was indented by the vertebral column (see fig. 6.4B). The presence of a large, unilocular ovarian cyst was confirmed on opening the abdomen. In another case, a very obese patient complained of heavy vaginal bleeding of six months' duration. Clinical examination proved unrevealing, even under anesthesia. Again ultrasound suggested the presence of a cyst, a finding that laparotomy confirmed.[42]

Sometimes, however, a cystic appearance could be misleading. A confident ultrasonic diagnosis of ovarian cyst was confounded when bilateral hydrosalpinx (fluid in the fallopian tubes) was discovered at laparotomy. On another occasion, a partial disagreement between the clinical and ultrasonic opinions was resolved in favor of the clinical. Physical examination had revealed the presence of a bilobal mass in the pelvis, suggesting a diagnosis of multiple fibroids. Ultrasonic examination confirmed the presence of solid masses but also detected a cystic structure between the two lobes. A revised diagnosis of multiple fibroids and ovarian cyst was offered. However, surgery revealed the ultrasonic diagnosis to be mistaken. Part of the bladder had become enveloped between two large fibromas, causing urine to be retained in the isolated portion. The persistence of a liquid-filled space within the pelvis after urethral catheterization had misled the ultrasound examiner.[43]

Donald and his colleagues derived much satisfaction from those instances in which they were able to successfully contradict opinions derived from physical examination. In one such case, a clinical diagnosis of ovarian cyst was cast into doubt by the ultrasonic findings. The scan indicated that, though the swelling was indeed cystic, there were solid masses interspersed within the fluid. A series of transverse ultrasonograms taken along the length of the abdomen revealed that the swelling tapered downward, suggesting that its origin did not lie in the pelvic region. The ultrasound investigators did not offer a diagnosis but suggested further radiological investigation. Pyelography revealed that the tumor originated from the kidney—hydronephrosis, with numerous calculi.[44]

Donald was convinced that the scanner would prove useful beyond the confines of gynecology and obstetrics. A series of investigations were undertaken of patients with suspected disease of the liver or spleen, but no worthwhile results were obtained. A male case of polycystic kidneys proved more revealing, and ascites was confirmed in another male patient with incompetence of the tricuspid valve.[45] Donald also tried to apply ultrasonic investigation to his other main research interest, neonatal respiratory distress. He examined the heads of neonates with breathing difficulties to try to ascertain the presence or absence of intraventricular bleeding. These pediatric investigations proved unfruitful, which is not surprising given the difficulty of applying the probe of the bed-table scanner to the fontanelle of a premature baby. However, by experimenting along these lines, Donald anticipated one of the most dramatic advances in neonatology of the early 1970s.

The majority of the significant early successes were gynecological. In one remarkable case, ultrasonic findings made a major difference to its clinical management. A young woman was admitted to Donald's wards because of irregular vaginal bleeding and an abdominal swelling of several months' duration. She had been in the same ward a year earlier with a similar complaint and was suspected to have a uterine fibroid. On physical examination the uterus was found to be enlarged, but the woman had no breast symptoms and did not think she could be pregnant. It was decided to proceed with surgical removal of the fibroid. But before the operation could take place, an ultrasonic examination revealed that the uterus was enlarged with fluid. Moreover, faint echoes could be discerned within the cavity, which Donald and MacVicar were convinced were those of a fetus. A pregnancy test was ordered and its results eagerly awaited. The ultrasonic diagnosis was confirmed. Bed rest controlled the bleeding and, in due course, the woman gave birth to a healthy baby. The happy outcome of this case gave Donald enormous satisfaction. It was also an impressive diagnostic coup for the bed-table scanner, since the best diagnosis that could have been arrived at by conventional clinical means was undoubtedly myoma. Further ultrasonic investigations of this patient after parturition confirmed the presence of a fibroid at the fundus (the part of the uterus farthest from the birth canal). Myoma had coexisted with pregnancy. But the most noteworthy feature of the case lay in the fact that the bed-table scanner had detected a fetus of only about fourteen weeks' gestation.[46]

The scanner could help confirm the absence of pregnancy as well as its presence. This promised to be a useful application in an era when the techniques of chemical testing for pregnancy were time-consuming and unreliable. Determination of pregnancy by physical examination was also uncertain in the early months. In 1958, a woman was admitted to Donald's wards who believed she was pregnant. She had amenorrhea of six months' duration and swelling of the abdomen of four months' duration. She was sick in the mornings and claimed to feel fetal movements. Palpation and percussion of her abdomen were unrevealing. She was so anxious and tense that it proved impossible to perform an internal examination. Ultrasonic imaging, however, indicated that her uterus was not enlarged. In other words, she was not pregnant, a finding confirmed by vaginal examination under anesthesia.

Thus, in the few months after the bed-table scanner arrived in the Western Infirmary, much had been achieved. Of the first series of 125 gynecological cases, the ultrasonic diagnosis was shown to be erroneous in only eight instances. Ovarian cyst could be identified with some confidence. An opinion could often be advanced as to the size, number, location, and type of cysts present. This information was of value in assessing the urgency, or otherwise, of surgery and might assist the surgeon in planning the operation. The diagnosis of fibroid was less certain, but, nevertheless, the ultrasonic images generally assisted in forming a clinical opinion. There was also the promise of useful applications in obstetrics. It seemed that whether or not the uterus was gravid might be reliably ascertained at an earlier stage by ultrasound than with conventional clinical or laboratory techniques. Later in pregnancy, the position of the baby's head could be identified with certainty. The condition of polyhydramnios, excessive volume of amniotic fluid, proved an ideal one to diagnose by ultrasound, since the size of the "cystic cavity" in which the solid fetus floated was increased. Since polyhydramnios is often associated with fetal pathology, its identification provided useful information.[47] But there had also been some disappointments, the most notable being the failure of the team's attempts to visualize the placenta. Donald decided, however, that the time had come to publish their results.

On June 7, 1958, a paper appeared in the *Lancet*, under the joint authorship of Donald, MacVicar, and Brown, entitled "Investigation of Abdominal Masses by Pulsed Ultrasound." The article began with a short account of the clinical use of A-scope, chiefly in detecting retention of urine after bladder surgery, followed by a brief (and arguably inadequate) description of the technique used to produce two-dimensional images.[48] Despite the title of the paper, the first compound B-scope image reproduced was a rather crude cross section of Brown's thigh (fig. 6.4A). A similar illustration of a healthy abdomen also featured a team member, in this case MacVicar. This image appeared to show several layers of tissue in the abdominal wall, but the authors admitted that these could not be precisely identified. These images of normal structure were accompanied by three striking pictures of ovarian cysts (two are reproduced here; fig. 6.4B and C). In each of these, a dark space is clearly seen in the center of the image, indicating the presence of a fluid-filled cavity. In two of the three, the far wall of the cyst can readily be identified.

Donald, MacVicar, and Brown particularly emphasized instances in which ultrasound scanning had made a significant addition to the understanding of the patient's condition beyond that achieved by history taking and physical examination. In one case, for example, only a single cyst had been diagnosed clinically, but the outlines of two were displayed ultrasonically. In another, a swelling had been clinically diagnosed as a fibroid, but "the ultrasonic characteristics of a fluid-filled cyst are here quite unmistakable." The authors placed great stress on the contrasting ultrasonic appearances of cystic structures and solid tumors, because the latter "tend to absorb and scatter ultrasound, with the result that only faint echoes can be recorded from the posterior surface of the mass" (fig. 6.4E).[49] Another remarkable image illustrated the deeper penetration of the ultrasound beam into the abdominal cavity that the team had identified as characteristic of ascites (fig. 6.4D). To emphasize their concern with safety, the authors gave considerable prominence to an account of Bacsich's experiments with kittens and their negative results.

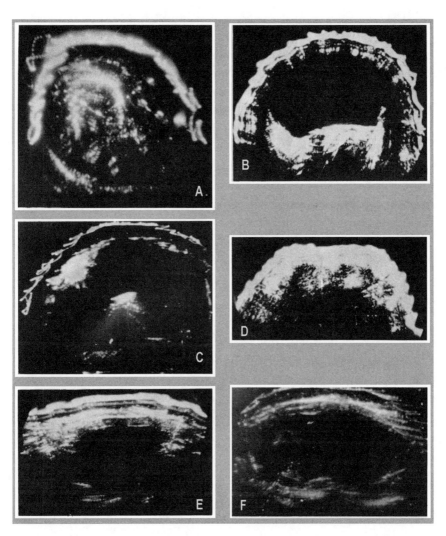

Figure 6.4. Cross-sectional images from Donald, MacVicar, and Brown's 1958 paper. *A*, transverse section of the anterior half of a thigh, showing the femur. *B*, large simple ovarian cyst with its posterior surface indented by the vertebral column and posterior abdominal wall. *C*, bilateral ovarian cysts; on removal, left cyst found to be 28 inches in diameter and right cyst 12.5 inches (70 and 32 cm). *D*, gross ascites due to cirrhosis of the liver; the ultrasonic beam can penetrate more deeply in random fashion because of fluid between the coils of intestine. *E*, multiple fibroids, showing progressive attenuation of ultrasound, with only faint echoes from the posterior surface of the mass, in contrast to ovarian cysts. *F*, uterus at 14 weeks' gestation, showing echoes from the fetus toward the left half of the uterus; the provisional clinical diagnosis had been that of fibroid. *Reprinted from I. Donald, J. MacVicar, and T. G. Brown, "Investigation of Abdominal Masses by Pulsed Ultrasound," Lancet, vol. 271, pages 1188–95, 1958, with permission of Elsevier Ltd.; legends as in the Lancet, with minimal editing*

The most historically significant images in the 1958 paper are those of the fetus. As the authors dryly observed, "the pregnant uterus offers considerable scope for this kind of work because it is a cystic cavity containing a solid foetus." A clear outline of a fetal skull, at thirty-four weeks' gestation, features in one image. Another picture shows twins at thirty-seven weeks—two pairs of buttocks can be discerned at the uterine fundus. There is a crude but vivid visualization of polyhydramnios. Possibly the most intriguing image of all is from the case described above, in which a fetus of fourteen weeks' gestation, with a coexisting myoma, was detected in a woman in whom pregnancy had not been suspected (fig. 6.4F).

Overall, the claims made in 1958 by Donald and his colleagues were strikingly modest.

> Our experience . . . indicates that ultrasonic diagnosis is still very crude . . . The fact that recordable echoes can be obtained at all has both surprised and encouraged us, but our findings are still of more academic interest than practical importance, and we do not feel that our clinical judgement should be influenced by our ultrasonic findings . . . further refinements in technique may provide a useful diagnostic weapon in cases in which radiological diagnosis with ionising radiation is either impracticable or undesirable.[50]

Similar disclaimers may be found in the conclusion to MacVicar's MD thesis, submitted in March 1959.[51] To a significant extent, this diffidence as to the value of diagnostic ultrasound must be seen as studied and tactical. Donald was not much given to modesty in the presentation of his scientific work. The statement in the 1958 paper that ultrasonic imaging had not yet meaningfully affected clinical decision making was certainly disingenuous. Donald's focus had been firmly on clinical application from the very beginning of his investigations, as the case histories described above exemplify. But Donald, MacVicar, and Brown all felt that some of the claims for ultrasonic diagnosis made by other workers were extravagant and unsustainable. They were aware, too, that Wild's assertion that he could distinguish malignant from benign tissue by ultrasound had been greeted by his peers with incredulity. Heuter, for instance, had expressed considerable skepticism about Wild's claims, on one occasion describing them as produced by "twiddling of the controls."[52] Challenging the status of histology as the gold standard in pathology was not a sensible approach for the proponents of a fledgling diagnostic modality. Nor would it have been tactical to suggest that traditional methods of clinical diagnosis were being radically superseded. Donald and MacVicar chose instead to proceed incrementally, to present themselves as cautious, open-minded, empirical investigators. "A plea must be made," MacVicar wrote, "for more honest experiment without haste to claim accurate diagnosis . . . What the eventual role of ultrasound as a diagnostic aid will be can only be left to conjecture."[53] Nevertheless, Donald shortly came to regard the *Lancet* paper as the most important he ever published. It has had very considerable impact, as the following chapters explore.

CHAPTER SEVEN

The Automatic Scanner and the Diasonograph

The first ultrasound images of the fetus were published in June 1958.[1] The *Lancet* article by Ian Donald, John MacVicar and Tom Brown occasioned a great deal of interest and comment, in Britain and abroad. However, the scanner that Brown had built for Donald was not much more than an experimental mock-up. The images it produced were of variable quality. Image resolution and definition left much to be desired. It was obvious, especially from Brown's engineering perspective, that much technical improvement remained to be accomplished. In this chapter, we follow the further development of the contact scanner, culminating in the production of a commercially marketable model. We are particularly interested in how technical problems were solved and how the technology became "black-boxed," so that a detailed knowledge of how the scanner worked was no longer required of its operators.

Donald was, by early 1958, intensely enthusiastic about the potential of compound B-scan to provide two-dimensional representations of the abdominal cavity. The new technique posed exciting challenges for the clinicians as they sought to interpret the images and relate them to clinical decision making. Brown, however, was often not happy with the way scanning was being performed. To achieve consistent results, the ultrasonic probe had to be moved steadily across the patient's abdomen. This motion was twofold: the probe was repeatedly swung through an arc of approximately 60 degrees, while slowly traversing the abdomen (see fig. 6.1). As noted in chapter 6, the bed-table scanner was formidably inconvenient to use. The operator had to crouch beside the patient's bed, turning his head to view the screen while simultaneously reaching upward, through the frame of the bed-table, to apply the probe to the abdomen. He was at considerable risk of bumping his head on the underside of the frame and would often have olive oil (used for acoustic coupling) running down his sleeve.[2] Achieving the necessary consistent motion of the probe was not easy under these circumstances.

When first put into service, the scanner was equipped with three oscilloscope screens. One was for A-scope, another was a short-persistence B-scan screen with a camera mounted in front, and the third, also B-scan, was a long-persistence screen with which the operator could monitor the echoes received from the patient's abdomen and follow the development of the image. The clinicians watched the third screen with fascination as the outlines of reflective surfaces gradually appeared. Such avid attention to the emerging image was often counterproductive. If some feature happened to catch the operator's interest, he tended to dwell on that part of the scan, eager to see as much detail as possible. Localized overexposure of the photographic film was often the result. This posed a serious problem because, at this time, the clinical usefulness of each scan greatly depended on the quality of the photographic record, if only because MacVicar and Brown needed to have concrete evidence to show Donald. After vigorous exhortation failed to remedy the clinicians' scanning faults, Brown responded by removing the B-scan monitoring screen from the apparatus. Henceforth, the operator would have to rely solely on the A-scan display for confirmation that echoes of sufficient strength were being received. MacVicar and Donald protested at the imposed modification, but Brown was adamant that the quality of the final image would be improved.[3]

It did improve—but not as much as Brown had hoped. Even after removal of the long-persistence screen, results remained uneven. Although conscious of the awkwardness of the prototype scanner, Brown "found it difficult to decide whether problems or apparent inconsistencies were due to equipment variations, or to operator-related causes."[4] He was also painfully aware that with clever manipulation of the electronic settings, the operator could make the oscilloscope image take on virtually any appearance that he wanted. This was one of the reasons why, when building the bed-table scanner, Brown had deliberately not put identifying labels on its control knobs. He wished to ensure that he had to be present during its use and so could standardize, to some extent, the electronic conditions of each scan. Nevertheless, Brown remained a frustrated spectator at the scanning sessions, a proud inventor unable to participate fully in the deployment of his own invention and feeling that, as a result, its performance was not optimal.

Ideally, Brown would have liked to undertake the scanning himself. But, as he recollected, "It *was* the middle 'fifties and I was a young medically-unqualified layman, and there was no way the rather Victorian establishment of the Western Infirmary could countenance me ever laying hands directly on patients, especially O&G ones." There had even been some discussion as to whether Brown could remain in the room while scanning was taking place. Donald attempted to save appearances by insisting that Brown wore a white coat. "So," Brown concluded, "if I was going to take control of the examination conditions, I was going to have to do so by some other stratagem."[5]

Brown's inability to regulate how the clinicians operated his prototype scanner led him to a radical rethinking. He conceived a new goal—a machine that would not need a clinician to operate it. He began, in other words, to design an automatic scanner. As described in chapter 5, Brown's first innovation in the field of ultrasonic technology had been the development of a mechanized industrial flaw detection system. This episode had taught him a great deal about scanning systems. There were enormous differences, both mechanical and electronic, between Brown's prototypal industrial device and the automatic diagnostic scanner he was eventually to design and build. Nevertheless, building the flaw detection system introduced him to the possibility of automation and impressed on him its potential for standardization and consistency of results. An automatically scanned image could be presented as intrinsically free from operator bias and thus, ostensibly at least, as more objective than one whose production was predicated on the skill of an individual operator.[6] As we have seen, at this time there was widespread skepticism surrounding the value of ultrasound as an imaging modality. Brown thus conceived of a system that would both free him from his dependence on his clinical colleagues to do the scanning and help deflect the criticism that the operator could visualize whatever he wanted to see. In these respects, Brown's experience with mechanized flaw detection prepared the way, cognitively more than technically, for automating a diagnostic scanner.

While building the Automatic Scanner, Brown made a significant modification to the bed-table instrument, which remained in use in the Western Infirmary. He replaced the Cossor oscilloscope camera with a Thompson Polaroid-Land camera—a major enhancement of the clinical utility of the scanner.[7] Results could now be obtained within a few minutes of the scan being performed, and the process repeated immediately if the images were not of adequate quality. It soon became apparent, however, that Polaroid film was less sensitive than the conventional stock used by the Cossor. Smaller echoes were being lost. By studying data supplied by Polaroid, Brown worked out that this problem could be overcome by a brief preexposure of the film before it was used for scanning.[8] He designed an illuminated box, mounted between the short-persistence screen and the Polaroid camera, that could perform a controlled preexposure.

By this time, the team was generating photographic records of scans at an ever-increasing rate. Brown appreciated that these photographs would have to be systematically annotated and catalogued, if their full clinical value was to be realized. Accordingly, he obtained a supply of customized record cards that could be placed into a slot in the illuminated box. Along the bottom edge were spaces for recording the frequency of the transducer used, the position and orientation of the scanning plane, and the sensitivity setting. When an exposure was made, this information appeared on the margins of the Polaroid image, unequivocally characterizing the scan. On the left margin of the card were spaces in which to enter, by hand, the patient's name and hospital number, the date, and the reason for scanning (see fig. 7.1I).[9]

The card system not only organized the records of individual patients but also facilitated retrieval of information across cases. Around the edges of the card were a series of holes that could be converted into slots with cutting pliers. Slots were created according to a number of clinical criteria. This allowed the records of all patients with a similar condition to be readily separated. To do this, a long pin was passed through the relevant hole in the card pack, so that when the pack was lifted, records of the desired category remained behind. Brown's simple but effective organization of photographic and clinical records was to contribute substantially to the success of the team's research.[10]

During this time, Brown also worked on improving the performance of the ultrasonic transducers. As described in chapter 2, the earliest Kelvin and Hughes flaw detectors used two probes, one transmitting and the other receiving. Later instruments used a single probe with two transducers. These arrangements protected the receiving amplifier from the transmission pulse. There was, however, another advantage. The beam patterns of the two acoustic elements progressively overlapped with increasing distance from the probe. This meant that the sensitivity of the system was relatively low close to the transducers and rose to a maximum some centimeters away. This increase in sensitivity with distance counteracted, to some extent, the fact that echoes coming from deeper in the target were weaker owing to attenuation of the beam by tissue.

In other words, twin-element systems rendered deep echoes more readily comparable with shallow ones. Because of these beneficial characteristics of the twin-element system, neither the early Kelvin and Hughes flaw detectors nor the bed-table scanner employed electronic swept-gain (as defined below). Overall, twin-element probes were not very sensitive, but this was acceptable in industrial application in the light of the poor performance of the single-element transducers then available.[11]

By the late 1950s, Kelvin and Hughes engineers were investigating the potential of single-element systems, whereby one transducer accomplished both transmission and reception. Brown was aware of these developments and concluded that the greater sensitivity of an improved single-element system might be beneficial in medical applications. Moreover, single-element transducers could be used with a lower power output, and Brown remained concerned to minimize the levels of ultrasonic energy entering the abdomen. Accordingly, he began to search for a transducer that could function as both transmitter and receiver, to incorporate into his new design.

In addition to the tendency for the receiver amplifier to be paralyzed by the transmission pulse, another difficulty with single-element systems was control of the "initial complex." The transducer element, referred to as the crystal, was a disk of piezo-electric material such as quartz or, later, barium titanate or lead zirconate-titanate. The disk was mounted on a block of supporting material. When pulsed electrically, the crystal emitted ultrasonic waves from both faces of the disk. The forward wave was directed into the target, and the backward wave had to be suppressed as much as possible, otherwise it would be reflected by the rear surface of the block, return to the disk, and cause unwanted vibrations in the transducer. It would be impossible to distinguish these retrograde echoes from those returning from the target. Accordingly, the mounting block was made from material that could absorb the backward wave. This material also served to damp the vibration of the disk, resulting in a shorter, sharper transmission pulse and a faster recovery of the transducer to a quiescent state, ready to receive the returning echoes. In practice, both control of the retrograde wave and efficient damping of the disk were difficult to achieve. In the industrial context, much effort had gone into devising backing materials that could perform these functions adequately.

Spurious signals could also be produced if reflective discontinuities, such as air bubbles, were present in the mounting block. These signals would appear on the oscilloscope screen as a collection of false echoes, apparently coming from just inside the target. In the medical context, this posed a problem.

> Although one might have thought that such artefactual signals would be constant, and therefore easily disregarded, Nature is rarely so accommodating. What happened in practice was that the amount of energy going back into the backing block was affected by the effectiveness of the forward acoustic coupling between the probe and the patient. Also, genuine echoes coming from the layers of tissue below the skin would interfere constructively or destructively, with the spurious echoes from the backing block, causing a very confusing pattern, within which it was very difficult to sort out anatomical structure from artefact.[12]

Backing blocks were usually made from an epoxy resin into which fine metal powder was mixed. Air bubbles often became trapped in the resin as the powder was added. In the industrial context, various methods had been tried to obviate this, such as degassing with a vacuum pump or compressing the mixture in a hydraulic press. Owing to the viscosity of the metal-epoxy mixture, the vacuum technique removed only some of the bubbles, and those that remained were larger, creating stronger artifactual echoes. Compression of the mixture eliminated the bubbles but reduced the acoustic attenuation of the backing block so that reverberation of the retrograde wave was increased.

Brown now worked on improving the backing block on which the piezoelectric disk was mounted, in collaboration with Clive Ross, a colleague at Kelvin and Hughes's Hillington plant. After much trial and error, they came to the conclusion that entrapment of air in the backing block was unavoidable. What was needed was some means of causing the bubbles to move to the surface of the mixture. Their solution was to spin the block in a high-speed centrifuge while it was setting. The centrifugal movement of the metal particles displaced all the air bubbles inward until they collected at one end. The block could then be placed in the probe with that end farthest from the disk. The other end, more attenuating because of the greater concentration of metal particles, would absorb most of the backward wave before it reached the bubbles. A further ingenious refinement was to centrifuge the blocks with their long axes at 45 degrees to the plane of rotation. This gave the block a reflective interface that was not perpendicular to its long axis. Thus, any backward wave that reached the interface was not reflected directly forward but was sent on a longer, more attenuating path. Brown and Ross were able to make "some quite respectable single-transducer probes," which Brown built into his new Automatic Scanner.[13]

Brown and Ross decided on a range of transducers operating at 1.5, 2.5, and 5 MHz, because those frequencies were standard in Kelvin and Hughes's industrial ultrasonic equipment. Brown later noted that "with hindsight it was unfortunate that we missed what has turned out to be possibly the optimum range-versus-resolution frequency of 3.5 MHz. However I don't think that was too significant with the other equipment limitations of the time."[14]

Although the Automatic Scanner was mechanically very different from the bed-table machine, its electronic circuitry was virtually identical, having been transferred from one machine to the other. However, a number of modifications were made simultaneously with the change to a single-element transducer probe. The amplifier of the Mk IV flaw detector was prone to paralysis and so was unsuitable for use in the new machine. Fortunately Brown's colleague John Woods, an electronic engineer with a background in radar, was an expert in the design of rapid recovery amplifiers. He had worked on the development of electronics for the Mk V flaw detector. Woods sought to optimize the performance of the single-element transducer system by designing amplifiers for use with specific transducer frequencies. Thus Brown built the Automatic Scanner to accept three different plug-in amplifiers, one for each of the 1.5, 2.5, and 5 MHz transducers.[15]

The plug-in amplifiers were adapted to incorporate a swept-gain control. Swept-gain increases amplification (gain) progressively as the time taken for echoes to return to the transducer increases. In other words, echoes originating from deeper inside the target are amplified more strongly than those from more superficial structures. Swept-gain compensated for the progressive attenuation of the signal as it passed through tissue and hence reduced the dynamic range of the echo signals (which could be greater than 60 dB) to more closely match the capability of the signal processor and display unit (~30 dB). In effect, swept-gain made possible the simultaneous display of stronger, nearer echoes and weaker, deeper ones.

Brown wanted to ensure that the only factor that changed when scanning the same tumor at different frequencies was the frequency itself.[16] In other words, transducers of different frequencies had to have similar ultrasonic characteristics, in terms of beam shape and sensitivity. This was a desirable general principle for the design of diagnostic instruments, but it also gave Donald the opportunity to investigate the relationship between frequency and the characteristics of tissue. In the late 1950s, Donald gave serious consideration, in private if not in his published articles, to John Wild's suggestion that different types of solid tumor might be distinguishable by means of their differential absorption of ultrasound.[17]

A crucial variable in transducer design is the length of the near-zone, the region adjacent to the crystal in which the sound is propagated as a parallel beam. The length of the near-zone varies with the diameter of the crystal's active surface and, in any given medium, with the frequency of its vibration.[18] By the late 1950s, Brown had become aware of the research being undertaken by Douglass Howry and his associates in Denver. They had learned to improve the resolution of their scanning system by placing a concave sonic lens on the face of the probe. Brown appreciated that lens profiles might be devised that would equalize the near-zone length between probes of different frequencies.[19] Working purely empirically, Ross devised a range of lens profiles that optimized the performance of each of the different transducers used in the Automatic Scanner. He concluded that a conical rather than a spherical lens gave the best results.

(((((It had become apparent by this time that building the Automatic Scanner would be an expensive undertaking. As noted in chapter 6, the medical research at Kelvin and Hughes had been kept going by the enthusiastic support provided by William Slater. However, in December 1959, Slater told Donald that he was having great difficulty protecting the ultrasound work in the face of increasing opposition from his fellow directors. Brown's initial budget of £500 had been spent many times over. The company's investment was now running into several thousand pounds, with no immediate return in prospect. Worryingly for Slater, Donald estimated that it might take a further fifteen years of research and development before diagnostic ultrasound would become fully accepted as a routine clinical procedure. In the light of the evident need for serious, long-term financial commitment, Slater reluctantly informed Donald that he could no longer support the project.[20]

Donald immediately went to see Sir Hector Hetherington, principal of Glasgow University. Eager to sustain the research effort of one of his key appointees, Hetherington responded positively and immediately to Donald's account of his difficulties, and £750 was found from university funds to enable the ultrasound work to continue. Hetherington also advised Donald to approach Dr. Johnston, of the Advisory Committee for Medical Research of the Scottish Hospitals Endowments Research Trust (SHERT). As a result, Donald and Slater were invited to lunch in Edinburgh with the Trust's chairman, Sir John Erskine, who was a friend of Hetherington.[21] SHERT promptly provided another £4,000. Erskine also briefed Donald on how to make an application to the National Research Development Corporation (NRDC). The NRDC was a semi-commercial organization set up to assist British industry to compete in the international marketplace. As well as providing development grants, the NRDC made strategic investments in R&D companies, on which it hoped to make a profit. Despite Donald's frankness about the long-term nature of any investment in diagnostic ultrasound, the NRDC came to a commercial arrangement with Kelvin and Hughes by which it committed a total of £10,000 to the company's development of diagnostic scanning over several years.[22] These monies enabled work on the Automatic Scanner to continue. With the assistance of persons such as Sir Hector and Sir John, influential, well-connected, and well-disposed toward his research, Donald had found it surprisingly easy to overcome his funding problem. (Erskine was later to say that his decision to back Donald at this time gave him more satisfaction than any other in his long career in public life.)[23] If Donald had not enjoyed Hetherington's ready moral and financial support and the benefit of his contacts within British public administration, the project to develop an ultrasound scanner in Glasgow might easily have failed at this point.

(((((With financial backing secured, Brown could now complete the construction of the new scanner (see fig. 7.2 and fig. 5.1D). In this machine, the transducer was contained in a metal sphere, the "silver ball."[24] The ball was mounted on a vertical column, which moved up and down, keeping the face of the transducer in gentle contact with the patient's abdomen while scanning was underway. A pressure switch prevented the transducer from pressing too heavily on the skin. Driven by a system of cranks and connecting rods, the ball also rocked backward and forward in the plane of the scan. Sensors built into projections on either side of the ball detected when it had rotated about 30 degrees. The ball was then rotated 60 degrees in the opposite direction. Each time the rocking motion of the probe reversed, the vertical column moved horizontally about 15 mm. This pattern of rotation and forward movement was repeated, thus advancing the ball across the abdomen.

To enable it to work properly on the steep flanks of often rather rotund ladies . . . an automatic changeover mechanism operated at about the 45 degree point on either side of the patient, so that the horizontal drive then controlled the pressure, and the vertical drive did the "inching" . . . Nowadays it would all be done by microprocessor, but then it had to depend on cams, switches and relays . . . which would have delighted Heath Robinson.[25]

The operator positioned the probe at the start of each scan by means of a joystick controller. Otherwise, the scanning was wholly automatic. The overall result was what Brown sought: a truly consistent compound scan (fig. 7.1B, C, E, and F).[26]

Most of the scanner's working parts were built into a metal box, the main enclosure, which was supported by a gantry (fig. 7.2; see also fig. 5.1D). The gantry was large enough to allow a hospital bed to be positioned beneath the scanning apparatus. Ill patients could thus be examined without being moved from their beds. The motors that controlled the vertical motion of the column and the rocking motion of the probe were mounted on a turntable within the main enclosure, enabling the column to be turned through 90 degrees. Scanning could thus be done longitudinally as well as transversely. Also, the main enclosure was supported on pivots within the gantry so that it could be tilted from the vertical, enabling the ultrasonic beam to be directed under the rib cage or into the pelvic cavity. At this time, however, oblique scanning was seldom undertaken for clinical purposes, since images taken at unusual scanning angles proved difficult to interpret.

When Slater first saw the Automatic Scanner, he was concerned about the safety implications of the heavy apparatus of relays, switches, and motors suspended over a vulnerable patient. But Brown had incorporated safety devices, rather like those in an elevator—the chains that raised and lowered the main box were fitted with cams and a ratchet so that, if one broke, the box could fall only a few millimeters. Nevertheless, there were occasions in the first few days of the scanner being used in the Western Infirmary when it appeared that the silver ball was attempting to burrow into the flesh of some particularly adipose patient. The emergency stop button had to be hurriedly pressed and modifications made to the mechanism's settings. As was soon discovered, however, this burrowing effect was caused by the patient drawing away from the ball, and the probe attempting to follow her. What solved this unanticipated problem was securing the cooperation of the patient, by explanation and reassurance.

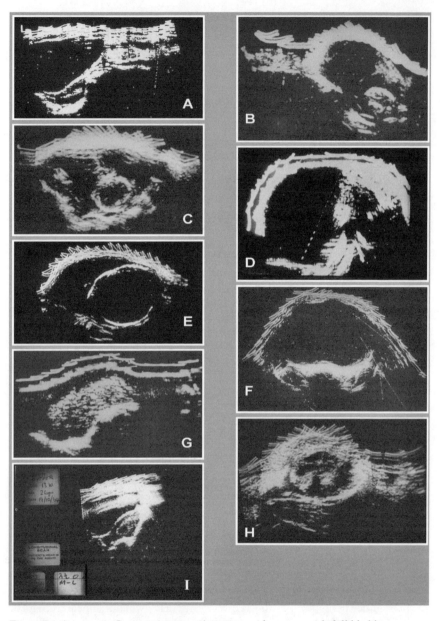

Figure 7.1. Automatic Scanner images. *A*, non-gravid uterus, with full bladder. *B*, fibroid and pregnancy, 17/52; fetus dead? *C*, cyesis, 18/52; pregnancy continues normally. *D*, ovarian cyst and pregnancy at 30/52. *E*, hydrocephalic fetus. *F*, ovarian cyst. *G*, hydatidiform mole. *H*, cystadenocarcinoma of the ovary. *I*, single early pregnancy, below and to the right of a full bladder; the record card gives position and direction of the scan—annotated by John Fleming, October 1964. Images *B*, *C*, *E*, and *F* clearly show that a "truly consistent" scanning pattern was achieved. *Reproduced with permission of the BMUS Historical Collection*

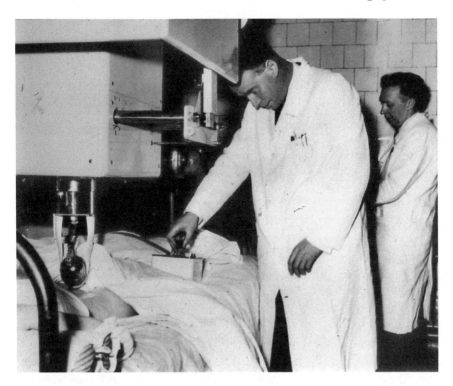

Figure 7.2. Donald and MacVicar operating the Automatic Scanner, Western Infirmary, Glasgow, ca. 1960. *Reproduced with permission of the BMUS Historical Collection*

Later, a white nylon ring was placed around the ball to increase its surface area and make it seem less oppressive.[27]

It was vital for Brown and his colleagues to realize that removing the clinician's hands from the probe had not eliminated human agency from the scanning process. Ultrasonic scanners interfaced with patients' bodies and emotions, as well as with clinicians' hands and arms. The real working unit, that which actually accomplished the diagnosis, was not the scanner alone but a more complex entity, a hybrid of operator, machine, and patient. Eventually, the system worked so smoothly, and Donald and MacVicar developed such confidence in its operation, that Brown found it necessary to install a bell that rang when a scan was completed, to summon the clinician back to the patient.

In July 1960, Brown demonstrated the Automatic Scanner at an exhibition of medical technology, held at Olympia in London (see fig. 5.1D).[28] It was on this occasion that Donald and Brown first met Douglass Howry.[29] Howry was favorably impressed with the Automatic Scanner and, in particular, with Brown's achievement in making contact scanning work effectively. This was the start of a long and mutually supportive interaction between the ultrasound teams in Glasgow and Denver. Howry learned a great deal from Brown, and Donald visited the University of Colorado several times in the 1960s and 1970s to lecture on diagnostic ultrasound and its clinical applications.

The Automatic Scanner was a complicated piece of machinery, and inevitably, despite Brown's best efforts, it sometimes functioned less than optimally.

> Because the Automatic Scanner ran on DC motors it was inclined to produce electrical hash, electrical interference. When the contacts started sparking you got a snowstorm across the screen and you had to send somebody up to clean the contacts and put the suppressors in and make sure the wires were properly shielded and so on. There was an ongoing problem with it. It was episodic.[30]

Sometimes, the olive oil used for acoustic coupling congealed around the transducer, preventing it from moving easily within its housing in the silver ball. The transducer would then press harder on the patient's abdomen than was intended. But, crucially, the automatic nature of the apparatus substantially freed the clinicians from the need to concern themselves with the electronic or physical conditions of the scanning process. They could concentrate on setting up the scan, ensuring the patient's comfort, and interpreting the ultrasound images in the light of their growing experience with the modality. The Automatic Scanner, in other words, began the process of black-boxing the technology. Clinicians could use the apparatus without having to think constantly about how it worked. Diagnostic ultrasound was moving toward becoming a technique that an obstetrician-gynaecologist who, unlike Donald, had little interest in engineering could happily adopt.

(((((In the process of becoming, metaphorically speaking, a black box, diagnostic scanners went, literally, white. The bed-table prototype had been painted in whatever color happened to be readily available in the Hillington factory. Its drab gray is explicable by the company's large amount of work for the Admiralty. The outer framework of the Automatic Scanner was, by contrast, finished in white enamel, which in the late 1950s was becoming typical for large items of commercial medical equipment. In other words, although the Automatic Scanner was built, by Brown and a small group of engineers, using the craft mode of production, elements of its design represented a step toward the diagnostic scanner becoming a commercial commodity.[31] Brown certainly hoped that his Automatic Scanner would form the basis of a marketable product for Kelvin and Hughes.

It was therefore an enormous boost to the morale of the team when the first commercial order was placed. Here again, the sequence of events hinged on happenstance and personal connections. Ever enthusiastic about innovative medical technologies, Donald had been closely following the development of the laparoscope.[32] Laparoscopy is a technique for the direct visualization of the contents of the pelvis and abdomen by insertion of a flexible optical device through a small incision in the abdominal wall. One of the leading pioneers of laparoscopy in gynecology was Alf Sjövall, professor of obstetrics and gynecology in Lund, Sweden. Donald went to Sweden to spend a week with Sjövall, learning how to use the new diagnostic tool.[33] Donald believed that laparoscopy and ultrasound would complement one another. Abnormalities suspected on ultrasound examination might be further investigated by the laparoscope, without the full surgical procedure of laparotomy being resorted to.

By coincidence, Lund was one of the few European centers where research into diagnostic ultrasound was underway. By 1957, the investigations by Leksell on the detection of brain lesions and by Edler on echocardiography were well known throughout the University of Lund Medical School. The possibility of diagnostic applications of ultrasound within their own field was a frequent topic of discussion among the staff of the Department of Obstetrics and Gynaecology. Interest was such that a young resident, Bertil Sundén, was encouraged by his senior colleagues to investigate its potential. Sundén acquired a Krautkrämer flaw detector, with which he examined a number of pregnant women.[34] He readily obtained echoes from within the gravid uterus but was unable to interpret them with any confidence. Donald's arrival in Lund, with news of the invention of a two-dimensional contact scanner, revived Sundén's interest in ultrasound. Donald invited him to visit Glasgow to learn more about the technique. Late in 1958, Sundén spent three weeks in the Royal Maternity Hospital and the Western Infirmary, observing Donald's use of the bed-table scanner. On his return, Sundén secured a grant from the Staten Medicinska Forskningsråd, Sweden's Medical Research Council, and persuaded the University of Lund to purchase a scanner like the one he had used in Glasgow. The order was placed in 1959.

By this time, the Automatic Scanner had been built and was in regular use in Donald's clinic. But Sundén had been taught on the bed-table scanner and he wanted to obtain a similar machine. In particular, he wished to be able to do the scanning himself, rather than delegating this key function to a mechanical system. In accordance with Sundén's wishes, the order placed with Kelvin and Hughes by the University of Lund was for a manual rather than an automatic instrument. Sundén, Brown recalls, "would have been quite happy to have a replica of Donald's original [bed-table] scanner but we thought we could do better than that. So I decided that I was going to make a prototype of a hand machine and set about designing it."[35]

Brown's plan to base commercial production on the Automatic Scanner was thus thwarted. His intention to remove the clinicians' hands from the probe was defeated by the clinicians having their hands on the purse strings. Paradoxically, by this time, the high quality of the images obtained by the Automatic Scanner had to some extent helped convince Brown that automatic scanning was not essential. The Automatic Scanner provided a benchmark by which the standard of the images obtained by manual scanning could be objectively judged. As had become evident, manual scanning by properly trained and experienced personnel was adequate for clinical purposes. Furthermore, manual systems would be considerably cheaper and easier for Kelvin and Hughes to build and maintain.

With an eye to further development, Brown had designed the Automatic Scanner so that it was potentially capable of scanning in three dimensions. The vertical column was motor-driven in three directions, orthogonal to one another. Thus it would have required only a minor modification of the mechanism to enable the silver ball, having finished one traverse of the abdomen, to begin a parallel scan in another plane, adjacent to the first. In this way, the silver ball might gradually have traversed the length and breadth of the abdomen, or as much of it as the operator wished. All three translational movements could be measured. The obstacle was that no imaging system then existed that could display three-dimensional information in a practically useful form. Brown regarded a suitable method of three-dimensional display as a project for the future. Later, in 1962, when John Fleming joined the staff of the Hillington factory, Brown instructed him to work on the problem.[36] But no immediate solution was found.

The Automatic Scanner was effectively a cybernetic device. Cybernetic systems are characterized by servomechanisms, or feedback loops. In the public mind, cybernetics was the science of robotics and, as such, it had an aura of popular glamour in the 1950s and 1960s. One of Britain's leading cyberneti-cians was Grey Walter, who was, from 1939, director of the Physiology Depart-ment of the Burden Neurological Institute in Bristol. Walter's most famous creations were his "tortoises," small, mobile devices with two motor-driven wheels at the rear.[37] Their direction of travel was determined by a third wheel at the front, which was connected to a photoelectric cell. When the photoelec-tric cell detected a light source, the drive motors switched on, and the device steered itself toward the light. The design of the tortoises incorporated the essential cybernetic connection between goal and feedback, but their behavior was unexpectedly lively and intriguing. Brown admired Walter's work and, as a young man, had been fascinated by the tortoises.[38] While the amount of feedback control built into the operation of the Automatic Scanner was rela-tively small, the scuttling, crablike motion of the silver ball across the abdo-men, independent of any direct human guidance, is oddly reminiscent of the performance of one of Walter's tortoises.

The significance of Brown's Automatic Scanner in the history of obstetric ultrasound is a moot question.[39] Manual scanning came to represent the main line of development. The principle of fully automated scanning was rejected by the first clinician to buy an ultrasound scanner, and no other such scanners have been built.[40] However, it could be argued that automated scanning played a cru-cial role in gaining acceptance for the new diagnostic technique. It appeared at a time in the modality's development when its usefulness remained the subject of some skepticism. The Automatic Scanner was Donald's principal machine dur-ing the critical period, between 1959 and 1965, in which he and his colleagues were largely responsible for establishing, beyond any reasonable doubt, the clini-cal value of ultrasound scanning in obstetrics and gynecology.[41] That the motor-ized driving of the probe ensured a high degree of consistency, within each scan and between one scan and another, undoubtedly did much to reinforce Donald's own confidence in diagnostic ultrasound. Furthermore, that the thousands of images produced by the Automatic Scanner were generated independently, at least ostensibly so, of the individual predilections of the operator undoubtedly increased their rhetorical force within Donald's advocacy of the technique. And, as we have seen, the Automatic Scanner provided, initially at least, a benchmark against which the quality of manual scanning could be judged.

(((((The arrival of the order for a manual scanner in 1959 imposed a fresh set of requirements on Brown and his colleagues at Kelvin and Hughes. Although the Automatic Scanner had a higher level of design refinement than the bed-table machine, it was still below the standard required in a commercial product. The services of a professional designer were evidently needed. But Brown did not have a high opinion of the designers employed at Hillington—most of whom, it is only fair to note, were accustomed to working on heavy industrial, military, or marine equipment. Something more refined was desirable, Brown thought, for a medical instrument. Here again, a chance encounter was to have a crucial impact on the story of ultrasound in Glasgow.

Dugald Cameron was a final-year industrial design student at the Glasgow School of Art.

> In the Art School when I was in my final year . . . there was an attractive young lady in the first year, who we all used to chase after. She was Tom Brown's sister-in-law and I can remember her saying to me . . . that her brother-in-law was doing this sort of development and he really didn't think much of industrial designers, which I was rather keen about and studying at the School of Art and I said "Well, that's really an awful pity, I better meet him."[42]

Miss Stevens introduced Cameron to her brother-in-law, and the two men met in Brown's flat to discuss design issues. Brown showed Cameron preliminary drawings made by one of Kelvin and Hughes's industrial designers. Cameron agreed that both the ergonomics and the aesthetics of the design left something to be desired. Moreover, whereas the bed-table scanner was best operated with two people in attendance—one to manipulate the probe, the other to set the controls and open the camera shutter—Cameron was convinced that an improvement in the layout of the apparatus would allow scanning by a single operator. Brown thought that the operator ought to be able to choose whether to sit or stand while using the machine. But Cameron persuaded him that to optimize the ergonomics, they needed to decide whether scanning was to be undertaken standing or sitting. Brown chose standing, and Cameron arranged the units accordingly. Cameron also incorporated into the design of the Lund machine several features to improve ease of use, such as convenient holders for spare probes and for bottles of olive oil.

Cameron's concern extended beyond the convenience of the operator or the cosmetics of the machine. Committed to the new consumer-oriented outlook that was revolutionizing industrial design in the early 1960s, Cameron recognized that two groups of users, with radically different relationships to the machine, had to be considered. He was aware, in other words, that the scanner's clientele consisted of patients as well as clinicians. Therefore, he set out to design a scanner that would not be intimidating to a woman undergoing an unfamiliar and potentially anxiety-making form of medical examination. As noted above, when the Automatic Scanner was in use, a heavy and bulky (54 × 50 × 43 cm) box hung over the patient, in a way that some found menacing. In Cameron's design, this box was replaced with a slim, elegant, rectangular enclosure, supported by a sturdy, hinged arm. The arm was attached to a central pillar, the tree-trunk-like dimensions of which were calculated to allay a patient's fears that the apparatus might topple over on top of her.

The modular layout of the bed-table scanner and the Automatic Scanner, with the electronic and mechanical components contained in different units, was retained in Cameron's design. Brown and his colleagues developed an ingenious differential drive system that enabled positioning of the sine/cosine potentiometer in the measuring frame, some distance away from the transducer. This modification contributed to the smaller, neater design of the probe head.

The Lund scanner was equipped with two displays, short-persistence and long-persistence. The short-persistence screen had the Polaroid camera mounted in front of it (fig. 7.3A). The long-persistence screen enabled the operator to monitor whether echoes of sufficient strength were being received and to follow the development of the image. In deference to the clinical customer, Brown had reinstated the long-persistence display, which he had removed from the bed-table scanner. A separate A-scan screen was no longer considered necessary, but A-scan images could be displayed on either of the two screens, if required.[43] Brown's attitude to the safety of the modality remained a cautious one, and accordingly, besides retaining the arrangement whereby the amplifier was set to maximum gain and the transmitter to minimum power, he reduced the pulse-repetition rate of the new scanner from 50 to 25 per second. This gave the images produced by Sundén's machine a characteristic spotty appearance (fig. 7.3B).

After extensive testing by MacVicar and Donald in the Western Infirmary, the scanner was delivered to Sundén on March 30, 1962, with Clive Ross traveling to Lund to install it in the Department of Obstetrics and Gynaecology.[44] Sundén scanned five patients on the first day the scanner became operational, and within two years he had conducted an extensive series of investigations.[45] His MD thesis was examined by Donald in 1964—the first MD to be awarded for work with diagnostic ultrasound by an institution other than the University

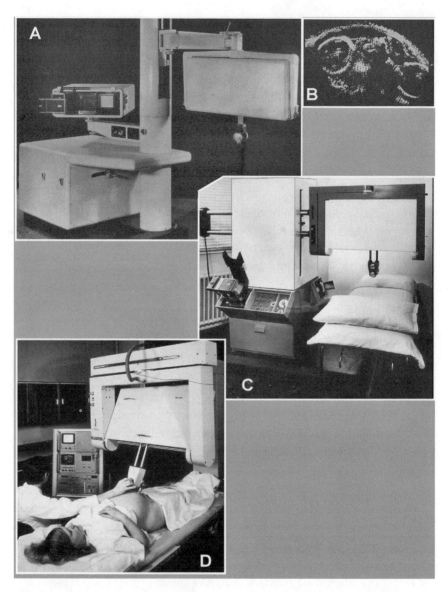

Figure 7.3. The first commercial scanners. *A*, ready for delivery to Dr. B. Sundén, Lund, Sweden, 1962. *B*, image showing twins, cephalic and breech. *C*, Smiths Diasonograph in the Queen Mother's Hospital, Glasgow, soon after installation, 1964. *D*, Nuclear Enterprises Ltd. NE4102, in use by the late Dr. B. Buttery in the Queen Mother's Hospital, ca. 1975. *Reproduced courtesy of the BMUS Historical Collection; B, ultrasound image reproduced courtesy of the late Dr. B. Sundén*

of Glasgow. Sundén acquired his machine for the nominal price of £2,500. There was no profit in this transaction for the manufacturer, but the Kelvin and Hughes management was greatly encouraged by having secured an order. In September 1962, another development engineer, John Fleming, was engaged to work on the design of a scanner that could go into full-scale production and to continue the day-to-day support of Donald and MacVicar. Fleming was recruited from Ferranti, a large electronics manufacturer in the south of England that was heavily involved in the arms industry. He had disliked working on military projects and warmly welcomed the opportunity to change to medical applications.

The Sundén machine represented a considerable refinement of scanning technology, when compared with the Automatic Scanner. However, although Sundén achieved impressive clinical results, the machine did require some regular attention, and it was fortunate that engineering assistance was available in Lund. In March 1964, the manufacturer arranged for Fleming to undertake a major overhaul. He was by this time familiar with the layout of the machine, having formalized the circuit diagrams as a step toward the design of the next generation of scanners. It was nevertheless, as Fleming recalls, a valuable exercise to deal with the Sundén system "in the flesh." As well as performing routine maintenance, Fleming replaced the sine/cosine potentiometer.[46] The "sine/cos pot" was proving to be a regular cause of trouble. In these potentiometers, the resistive element consisted of fine wire wound over a flat, nonconducting frame. Electrical contacts slid over the wire's surface, giving the device an inherently limited lifespan, which the oscillatory movements of the diagnostic scanners further shortened. In the early 1960s, moreover, this reliability problem was getting worse—owing, it was suspected, to falling standards of manufacture. Wear in the sine/cos pot caused echoes to become misplaced, quite unpredictably, on the diagnostic image.

In the late 1950s, Kelvin and Hughes was rebranded as a division of its parent company, Smiths Industries Ltd. The change of name did not directly affect the ultrasound R&D, but Brown's work was shortly to have a hiatus imposed on it. Brown's prototype of a mechanized industrial flaw detector system had been transferred to the company's factory at Barkingside for commercial development. On the basis of Brown's success, Alex Rankin had encouraged sales staff to secure advance orders for mechanized detectors. Many of these industrial customers were important enough for Smiths Industries to be unwilling to disappoint them. Unfortunately, the team charged with providing a marketable product had found it difficult to emulate the performance of Brown's prototype. Orders were not being delivered on time; a situation deeply embarrassing to Smiths was developing. Eventually, the project was transferred back to Hillington, together with the rest of the company's ultrasound R&D. Shortly afterward, Rankin died unexpectedly, and Brown took over as department head.[47] He was no longer able to devote a great deal of his attention to the medical project, but he and Fleming continued to work on developing a scanner that could be marketed commercially. Fleming revised the electronics, whereas Brown oversaw the redesign of the mechanical systems. In particular, he sought an alternative to the folding arm that supported and controlled the measuring frame. Its original design was elegant but had proved expensive to manufacture.

To some extent, the delay caused by Brown's other work commitments gave time for the problems of the Automatic and Lund scanners to reveal themselves and for solutions to be incorporated in the next generation of manually operated machines. As Fleming recalls:

> The circuits were very similar to the Sundén machine and a lot of the problems were weaknesses in the circuit design in that they were dependent on unspecified characteristics of the valves. If you buy an electronic component it has lots of parameters held within limits. There may be other parameters, which are not regarded as important, that nobody cares much about but if you try to design a circuit that depends on those, you can be in trouble. A lot of it [redesign work] was that sort of thing because I inherited this circuit. I wouldn't say that I did much actual new circuit design on the principal parts of it. The whole power supply I changed . . . but a lot of it was a given, like "Make that work!" It's a common problem if somebody lashes up a circuit and it works and you think "Fine," then you try and make 3 of them and they don't work![48]

In building the electronics for the bed-table scanner, Brown had used an ingenious, if unorthodox, arrangement of two triode valves connected in reverse. (Brown was here using a trick much like that of a clinician exploiting the side effect of a drug.) This arrangement functioned, in effect, as a very fast switch. It was used to set the initial conditions of the integrators that generated the time-base waveforms that, in turn, produced the line representing the sound beam on the display. The same circuit was retained in the Automatic and Sundén machines. But stabilizing this system to production standards caused Fleming a lot of problems, and he thought a radical solution was available.

While at Ferranti, Fleming had worked with state-of-the-art semiconductor electronics. Solid-state components were particularly valued in military applications because of their small size and low power consumption. They were also more robust than thermionic valves, which had delicate glass envelopes and electrically heated cathodes. Fleming offered to transistorize the circuits of the new scanner. But Brown considered that a redesign of this magnitude would be expensive and time-consuming. Eager to proceed toward production without further delay, he insisted that Fleming continue with adapting and improving the valve circuitry.

In refining Brown's design, Fleming was able to employ circuitry from the latest model of Kelvin and Hughes's series of flaw detectors, the Mk VII.[49] (Industrial ultrasound was developing in parallel with diagnostic ultrasound throughout this period.) Fleming adapted the switchable amplifier from the Mk VII to replace the three plug-in units used in the Automatic Scanner. In addition to improving performance, this overcame the problem of the vulnerability of the plug-in units to contamination while not in use. The transmitter and timing circuits from the Mk VII were also deployed.

(((((In late 1963, Hetherington's long-cherished plan for a new maternity hospital in Glasgow finally came to fruition. In December, the Queen Mother's Hospital took delivery of the first Diasonograph (fig. 7.3C), as the new machine was dubbed. In January 1964, the first patients were admitted and clinical trials of the new scanner began. By the time the hospital was officially opened in September 1964, a "sonar" department for ultrasonic diagnosis and research was already established.[50]

Dugald Cameron had again been involved, as "industrial design consultant." The original, elegant plan of the Sundén machine was considerably modified, in consultation with David McNair, who undertook some mechanical design work while Brown was occupied with the industrial project.[51] The new scanner had a simpler, more linear layout. It was also bigger, its slablike sides and massive boxed superstructure proclaiming the factory's industrial heritage. The Diasonograph was Clyde-built, at a time when that epithet still alluded to an admired tradition of heavy engineering. The scanner was certainly heavy, weighing approximately one ton. It rapidly acquired the nickname Dinosaurograph.

The Diasonograph's industrial provenance was not the only reason for its bulk. Cameron's concern that a patient should not feel threatened while lying under the scanning arm continued to influence the thinking of the design team. The machine was made reassuringly large and stable. Moreover, while the Diasonograph was designed to be operated manually, Brown had not wholly abandoned his aspiration toward automatic scanning. He insisted that the counterweight mechanism have sufficient capacity to allow for the movements of the probe to be motorized at some later stage.[52] Brown also envisaged that, during automatic scanning, the patient would be moved longitudinally relative to the probe. Cameron's original drawings incorporated an elegant motorized platform to achieve this. This feature was abandoned when the scanner went into production, on the grounds of cost, and was replaced with a modified hospital trolley.

After the Diasonograph came into service, an engineer or technician was still often in attendance while scanning was underway, to adjust the controls and offer support to clinicians only gradually gaining competence in the operation of the machine. As Fleming recalls, "I suppose there were two people involved quite a lot because it was such a new thing and people were learning a lot . . . Perhaps the likes of me just operating the camera and saying 'Well, Professor Donald, do you want a bit more power,' . . . Or perhaps 'I need to adjust the swept gain for you.' Which was difficult, it was all hidden away."[53]

Brown was still uneasy about the freedom with which clinicians could manipulate the image in ways that were detrimental either to image quality or to the objectivity of the diagnostic process. Accordingly, to ensure that engineers retained some degree of supervision over the scanning, he had incorporated a hierarchical control system into the Diasonograph. The controls governing the simpler functions such as frequency and transmitter output level—"the doctors' controls," as they were called—were located at the right-hand end of the main control panel and were thus readily accessible to the operator. To the left was a second panel with switches for the various scanning modes. A moveable cover could be positioned to hide both panels, or to reveal only the right-hand panel, or to reveal both panels. Access to the controls could thus be suited to the capability of the person operating the scanner. Below the main panel, and behind a hinged flap and hence relatively inaccessible, was a third set of controls, where such functions as swept-gain and calibration velocity were adjusted. Use of these controls required a screwdriver and a knowledge of the circuits and calibration processes. This "third level of control" was intended to be uniquely the engineer's province. Brown sought, as he put it, to make the Diasonograph "doctor-proof."[54]

Donald, however, enjoyed playing with the controls of the machine almost as much as he enjoyed scanning the abdomen. As a result, he later substantially switched the role he undertook in operating the Diasonograph. In the Western Infirmary, he had enlisted a nurse, Mrs. Helen Sawers, to help him use the Automatic Scanner. Later, in the Queen Mother's Hospital, he trained Mrs. Ida Miller to scan with the Diasonograph, while he operated the electronics. Mrs. Miller was the wife of a well-known Glasgow general practitioner, Dr. Jack Miller. During a conversation at a medical dinner, Dr. Miller remarked to Donald that his "very efficient" wife was looking for work.[55] On this recommendation, Donald employed her, initially as a clerk to organize the large number of clinical records the Diasonograph was generating. However, Ida Miller shortly became, in effect, the world's first ultrasonographer. Initially working alongside Donald, she gradually took over a major role in the operation of the machine, doing many hundreds of initial or routine scans and working productively for several years in the Queen Mother's Hospital. Donald circumvented the issue of her lack of formal qualifications by having a television link installed between her scanning room and his office, so that he could, nominally at least, supervise her work from his desk.[56]

That Donald encouraged Miller to undertake diagnostic scanning, whereas he had prevented Brown from having any direct contact with his patients, might be regarded as surprising. However, it is indicative of a prevailing attitude among older members of the medical profession at this time that the wives of general practitioners, accustomed as many of them were to assisting with their husband's practices, were a category of layperson to which certain responsibilities might be readily devolved.[57] Being female, doubtless, also made Miller more acceptable in obstetric and gynecological clinics. Donald's willingness to delegate scanning to Miller was also a measure of his growing confidence in ultrasonic diagnosis and an indication that it had gained the status of a routine procedure in his clinic. Donald was, as he acknowledged, notoriously impatient with routine investigations.[58] He was appalled when, on her husband's election as treasurer of the British Medical Association, Miller resigned her post so that she could be his hostess at official functions. Donald, who otherwise had traditional views on the employment of married women, saw this as a waste of the abilities of a trained and talented member of his staff.[59]

The Diasonograph produced images that were more revealing of anatomical detail than those provided by its predecessors (fig. 7.4 shows examples).

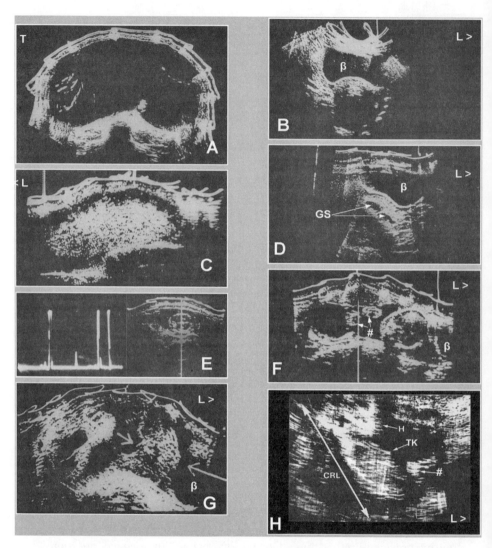

Figure 7.4. Images from the Diasonograph and NE4102. *A*, pseudomucinous cystadenoma of the ovary. *B*, fibroid. *C*, hydatidiform mole. *D*, twin gestational sacs at 7/52. *E*, fetal cephalometry; this A-scan shows echoes from the two sides of the skull, the midline, and far wall of the uterus. *F*, fetus at 24/52, head to the right; hydramnios; upper anterior placenta, two limbs near vertical marker line. *G*, pregnancy at 36/52, central placenta (*arrows*). *H*, NE4102 image—normal fetus at 14/52; CRL = 80 mm. Abbreviations: T, transverse scan; L>, longitudinal scan, with feet to right; <L, feet to left; β, bladder; GS, gestational sac; #, limb; TK, trunk; H, head; CRL, crown-rump length. *Reproduced with permission of the BMUS Historical Collection*

However, if one compares its design with that of other, later instruments, it can be seen as the fullest expression of an engineer's, as opposed to a clinician's, conception of what a diagnostic scanner should be. In the Diasonograph, the large box that hung over the patient was, in effect, a very precise measuring frame. In compound scanning, each reflective surface was scanned from a number of different angles. It was essential that both the position of the transducer and the angle of the beam were precisely determined, allowing the same reflecting point to be imaged in exactly the same position on the screen from whatever angle it was scanned. This parameter was known as registration. In addition to the electronic system of registration, metal measuring rules were fitted to the outside of the main enclosure and gantry of the Diasonograph, so that the position of the scanning plane within it could be specified precisely, relative to an orthogonal grid. This was an engineer's mode of recording location, analogous to that used on a draftsman's drawing board, but in three dimensions rather than two. However, clinicians preferred to locate the scanning plane relative to the anatomical landmarks of the patient's body. Thus expressions such as "two centimeters below the umbilicus," already common in the recording of clinical findings, were adopted to record the details of ultrasonic examinations. To accommodate this, the measuring frame of the scanner could be zeroed to a particular anatomical reference point.

(((((In 1965, Smiths Industries underwent some changes in organization that Brown did not find congenial, so he left to join another electronics manufacturer, Honeywell.[60] Brian Fraser took over the leadership of Smiths' ultrasound department, and he and Fleming saw the Diasonograph into commercial production. In 1966, however, another crisis loomed for Donald and his colleagues in Glasgow. By this time, Smiths had sold twelve Diasonographs, to hospitals in England, North America, and Iraq as well as Scotland, but the Hillington factory was losing money. Smiths was also engaged in a damaging legal dispute with Automation Industries in the United States over the global patent rights to contact transducer systems. On losing the case, Smiths decided to close the Hillington factory, abandoning its investment in medical ultrasound. Donald was aghast: "Sonar as a subject, at least in this country, seemed finished and it looked as though America would inherit the lot, and we ourselves would be faced with the dust-sheet."[61] This possibility affronted Donald not only as a user of ultrasound but also as a patriotic champion of

British industry. He sought another financial backer, initially without success. Desperate recourse was again made to the principal of the University of
Glasgow, now Sir Charles Wilson. Donald tentatively sought permission to engage electronic engineers on an ad hoc basis to maintain the ultrasound equipment in the Queen Mother's Hospital. To his amazement, Wilson immediately
authorized him to set up a University Department of Ultrasonic Technology
and to engage two full-time staff at competitive rates of pay. Fleming enthusiastically accepted the offer of a position as "research technologist" in Donald's
new department and encouraged Angus Hall, who had left Smiths a few months
earlier, to join him. Thus Donald was provided with a talented and experienced
in-house team of ultrasound engineers. A large quantity of instruments and
electronic components was also acquired from Smiths for a nominal sum.

Delighted by this outcome, Donald described his project as now being
"gloriously independent" of the "vagaries of commercial balance sheets and
the whims of industrial profits."[62] Fleming and Hall could now assist the clinicians on a more regular basis, publish research papers on the physical and
technical aspects of diagnostic ultrasound,[63] and make some improvements to
the Diasonograph that had not been feasible at Smiths.

> Angus and I [Fleming] . . . had a Diasonograph in the Western Infirmary that
> wasn't quite complete so we completed it and by that time we were aware that the
> sine/cos pot was an absolute pain and we just set about finding an alternative.
> There weren't many but we eventually found one that was made with a plastic
> conductive track . . . it's a solid material loaded with carbon, rather than a piece
> of "cardboard" with wire wrapped on it, which is what the Smiths one was. We
> found this better one . . . they were being manufactured in the States. They were
> quite expensive but they completely solved the problem.[64]

Fleming and Hall identified another problem in particular need of attention.
Electrical feedback between the transducer and the amplifier produced unpredictable, transient, and very annoying corruptions of the image. To prevent
this, the earthing of the amplifier and the probe was improved. This modification allowed the amplifier of the Diasonograph to be operated at higher gain,
and thus overall sensitivity was enhanced.[65]

In 1967, after some tense negotiations, including a direct appeal by Brown
to the Ministry of Health, Smiths' interest in medical ultrasound was sold to
Nuclear Enterprises (NE), a small but successful Edinburgh-based medical
electronics manufacturer. Nuclear Enterprises promptly hired Brown. Fraser

was also employed by NE, having been made redundant by Smiths. Development of the Diasonograph continued, with Donald as a consultant.[66] (Fraser and Donald had become friends, partly through a common interest in sailing.) Shortly afterward, Nuclear Enterprises marketed the NE4101 (fig. 7.3C), a scanner virtually identical to the Diasonograph, but with performance improved through better-quality components and more careful assembly. Attention to detail paid considerable dividends in the functioning of a compound scanner: "Everything you could do to get registration that little bit better was worth having," as Fraser put it.[67]

Nuclear Enterprise then set out to improve the design further. Alan Cole was given the task of redesigning the electronics, using solid-state integrated circuits in place of the, by then, outdated thermionic valves of the NE4101. When the next model, the NE4102 (fig. 7.3D), first went on sale, only a single valve remained, the thyratron in the transmitter, and this was shortly replaced when a suitable solid-state alternative, a silicon controlled rectifier developed for the television industry, became available. The electronics of the NE4102 were put in a separate, moveable console so that the operator could sit next to the patient while facing the screen, a more satisfactory arrangement in clinical use.

In the mid-1960s, electronics manufacturing was moving toward modularization, and the design of the NE4102 reflected that change. When building the Diasonograph, Fleming had designed its power supply from scratch. Its oscilloscopes were likewise built at Smiths around cathode-ray tubes bought from General Electric. Cole now bought fully assembled oscilloscopes from Hewlett Packard, acknowledged to be among the finest available, and designed a small plug-in module that adapted the unit to perform those functions specifically required for use with ultrasound. Power supply units were also bought ready-made, from STC Ltd. The use of modularized components produced noticeable refinements in the resultant images. As Fleming reflected:

> You bought the tube and you built your electronics to go around it, which was alright but with the engineering effort available—me—they wouldn't have been up to Hewlett Packard or Tektronix standard because they'd have a whole team of guys working on getting the absolute best you could. There were all sorts of little compromises you make and little adjustments; we get another half a percent here if we do this, and so on.[68]

The craftsmanlike mode of production that had characterized the development of medical ultrasound in Scotland since its inception by Brown in 1956 had now been superseded. With the launch of the NE4102 in 1972, the ultrasound scanner had undergone a complete transformation into a commodity in the modern medical marketplace. The NE4102 was a most successful product. The images it produced were significantly better than those of any of the earlier machines (fig. 7.4H). It was bought by many British hospitals, often as their first ultrasound scanner, and was also sold widely throughout the world.[69]

CHAPTER EIGHT

Behind the Iron Curtain
Ultrasound and the Fetus

Ian Donald's earliest clinical investigations with the ultrasonic scanner were in the field of gynecology, but there is no doubt that his imaging research achieved its greatest impact through its application to the gravid uterus. During the early 1960s, in a series of publications, Donald and his colleagues revealed the developing fetus and its disorders to clinical and scientific scrutiny to a remarkable and wholly unprecedented extent. This chapter explores this period of intense innovation. We also examine how ultrasound scanning became incorporated into routine clinical practice, and how that incorporation changed not only the status of the fetus but also the significance accorded to the pregnant woman's experience of pregnancy.

In their 1958 paper in the *Lancet*, Donald, MacVicar, and Brown announced that they had visualized a fetus of only fourteen weeks' gestational age. The discovery was made accidentally when examining a woman with uterine enlargement, thought to be due to fibromyomata.[1] After this case, Donald became interested in whether the fetus could be identified at still earlier periods of gestation. He also sought to explore ultrasound's potential for investigating the complications of early pregnancy. By 1963, he and his colleagues had used the Automatic Scanner to examine more than 130 women whose pregnancies were of less than twenty weeks' duration.[2] A standardized procedure had been developed for the examination of such patients. First, a longitudinal scan was taken, from the xiphisternum to the symphysis pubis, with the probe working at a frequency of 2.5 MHz. If the patient was indeed pregnant, both the outline of the uterus and fetal echoes within it could, in most cases, be readily demonstrated. A transverse scan was then taken, to try to visualize the fetal head. This was usually possible if the fetus was sixteen weeks or older. If the uterine outline could not be found, the longitudinal scan was repeated at 1.5 MHz. The deeper penetration afforded by the lower frequency often allowed the uterus to be located, even if it was retroverted or lying under coils of bowel. Under these circumstances, it should be noted, the uterus often could not be found by abdominal palpation. If the outline of the uterus was visible on the scan but no fetal echoes could be identified within, the longitudinal scan was repeated at a slightly increased power output to try to locate a fetus.

MacVicar and Donald were now able to report that they could find fetuses of twelve weeks' gestation, generally without great difficulty. At earlier gestational ages, the small size of the fetal sac relative to the enlarged uterus made location more difficult. But if the operator made several passes with the probe angled into the pelvic cavity, fetal echoes could often be identified. The youngest fetus whose presence MacVicar and Donald were able to confirm by ultrasound had a gestational age of between eight and nine weeks.[3]

There can be little doubt that Donald and MacVicar's motivation to pursue this work sprang, to some extent, from their eagerness to explore the imaging possibilities of their new equipment, the Automatic Scanner. But even their first series of investigations of early pregnancy promised considerable clinical utility. At that time, the confirmation, or otherwise, of continuing pregnancy was not straightforward. This was a matter of great emotional and practical significance to patients. In Donald's wards, a woman in early pregnancy who displayed the symptoms of threatened abortion—vaginal bleeding and intermittent pain—would be confined to bed and sedated, for several days, until either the bleeding stopped or spontaneous abortion occurred. If she expelled identifiable products of conception, the failure of the pregnancy was unequivocally confirmed, and steps could be taken to control further bleeding and address any remaining clinical concerns. However, if the products of conception were not found, the obstetrician was often uncertain as to whether or not fetal death had occurred. The pregnancy tests available in the early 1960s were slow to report a result and were sometimes unreliable.[4] Gonadotropins, on which some tests were based, can persist in the bloodstream for several days after the death of the fetus. Diagnosing a missed abortion when, in fact, pregnancy was continuing was, as Donald put it, "the greatest pitfall" a clinician needed to avoid under these circumstances.[5] Most obstetricians who practiced in the 1950s had experienced the "horror," as one of our interviewees expressed it, of finding an apparently normal fetal sac in material evacuated by curettage from a patient who had seemed to show all the clinical signs and symptoms of missed abortion.[6]

Under such conditions of uncertainty, the only safe option was to wait for an unequivocal sign of a failed pregnancy, such as a sustained diminution in the size of the uterus. This might take two or even three weeks, during which the woman could suffer considerable anxiety and distress, not to mention serious inconvenience if she had family or other responsibilities. Moreover, her clinician might be concerned that her symptoms were suggestive of a pathological condition for which prompt intervention was advisable. Ultrasonic confirmation that pregnancy was continuing could offer considerable reassurance to both parties.

By the end of 1963, MacVicar and Donald had ultrasonically examined sixty-five cases of doubtful pregnancy. In fifty-five of these, they identified fetal echoes within a fluid-filled uterus and diagnosed a continuing pregnancy. Fifty-four of these women went on to have a normal pregnancy or later aborted a fresh fetus. There was, in other words, only a single false positive. There were, however, three false negatives: cases in which a fetus had not been found but the woman had later exhibited unequivocal signs of continuing pregnancy. Although these cases either occurred early in the series of sixty-five cases or had presented exceptional difficulties in examination, MacVicar and Donald cautioned that, in instances of suspected missed abortion, a repeat ultrasound examination should be carried out after a lapse of fourteen days. The second scan would concentrate on the more easily visualized anterior and fundal surfaces of the uterus. If the uterus had not increased in size over that time, a diagnosis of noncontinuance of pregnancy could be arrived at with confidence.[7] Thus, at this stage in its development, diagnostic ultrasound could, in most cases, usefully confirm the existence of a continuing pregnancy, but failure to find fetal echoes did not yet sustain a confident conclusion that a pregnancy had ended. However, ultrasonic determination of the size of the uterus was certainly more precise and objective than abdominal palpation. In effect, at this time, the impact of ultrasound was to complement and refine rather than replace orthodox clinical procedures.

(((((One of the differential diagnoses that the obstetrician has to consider when presented with a case of persistent vaginal bleeding in a woman who appears to be pregnant is hydatidiform mole. This disease, in which a disorganized mass of cells forms in the uterus, is potentially serious. The mass may perforate the wall of the uterus and cause intra-abdominal hemorrhage.

Hydatidiform mole is also associated with hyperemesis, preeclampsia, and increased risk of malignancy. Early diagnosis followed by prompt clearance of the uterus by dilation and curettage (D&C) is therefore desirable. But, of course, clearance should not be resorted to until the obstetrician is absolutely sure that a viable fetus is not present.

Hydatidiform mole is characterized by vesicles in the tissue mass and by hydropic enlargement of the chorionic villi. Surmising that the presence of a considerable number of small cystic objects within the uterus should provide recognizable reflections, Donald began a systematic study of the ultrasonic characteristics of hydatidiform mole.[8] He alerted the local gynecological community to his interest, and suspected cases were referred to the Western Infirmary from units around Glasgow.[9] By the end of 1963, fifty patients had been examined.[10] In sixteen, ultrasonic examination corroborated the clinical suspicion of hydatidiform mole, a diagnosis confirmed on evacuation of the uterus. In twenty-nine cases, MacVicar or Donald was able to reassure the patient and her obstetrician that a normal pregnancy was continuing.

One such case evidently gave Donald considerable satisfaction.[11] A woman had undergone, in successive pregnancies, a stillbirth, a spontaneous abortion, and a hydatidiform mole. In her late thirties, she became pregnant again, but in the first trimester she bled persistently and was admitted to a hospital in Accra, where she was living. Her doctors informed her that she had passed a hydatidiform vesicle and that there was therefore no doubt that her pregnancy was again molar. Advised to have a uterine evacuation, she decided to return to Scotland, for the procedure to be performed in the Western Infirmary. She was admitted to Donald's wards in considerable distress, despairing over her chances of achieving motherhood. Ultrasound examination demonstrated fetal echoes. Donald treated the patient conservatively, and she eventually gave birth to a normal child.

On the other hand, in Donald's first series of fifty cases, he made the diagnosis of hydatidiform mole in error on three occasions. Fortunately, in each case, Donald offered the diagnosis only tentatively and no action was taken. Two women eventually delivered normal babies and the third aborted twin fetuses. These cases were all early in the series and show the complexity of the learning course on which Donald and his team had embarked. At the ultrasonic power levels that Donald and his colleagues normally used, if a hydatidiform mole were present, the contents of the uterus appeared to be "a confluent mass of 'dots.' "[12] But sometimes, particularly if more than one fetus was present, the appearance of a gravid uterus might be superficially similar. By chance, the team discovered that in cases of molar pregnancy, the dotted appearance became less obvious at lower levels of sensitivity. Fetal echoes, on the other hand, tended to persist. So, if intrauterine echoes were not readily suppressed by reducing the transmitter output, then the presence of a fetus rather than a mole could be assumed.[13]

With experience, operators soon learned to recognize the ultrasonic appearance of hydatidiform mole more directly. (Mistakes were still made, however, as we shall see later in this chapter.) But the rule—if intrauterine echoes disappeared when the sensitivity was reduced, while the outline of the posterior wall of the uterus could still be visualized, then a hydatidiform mole was probably present—is a good example of the informal guidelines Donald and his colleagues developed to help them interpret B-scan images. As noted above, Donald and MacVicar looked for the outline of the surfaces of the uterus as key landmarks. Early in pregnancy, the uterus clearly displays the ultrasonic characteristics of a cystic structure, since most of its increased volume is occupied by amniotic fluid. The interface between uterine wall and its fluid contents provides a strongly reflective surface. This was, in itself, a useful indicator of pregnancy. A uterus enlarged owing to causes other than pregnancy generally lacked the fluid content of the gravid uterus and so did not present such a definite echoic outline.

Early in 1963, a chance discovery was made that was to render the application of diagnostic ultrasound considerably more straightforward, for gynecological patients and obstetric patients in the first trimester. A woman in the early weeks of pregnancy had been inadvertently kept waiting much longer than usual for her scan. She had been too nervous to ask to go to the toilet and presented herself for examination with a very full bladder. On viewing the Polaroid images, the operators realized that her enlarged bladder had displaced the bowel from above the uterus and provided a clear, sonic window into the abdomen. This was a major breakthrough.

The discovery of the full-bladder technique was fortuitous. It was also embarrassing for MacVicar. In the 1950s, he and Brown had done a series of experiments in which they scanned each other's bladders in various degrees of fullness, but they had not noticed the extent to which the enlarged bladder afforded a clearer view of the underlying structures. MacVicar had also used ultrasound extensively in monitoring bladder function after pelvic surgery. He had guessed, moreover, the advantages that a large fluid-filled structure in the abdomen might provide and had even suggested to Donald that they experiment with inflating the rectum with water. "One of the things which was the most simple," MacVicar recalls, "was using the full bladder technique, really we were very stupid not to have thought of it before. You know, it's so simple . . . why we didn't think of using it to see a pregnancy behind it I don't know. It was one of those things where there is just a blank."[14]

The full-bladder technique was first reported in the medical press in late 1963.[15] It soon became standard practice for women who were waiting to be scanned to be provided with orange juice. Donald liked to scan with the bladder just at the point at which distension was becoming uncomfortable, and Fleming recalls how, after the examination, Donald delighted in saying to his patient, "And now, my dear, you can go and enjoy one of life's simple pleasures." As was later noticed, however, even the full-bladder technique was not without its limitations. A bladder that was overfull could press upon and distort an otherwise normal gestational sac, leading an unwary obstetrician to suspect a malformation.

In Donald's account of these early cases, it is clear that a complementary relationship pertained between clinical diagnosis and ultrasound scanning. Nevertheless, he and MacVicar evidently took considerable pride in those occasions when ultrasound provided crucial diagnostic information that could not have been obtained by any other form of examination. One patient was referred from another hospital because her uterus was enlarged to the size commensurate with thirty weeks' gestation, whereas the period of amenorrhea had been only sixteen weeks.[16] A clinical diagnosis of twins with polyhydramnios had been made, but radiological investigation revealed no fetal parts. An ultrasound scan showed what appeared to be a single fetus within a uterine cavity that was about the normal size for a pregnancy of sixteen to twenty weeks' duration. At the fundus, however, there was an area through which the ultrasound beam could not penetrate. A diagnosis of fibroid coexisting with a normal pregnancy was made, which was eventually confirmed on cesarean section.

Cases like this vividly exemplify that the uterus was no longer quite the mysterious object it had previously been. The ultrasound beam had allowed the medical gaze to breach the "iron curtain of the maternal abdominal wall," to use Donald's phrase. But learning to interpret what could now be seen within remained an intricate and challenging process. Donald remained cautious in his public claims regarding clinical application. In 1965, he described ultrasound as "a subject hovering between research and routine diagnostic practice," admitting, for instance, that twin pregnancies could not yet be reliably diagnosed in the first trimester—the greater number of reflective surfaces within the gestational sac leading to the danger of confusion with intrauterine pathological structures, as we have seen in his false-positive diagnoses of hydatidiform mole.[17]

Improvements in the clinical application of ultrasound scanning often derived from the learning experience provided by unusual cases. On one occasion, Donald made the "calamitous mistake" of diagnosing a hydatidiform mole when in fact the patient had a missed abortion coexisting with a large fibroid. To Donald's great embarrassment, the woman underwent unnecessary laparotomy and hysterotomy: "I was at a loss to explain our error until [on a later occasion] I came upon a large fibroid which had undergone acute myxomatous degeneration in a non-pregnant woman whose ultrasonogram was very similar to that of hydatidiform mole."[18] Donald thus learned to first exclude the possibility of fibroid degeneration before confidently diagnosing hydatidiform mole.

(((((During the subsequent decade, the unveiling of the contents of the gravid uterus gathered pace and intensity. In the early 1960s, Donald initiated several different programs of ultrasonic research into fetal structure. As leader of the research team, he was greatly assisted by his position as professorial head of a large department of obstetrics and gynecology, providing easy access to large numbers of patients—the Western Infirmary and the Royal Maternity Hospital were major teaching hospitals and served as regional centers for western and central Scotland. He could readily draw on the services of younger colleagues who were eager to advance their careers by developing research interests. The next obstetrician-gynecologist to join his team was Dr. James Willocks, senior registrar at Rottenrow.

Whereas the work that Donald undertook with MacVicar concentrated mainly on the first trimester, the investigations he did in collaboration with Willocks were focused on the last few weeks of pregnancy. This difference reflected the geographic separation of Donald's gynecological wards, in the Western Infirmary, from his Obstetric Unit, in the Royal Maternity Hospital. In 1959, Donald and Brown, noting that clear echoes could be obtained from the fetal skull, had decided to try to develop an ultrasonic method of measuring the head. To do this, they reverted to an A-scan technique, since it was the magnitude of the echoes and the distance between them that were the key variables, rather than their positions relative to other reflective surfaces. Moreover, the hand-held probe of a flaw detector was easier to locate precisely against the relevant area of the maternal abdominal wall.

The technique relied on the observation that the fetal skull, roughly ovoid in shape, has only two sets of approximately parallel surfaces. The brow, in the front of the skull, and the occipital region, at the back, comprise one set; the other is formed by the two parietal eminences, which are the rounded protuberances on either side of the head, above the ears. The echoes received from a reflecting surface are strongest when the ultrasound beam is perpendicular to that surface. Thus maximal echoes will be obtained from the two sides of the head simultaneously only when the beam meets the skull at right angles on both sides. In other words, a pair of strong signals will be received when the beam traverses the skull through one of the sets of parallel surfaces, along either the occipitofrontal diameter or the biparietal diameter, as they are called. On any other traverse through the skull, either one echo will be noticeably weaker than the other or both echoes will be less than optimal, owing to the beam meeting one or both surfaces at an angle other than 90 degrees.

Brown and Donald were interested in measuring the biparietal diameter (BPD). During the later stages of pregnancy, the fetal head generally lies with the BPD roughly at right angles to the maternal abdominal wall and thus conveniently aligned to be traversed with the beam of a transabdominal scanner. Moreover, the parietal eminences can usually be located by palpation, thus identifying the BPD before scanning takes place. The greater length of the occipitofrontal diameter also helps obviate any danger of confusion between the two.

In endeavoring to measure the fetal skull, Donald was addressing a long-standing problem. The BPD is the dimension of the skull that, during labor, must pass through the narrowest part of the pelvic inlet. Its size is thus a crucial consideration in cases where disproportion between fetal head and maternal pelvis is suspected. Obstetricians had been trying to find a reliable method of estimating the size of the pelvic inlet since the late eighteenth century, and of the fetal head since the late nineteenth.[19] In the first half of the twentieth century, a sustained attempt had been made to predict disproportion by means of X-ray imaging. Chassar Moir was an enthusiast. There was, however, no consensus among obstetricians as to the value of his technique or any other that employed X-rays.[20] Donald was particularly dubious of X-ray cephalometry, maintaining that it was difficult to measure accurately the distance of the fetal head from the X-ray tube and that, owing to the geometry of shadow images, small errors were greatly magnified on the photographic plate.[21] Radiological cephalometry also entailed repeated measurements and, as noted in earlier chapters, by the mid-1950s, obstetricians' attitudes toward ionizing radiation were becoming increasingly cautious. There was evidently a need for a safer and more accurate method of estimating the size of the fetal head. Furthermore, disproportion was a particular problem in Glasgow, because of the number of women whose pelvis had been distorted by childhood rickets.

To obtain an estimate of the BPD by ultrasound, it was necessary to measure the time interval between the echoes obtained from the near and far sides of the skull. At first, Donald and Brown took measurements from a still photograph of the A-scope display. However, the photographic process introduced several sources of possible error, and the time-bases on industrial flaw detectors proved insufficiently accurate for this application. The method was also time-consuming. Brown managed to speed up the process and improve its accuracy by devising a system whereby the camera shutter was triggered automatically whenever two echoes were received that exceeded a preset threshold. But he was aware that further refinement of the measurement of the BPD was possible and desirable.

With Brown preoccupied with his responsibilities at Smiths, Donald sought some further technical input. Tom Duggan was a physicist and engineer who had been employed by Donald, with a grant from the Scottish Hospitals Endowment Research Trust, to assist with his work on neonatal respiratory distress. Despite SHERT making it an explicit condition of this funding that no monies were to be diverted to ultrasound research, Donald recruited Duggan to assist with fetal cephalometry. By this time, James Willocks had taken over the bulk of the clinical investigations in this area and was examining considerable numbers of patients in the Royal Maternity Hospital, using a Mk IV flaw detector. Working in cooperation with Willocks, Duggan set out to improve the measurement technique. Employed under university conditions, and based in the Department of Clinical Physics, Duggan was favorably placed to do the development work.

> I remember talking with Tom Brown discussing how we might do it. He knew perfectly well how to do it. He didn't have the [resources] for Smiths to have done a development on it [and] he would have had to raise money somehow and

there wasn't any. If I did it, it wouldn't cost anything except effort and what we could scrape off the grant so I discussed the idea with him and we then decided on some fantastic electronics.[22]

Duggan's solution to the problem of fetal cephalometry was an electronic caliper, designed around two Phantastron pulse generators.[23] The Phantastron was a sophisticated piece of circuitry originally devised, during the Second World War, for use in radar.[24]

Duggan's cephalometer enabled the operator to superimpose two bright dots on an A-scan display, and then position them to accurately mark the echoes obtained from the parietal eminences. One control moved the pair of dots along the trace while another altered their distance apart. The method required considerable dexterity on Willocks's part, but the cephalometer allowed precise measurement of the time taken for the beam to travel between the two marked points. By assuming a value for the speed of sound through the fetal head, the distance between the eminences could be calculated. The cephalometer also had the advantage of providing the operator with a measurement in millimeters that could be read, conveniently and directly, from a visual display. As a physicist, Duggan would have preferred to express the results in units of time, but he could not convince his medical colleagues to allow him to do so. Donald "wouldn't take it. I tried to persuade him at that time . . . I've got a note from him saying 'I don't understand microseconds, tell me centimetres.'"[25] Donald knew that if the technique were to be generally accepted, the length of the BPD would have to be expressed in terms that clinicians could readily understand and apply.

Converting microseconds into units of length was not a straightforward task. Initially, Willocks and Duggan accepted the received wisdom that the speed of sound in tissue was roughly the same as that in water at 20°C. However, when they compared ultrasonic measurements of fetal head size with measurements taken by mechanical caliper shortly after birth, they found that the ultrasonic method was consistently underestimating the length of the BPD. On reviewing the literature, they noted that whereas the speed of sound in water at 20°C had been accurately measured at 1,480 m s^{-1}, both Ludwig and Edler had estimated the speed in brain tissue to be 1,515 m s^{-1}. Moreover, Theismann and Pfander in 1949, and Fry and Dunn in 1962, had arrived at the significantly higher figure of 3,360 m s^{-1} for the speed in bone.[26] Duggan cal-

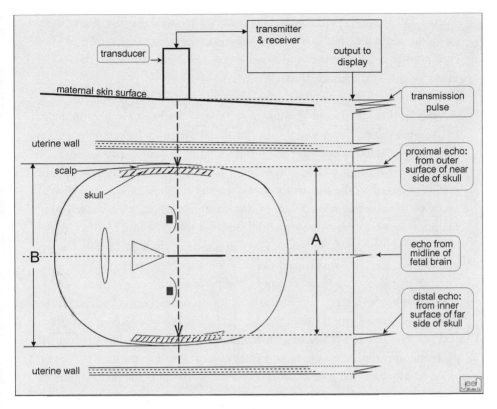

Figure 8.1. Diagram showing measurement of the biparietal diameter (BPD). A, intrauterine BPD—measured by ultrasound; B, postnatal BPD—measured by mechanical caliper. *Drawn by jeef*

culated that, assuming normal thicknesses of skull, the average speed of sound through the entire width of the head would be approximately 1,600 m s^{-1}.[27]

A second important source of error was shortly identified. The most strongly reflective surfaces in the head are the interfaces between soft tissue and bone. Thus, when the ultrasonic cephalometer was applied to the maternal abdominal wall above the fetal head (fig. 8.1), the strongest echoes were received from the outer surface of the skull bone nearest the probe and the inner surface of the skull bone farthest from the probe. But this meant that the ultrasonic cephalometer was not measuring the total distance between one side of the head and the other. The ultrasonic measurement was short, by the thickness of the scalp at the near side of the head and the thickness of the skull and scalp at the far side. Initially, Willocks and Duggan had assumed that this discrepancy would be negligible, but further investigations suggested that skull and scalp each constituted between 1 and 2 percent of the BPD. Allowance had to be made for this in the final estimate.

Willocks and Duggan also gauged the accuracy of their intrauterine measurements of the fetal head by comparing them with ultrasonic measurements of the same subject taken shortly after birth. (Babies born by cesarean section were the best subjects because their heads were not molded by passage through the birth canal.) Again they discovered a systematic difference between the results obtained by the two methods. When an ultrasonic probe is applied directly to the side of a neonate's head, the strongest echoes are obtained from the interface of the transducer and the skin and from the inner surface of the skull on the far side of the head. (The magnitude of the signal created as the pulses leave the transducer makes echoes from the near surface of the skull difficult to recognize.) In other words, the postnatal ultrasonic measurement is longer than the intrauterine equivalent by a single thickness of scalp. On the other hand, a mechanical caliper measures the entire distance from outside of scalp on one side to outside of scalp on the other and is thus longer than the postnatal ultrasonic measure by one thickness of skull and scalp.

Gradually, the two investigators learned how to allow for these factors. A formula was arrived at, $d = 0.08t_{of}$, by which the actual biparietal diameter (d) could be calculated, in centimeters, from the time measurement (t_{of}= time of flight in microseconds) with reasonable accuracy and consistency.[28] Duggan and Willocks eventually came to regard a difference between calculated and observed BPD of more than 2 mm as a bad result.[29] The cephalometry research was published first in Willocks's MD thesis in 1963 and then in a paper jointly authored by Willocks, Donald, and Duggan in the *Journal of Obstetrics and Gynaecology of the British Commonwealth*, in the following year.[30]

An unexpected outcome of the careful work done by Willocks on measuring fetal and neonatal skulls was the discovery that the skull might shrink somewhat in the first few days of life. This had not been known or suspected beforehand and was another reason that Willocks's initial estimates of the BPD late in pregnancy had consistently failed to correspond exactly with the measurements taken by mechanical caliper shortly after birth. The sequence of events by which this discovery was made is interesting in that it reveals the investigators' growing confidence in their technique. At first, an apparent discrepancy between calculated and observed BPD had been ascribed to shortcomings in the method of measurement. Later, the measurement was trusted and the discrepancy accepted as the discovery of a real physiological change in the object under study.

Donald and Willocks were aware that knowing the precise size of the fetal head had another clinical application, potentially even more important than the prediction of disproportion. They postulated that the length of the BPD correlated closely with the weight of the fetus. Thus, if the BPD could be accurately gauged, comparison of measurements taken over a period of time, say from twenty weeks' gestation onward, could give an indication of how well the fetus was growing. From his own investigations, Willocks estimated the normal rate of increase of the BPD to be 0.23 mm per day. He suggested that, if the fetus was not maintaining this rate of increase, this might be taken as an indication that its overall growth was faltering. Confident that it was safe to scan the fetal head repeatedly, Willocks constructed standardized growth curves for the BPD against which the progress of individual fetuses could be compared.

Willocks's method of cephalometry provided obstetricians with their first reliable indicator of fetal growth. This was an important aid to the effective management of pregnancy if the mother was suffering from a disorder, such as hypertension or nephritis, that was associated with the possibility of placental degeneration. In these conditions, the ability of the placenta to nourish the growing fetus might be compromised, possibly endangering its life. Thus, if fetal growth began to slow in the third trimester, this was an indication to the clinician that it was time to consider whether it was in the best interests of the fetus to be delivered electively. Similar considerations applied to other conditions, such as diabetes and severe antepartum hemorrhage. Ultrasound cephalometry could also help determine the age of the fetus when there was uncertainty about the duration of the pregnancy—for instance, if the mother was unsure of her dates. Mrs. M, for instance, was admitted to the hospital with severe preeclampsia when she was supposedly only five months pregnant. However, the uterus was enlarged to a size consistent with thirty-six weeks' gestation, and Willocks's estimate of the BPD was 9.3 cm, suggesting fetal maturity. Her condition deteriorated and labor was accordingly induced. She was safely delivered of a live child, weighing 6 pounds 9 ounces (3.0 kg).[31]

Willocks documented several instances in which cephalometry had appreciably assisted in the clinical management of problematic cases. Mrs. C, thirty-three years old, was pregnant for the tenth time but had only one living child, from her first pregnancy. All her subsequent pregnancies had ended in miscarriages between the sixteenth and twenty-eighth weeks. Her cervix was sutured at twelve weeks, but she had to be admitted to the Maternity Hospital at twenty-six weeks because of bleeding and abdominal pain. She had several episodes of light bleeding while in the hospital, but these settled and she was allowed to go home at thirty-one weeks. Ten days later, while attending an outpatient clinic, she suffered a more serious hemorrhage and was readmitted. Later that day, the fetal heartbeat seemed to slow, and it was decided to deliver the baby by cesarean section. The obstetricians had the confidence to proceed promptly to delivery, even though the mother was not in immediate danger, because the cephalometric data suggested that the fetus, though premature, was sufficiently developed to have a good chance of survival. As Willocks had predicted, the birth weight was about 4 pounds (1.8 kg). Both mother and baby did well.[32]

It soon became the practice in the Maternity Hospital to measure the fetal head after every episode of antepartum bleeding, to inform the decision whether or not to proceed to elective delivery. But Willocks's work was important not just for its direct clinical applicability. Enhanced ability to follow intrauterine growth changed the scientific understanding of the fetus. For instance, in the early 1960s, there was a growing conviction among obstetricians that many babies who were classified as "premature by weight" were, in fact, of mature gestational age. In 1962, Butler had estimated that as many as one-third of all "premature" neonates, weighing 2.5 kg or less at birth, were of thirty-nine weeks or more gestation.[33] These babies had a mortality rate more than twice the average. Their low weight was caused, it came to be understood, by placental insufficiency and undernourishment. Willocks's serial measurements of head size revealed, more directly than had previously been possible, the dynamics of this process. He was able to chart fetal growth slowing down and eventually stopping. In some cases, he recorded actual shrinkage of the head as the fetus literally starved in utero. Willocks's technique vividly revealed the continuity between events happening in the uterus before birth and the live, undernourished neonate, or indeed the stillborn baby—the ultimate consequence of placental insufficiency.

Initially, Willocks had been extremely puzzled by these cases in which the skull appeared to diminish, and they had again caused him to doubt the accuracy of his new technique. It seemed counterintuitive that the head of a living fetus could shrink. Gradually, however, with increased confidence in the electronic cephalometer, the interpretation of shrinkage as revealing placental insufficiency was arrived at. Again, a move was made from doubting the authority of the investigative technique toward a revised understanding of the object under study.

(((((In the early 1960s, Donald's success with ultrasonic diagnosis began to attract national and international attention. In 1961, he was invited to give the Charles J. Barone Lecture at the University of Pittsburgh. In 1963, he returned to the United States to present his work at a symposium organized in his honor by the SmithKline Corporation. On this occasion, he seems to have talked for several hours, showing hundreds of slides and a cine film, as well as conducting an extensive question-and-answer session.[34]

Donald's public presentations were not always so successful. In 1961, Donald, Brown, MacVicar, and Willocks were all invited to address the Royal Society of Medicine.[35] They prepared a film to complement their presentations. The meeting took place in November, shortly after Donald's first major heart operation. Although still an in-patient in the Western Infirmary, Donald was, characteristically, determined to attend the meeting. He discharged himself from the hospital and traveled, "blue and breathless," to London. Speaking after Brown, Donald got through less than half of his paper, when his breathing became so distressed that he had to stop. There was, Willocks recalled, "every sign of a medical crisis."[36] He and MacVicar tried valiantly to fill in the missing sections of their chief's presentation, as well as giving their own papers. Their difficulties were confounded when the film broke into several pieces and only a part of it could be shown. It is perhaps understandable that the reception accorded to the Glasgow presentations on this occasion was decidedly muted.[37] The discussion that followed, as recorded in the *Proceedings*, centered around another paper, on the location of the placenta with radioisotopes, given by a speaker from the University of Liverpool.[38]

In continuing to use the flaw detector for his work in the Maternity Hospital and claiming that A-scan had advantages in cephalometric applications, Willocks was making a virtue out of a necessity. At this time, Donald's team had only one compound B-scan machine (the Automatic Scanner) and it was housed in the Western Infirmary. But when the Queen Mother's Hospital opened in 1964, Donald's obstetric unit was transferred to the new facility, with Willocks appointed as a consultant. The Queen Mother's had a dedicated Ultrasound Department, equipped with a Diasonograph. Compound B-scan techniques could now be applied to cephalometry. Stuart Campbell, a Hall Research Fellow, joined Donald's team and took over most of the cephalometric research.

Initially, Campbell used two machines side by side, the Diasonograph and a Mk VII flaw detector, to which Duggan's cephalometer was attached. This arrangement was cumbersome, and he soon recognized the advantage in combining the two pieces of apparatus. Fleming modified the Diasonograph to accommodate the cephalometric circuitry. The electronic cursors could now be placed on the screen with the Diasonograph in A-scan mode, and the display rapidly switched between A-scan and B-scan modes.

With the modified Diasonograph, Campbell devised an improved method of cephalometry that involved the identification, in B-scan, of the echoes from the midline of the fetal brain. This allowed the biparietal diameter to be located very precisely. Once the echoes from the midline had been found, the Diasonograph was switched to A-scan. The electronic cursors were then put in place, one at either side of the skull, and a measurement was taken. Campbell's technique required considerable skill, as the cursors had to be placed very precisely and the switch between scanning modes made expeditiously. The operator had to be confident that the fetus had not moved in the meantime. But the combined use of the two modes of ultrasound allowed considerably more precise measurement of the BPD, especially earlier in pregnancy. This innovation was of considerable assistance in the monitoring of fetal growth, since it was found that the earlier a series of readings could be started, the more useful the results would be.[39] Following Willocks's and Campbell's publications, other obstetrics centers began to attempt ultrasonic cephalometry, but the combination of the imaging ability of the Diasonograph with the precision of the Duggan cephalometer, not to mention Campbell's dexterity in the use of the equipment and his ability to read ultrasonograms confidently, gave Campbell a clear technical advantage over his rivals. By 1967, Campbell could accurately chart the growth of the fetal head from the fourteenth week onward. His 1968 paper was a landmark in the acceptance of ultrasonic cephalometry as a standard procedure for the assessment of fetal growth and maturity.[40]

As Donald and his colleagues developed more finesse in ultrasonic diagnosis, they often had to revisit earlier certainties. One such revision was particularly ironic. As described in chapters 4 and 5, Donald's enthusiasm for ultrasound diagnosis was initially stimulated by the ease with which he could distinguish an ovarian cyst from a uterine fibroid, at first in vitro and later in vivo. However, Donald came to realize that in obstetric cases, the distinction might not be quite so straightforward. This was because, during pregnancy, the vascularity of the uterine wall increases. A greater supply of blood could change the ultrasonic characteristics of a uterine fibroid. "Cysts because of their watery content are normally more transonic than fibroids," he noted, "but the latter if scanned at normal incidence can in pregnancy look remarkably like cysts on ultrasonography." Even as late as 1965, Donald admitted to occasionally being mistaken in this application of the new modality.[41]

Looking back on the pioneering work undertaken by the Glasgow team, Willocks remarked that one of the reasons that diagnostic ultrasound developed so rapidly in his specialty was that obstetricians were trained to use the information gained by palpation of the abdomen to form a mental image of the layout of the fetus in the uterus.[42] This spatial awareness helped them interpret ultrasonic visualizations of the abdominal cavity. Willocks's observation is undoubtedly valid. But, on occasion, even an experienced obstetrician could be confused as to what he was looking at, with potentially devastating consequences. On one occasion, it was not noticed that an apparently normal image of a gestational sac had been taken on a plane some distance to the left of the midline.[43] A diagnosis of normal pregnancy was made. In fact, the pregnancy was tubal. The patient subsequently died of a massive hemorrhage. Donald was chastened by this tragedy and redoubled his efforts to achieve a reliable discrimination between intrauterine and extrauterine pregnancy.[44]

By exploiting the greater transonic clarity afforded by the full-bladder method, Donald and his colleagues were able to reduce still further the gestational age at which fetal echoes could be identified. Late in 1965, they reported the successful location of a fetus only thirty-five days after the presumed date of conception.[45] Donald presented this as an aid to the management of recurrent abortion, as precautionary measures could be instigated as early as possible. By 1967, twins could be reliably diagnosed at eight weeks' gestation, the ultrasonic appearance resembling, as Donald put it, "a double-yolked egg."[46] Again there was a danger of mistakes. Sometimes, a double-yolked appearance, strongly suggestive of twins, could be obtained as an artifact. By refraction, a second identical, but illusory, fetal sac might appear. The team had to guard against the danger of diagnosing twins when, in fact, only a singleton was present. A very high degree of similarity between the paired "yolks" alerted the operator to the possibility of a duplication artifact. This and other artifacts could usually be eliminated by taking multiple scans along different planes and at varying levels of sensitivity.

By 1967, the resolution of scanning had improved to the extent that even an unenlarged and empty uterus could be visualized, if it lay behind the bladder. This was valuable in ascertaining whether the products of conception had been retained after spontaneous abortion. With his intense pronatalist views, Donald had a strong dislike of unnecessary uterine evacuation, which, he thought, risked adversely affecting the woman's fertility. He compared the routine use of D&C after spontaneous abortion to "ritual cleansing by the high priest in the river Jordan."[47] Ultrasonic examination of the uterus allowed curettage to be targeted toward only those cases in which products of conception were indeed retained. Ability to identify the uterus, even when empty, also aided the recognition of tubal pregnancy.

As described in earlier chapters, Douglass Howry, based in Colorado, was an important pioneer of ultrasonic imaging. His technique had involved the use of water coupling, but, on seeing Brown's achievement with contact scanning, the Denver group had abandoned their water baths. Howry left Colorado in 1962, and the leadership of the ultrasound group was taken over by Joseph Holmes. Relationships between Glasgow and Denver remained cordial, Holmes and Donald becoming good friends. The two teams kept each other informed of developments, and Holmes's team was the first outside Scotland to take up the technique of fetal cephalometry developed by Willocks and Duggan.[48]

(((((A major focus of obstetrics research in the 1950s and 1960s was localization of the placenta. This interest was largely stimulated by the serious problem posed by placenta previa. In this condition, the placenta lies near or may overlap the uterine opening of the cervix. Bleeding may result. Moreover, as birth approaches and the lower uterine segment stretches to allow the fetal head to engage in the pelvic brim, the placenta may become detached, causing hemorrhage that may be serious enough to be life-threatening to both mother and baby. If a woman suffered vaginal bleeding after the first trimester, her medical attendants, without knowing the location of the placenta, could not exclude the possibility of placenta previa. Given the potential gravity of the condition, they would have to proceed very cautiously. It was standard practice, in the Queen Mother's Hospital as in many other centers, for the patient to be admitted to the hospital and kept there, under surveillance, until her pregnancy was in its thirty-eighth week. These elaborate precautions were extremely inconvenient for the woman, who might have other children at home. Beds and other resources were tied up for long periods, often unnecessarily. In the early 1960s, it was common for a maternity hospital to devote an entire ward to accommodating women who might or might not be at risk from placenta previa.

At the thirty-eighth week, when the fetus was deemed viable, a vaginal examination would be undertaken, with the patient under full anesthetic and a surgical team standing by. If the examination established the absence of placenta previa, the woman would be allowed to go home to await the onset of labor. If placenta previa were confirmed, she would have to remain in the hospital to await delivery by cesarean section. Sometimes disturbance to the cervix in the course of the examination provoked a serious hemorrhage, in which case an emergency cesarean was carried out.

Location of the placenta by soft tissue radiography could not be relied on, even in favorable cases, before the thirty-fourth week. Research into other methods of localization—arteriography, thermography, and the use of radioactive isotopes—was underway, but all these techniques only allowed the position of the placenta to be inferred indirectly from the position of the maternal vascular bed. Accordingly, they were imprecise, as well as invasive and slow. Again, concerns about the exposure of the fetus to ionizing radiation tended to discourage the prolonged or repeated use of X-rays or radioactive isotopes.

In the Queen Mother's Hospital, in cases of suspected placenta previa, radiographic localization of the placenta was generally attempted after the thirty-fourth week. Donald was painfully aware of the limitations of this technique, but he and his colleagues initially doubted that it would be possible to visualize the placenta using ultrasound. Willocks wrote in his MD thesis that it was unrealistic to hope that ultrasonography would reveal useful information about the placenta, given that the organ was "transonic and contained no pronounced discontinuities of density." In 1965, Donald was only slightly more optimistic: "It was hoped from our work on the echoes from hydatidiform mole that a satisfactory method of locating the placenta might be developed, but we have to confess that, so far, we have been more often wrong than right. The technical possibilities are still, however, being explored."[49] But, later that year, the Denver team stole a march on its Scottish counterparts. The arrival in Glasgow of a prepublication draft entitled "Ultrasonic Placentography" caused consternation.[50] Holmes and his colleagues claimed that the key to their success had been the incorporation into their apparatus of an extremely sensitive amplifier. But Donald quickly realized that the amplifiers he had been using were, in fact, already sufficiently sensitive. On the wall of a corridor outside his Ultrasound Department in the Queen Mother's Hospital, Donald had set up a display of ultrasonograms. Fraser recalls that when he visited Donald late in 1965, the professor left his desk and took him into the corridor. Walking along the line of images, Donald repeatedly pointed with his finger and exclaimed, "There's the placenta! And there! And there!" Now that he knew what to look for, Donald realized that the Glasgow team had been visualizing the placenta for some time. They had not been recognizing what they saw. Developing the educated eye that could interpret ultrasound images was indeed a long and arduous process.[51]

Donald began investigating the potential of ultrasonic placentography almost immediately, enlisting the assistance of another of his junior colleagues, Usama Abdulla. Donald had met Abdulla while on a lecture trip to Iraq in 1964 and had invited him to come to Scotland to learn ultrasound. Abdulla arrived in Glasgow in July 1965 and, by the end of the year, was working on the ultrasonic identification of the placenta.

In 1967, Angus Hall, with John Fleming, devised a modification of the Diasonograph to enhance its utility in this application. The Denver group had been able to identify the placenta only as a space-occupying transonic mass—a black shape on an ultrasonogram—and the earliest Glasgow localizations also took this form. But with the team's experience of the characterization of hydatidiform mole and Hall's modifications to the Diasonograph, which allowed finer adjustment of the level of amplification and improved the swept-gain facility, more detailed visualizations of the placenta were soon achieved. At high sensitivity, the image of the placenta developed a speckled appearance and its thickness could be determined. Most usefully, the fetal surface of the placenta could be visualized as a prominent white line.

Although Donald and Abdulla could, in most cases, confidently predict the placental site, checking the accuracy of these predictions was not straightforward. The position of the placenta could be verified with certainty only by direct observation during cesarean section or, in cases of vaginal delivery, by digital exploration of the uterus postpartum. Donald decided that it was not justifiable to invade the uterus for research purposes, in cases in which manual removal of the placenta was not clinically indicated. Thus, of their major series of 613 cases, the precise position of the placenta was established in only 151. Nevertheless, by mid-1968, Donald and Abdulla were able to publish their results.[52]

Of the 151 cases included in the study, the placental position had been accurately predicted ultrasonically, antepartum, in 142. There were seven undoubted errors and two dubious cases. The comparison with the principal alternative method, however, was telling. In 80 of the 151 patients, placental localization had also been attempted by radiography. Of these cases, thirteen placentas were located wrongly by X-ray but correctly by ultrasound, one was located wrongly by both, and only one was located wrongly by ultrasound but correctly by radiography. The crucial test of the method, however, was the accuracy of its diagnosis of placenta previa. In the series of 151 placental localizations, there were 30 cases in which placenta previa was confirmed clinically. Of these, in 2 cases the diagnosis was missed by ultrasound, and in another 2 cases the ultrasonograms were deemed inconclusive. In other words, 26 of the 30 cases of placenta previa were correctly identified by ultrasound. By contrast, soft tissue radiography of 15 of the patients with clinical indications gave false negatives in 4 cases.

By the time Donald and Abdulla's paper appeared, the technique had already begun to transform the management of placenta previa in the Queen Mother's Hospital. In the absence of other adverse indications, Donald was now prepared to send women home a week after bleeding had stopped, if he was reasonably satisfied that the placenta was wholly in the upper uterine segment. Vaginal examination under anesthesia, a stressful ordeal for both patient and obstetrician, was less frequently resorted to, since the procedure usually added little to the understanding of the position of the placenta that had been obtained by ultrasound.

Placental localization was to prove one of the most significant applications of obstetric ultrasound. Margaret McNay, later a consultant in ultrasound at the Queen Mother's, recalled the change that placentography made to her practice as a young obstetrician, when it was adopted in Glasgow's Royal Maternity Hospital.

> That was probably, although I was very sceptical about it at first, . . . one of the first steps forward and one of the landmarks in the early use of ultrasound. It was certainly my experience in the early 1970s at Rottenrow, when a patient came in with an antepartum haemorrhage, you didn't know whether it was from a low lying placenta. There was no good way of finding out for certain and she was literally kept in hospital until she was examined under anaesthesia at 38 weeks . . .

> The idea of somebody coming in at 28/30 weeks and having to remain for several weeks was, from a social point of view and using up a bed, from lots of viewpoints, just horrendous and the idea that you could have a modality that let you decide it was safe to let her home was really a great step forward . . . the recognition of placenta praevia, or of the absence of placenta praevia, was a major step forward.[53]

Ultrasonic placentography also made amniocentesis, the sampling of the amniotic fluid with a hollow needle, considerably less fraught, since it was now easier to avoid puncturing the placenta.

Unlike earlier workers, Donald and Abdulla were able to locate the placenta even if it lay on the posterior wall of the uterus. Their technique also allowed its macroscopic texture to be characterized, to some extent. For instance, they noticed that, in cases of severe hemolytic disease caused by rhesus immunization, the placenta was bigger, thicker, and less transonic than normal.

(((((Around this time, Donald also enthusiastically adopted another new technique, that of Doppler ultrasound. Use of the Doppler effect to detect blood flow in the fetus was first described in 1964.[54] With his usual technological enthusiasm, Donald quickly overcame some initial misgivings.

> It is possible to pick up the foetal heart very clearly long before quickening would occur and the fact that pregnancy is alive and continuing can be quickly determined in cases of doubt . . . The signals are presented on either a loudspeaker or through stethoscope earpieces. The patients always appreciate hearing the reassuring noise of their fetal circulation and learning that all is well.[55]

Donald did not, however, agree with his American counterparts that Doppler ultrasound could be reliably used to locate the placenta. He was satisfied with nothing less than the "display of the placenta in a pictorial sense"—in other words, a two-dimensional location and characterization such as could be achieved with good pulse-echo technique.

If an abdominal transducer was used, the Doppler method of detecting the fetal heartbeat was reliable after the twelfth week. Good results could be obtained earlier using a vaginal probe, but clinicians were understandably reluctant to impose vaginal examinations on patients with active bleeding or imminent threat of abortion. In 1965, another technique for ascertaining the presence of a living fetus became available. Siemens, a German manufacturer, marketed the Vidoson, a real-time pulse-echo scanner.[56] In skilled hands, the Vidoson allowed fetal movements to be detected around the tenth week, but the Glasgow team was not initially enthusiastic about this technology. For reasons we explore in chapter 9, they preferred to continue to rely on static B-scanning, complemented by Doppler.

In the early 1970s, together with two colleagues from the Western Infirmary's Department of Radiology, Patricia Morley and Ellis Barnett, Donald employed the Diasonograph in a detailed investigation of the complications of early pregnancy.[57] It was the success of this work that laid the foundation for the "simple and practical" fourfold classification of early pregnancy failure that was widely adopted in the late 1970s.[58] The categories were: blighted ovum (there is a gestational sac, but no fetus within it), missed abortion (a fetus is present, but is presumed to be dead), live abortion (the fetus is presumed to have been alive shortly before spontaneous abortion), and hydatidiform mole. The ability to classify noncontinuing early pregnancies systematically in this way exemplifies the extent to which ultrasound was revolutionizing the understanding of the fetus and its misfortunes. Nevertheless, as far as clinical decision making was concerned, Donald and his colleagues continued to stress the need for careful serial examinations of each patient with a problematic pregnancy. Under most circumstances, even after the introduction of Doppler, a series of observations spread over two or three weeks might be needed for a full understanding of the case to emerge.

By the time of the collaboration with Morley and Barnett, Donald and his colleagues had amassed several years of experience in using ultrasound to observe the characteristics and changing appearances of normal pregnancies during each stage of development. Despite being technologically mediated, their approach to the determination of gestational age and recognition of continuing pregnancy was essentially descriptive and subjective. By careful observation, Donald and his colleagues had developed a natural history of the fetus. Gestational age, for example, was estimated by using a number of clinical rules, based on the size and appearance of the gestational sac and the presence or absence of fetal echoes within it.[59] For instance, at five weeks of amenorrhea, the gestational sac should begin to be discernible in an enlarged uterus. At six weeks, the sac should have doubled in size, and at seven weeks, redoubled. At eight weeks, it should occupy half the uterine cavity, and fetal echoes should become visible. At nine weeks, the sac should occupy two-thirds of the cavity. At ten weeks, the cavity should be completely filled. In the eleventh and twelfth weeks, the intrauterine echoes had a distinctive "confused" appearance, but by the thirteenth or fourteenth week, it was normally possible to identify and measure the fetal head. From this time onward, the quantitative technique of biparietal cephalometry was the method of choice for determining the duration of the pregnancy. However, Donald and Willocks conceded that although cephalometry allowed accurate measurement of relative fetal growth, it was less precise in the absolute determination of gestational age.

Attempts were made, notably by Louis Hellman in New York, to base the estimation of gestational age, up to the twentieth week, on measurement of the relative sizes of the uterus and the gestational sac.[60] But the limits of accuracy of this method were admitted to be only "less than plus or minus two weeks." Donald remained content with his more subjective assessments.

By the early 1970s, Donald's work on diagnostic ultrasound was sufficiently well known and respected for him to secure a generous Programme Grant from the Medical Research Council.[61] He used the funds to employ two technicians, Jonathan Powell and Thomas Anderson, who would work with Fleming and Hall, and to support a "research registrar," Hugh Peter Robinson. As part of the requirements for the Membership qualification of the Royal College of Obstetricians and Gynaecologists, Robinson had undertaken an assessment of the clinical value of ultrasonic examination of patients with a history of bleeding in the first trimester. He gained his Membership in 1971 and began working with Donald in February of the same year. When Robinson arrived to take up his post in the Queen Mother's Hospital, Donald's only instruction to him was, "Oh, there you are, you've now got a job going. Do some research." Robinson was, in other words, given a free hand, the only effective constraint being Donald's expectation that his investigations should be relevant to the problems of early pregnancy.[62]

Shortly after Robinson took up his post, Nuclear Enterprises delivered to the Queen Mother's Hospital an improved version of the Diasonograph, the NE4102 (see fig. 7.3D), which Robinson adopted as his principal research tool. He was immediately aware that the new equipment would enable him to "see things that we couldn't see before."[63] He set out simply to characterize the early fetus more accurately than had previously been possible.

Novel features of the NE4102 were that it had a built-in electronic caliper, similar to Duggan's cephalometer described above, and that any two of its three modes of operation could be simultaneously displayed on its pair of oscilloscope screens. The operator could choose between A-scan, compound B-scan, and time-position mode, otherwise known as M-mode. In M-mode, the horizontal time-base trace is brightness-modulated and is moved down the screen at a speed of a few centimeters per second. Those echoes that originate from stationary structures appear as straight, vertical lines, whereas those that originate from rhythmically moving surfaces appear as regular waveforms. Irregular movements give disordered traces. M-mode was first used by Edler and Hertz in Lund, in 1954, as a technique for recording the motion of the valves of the adult heart. By the late 1960s, M-mode was widely employed in cardiology. In 1968, Hans Holms, in Copenhagen, demonstrated that fetal cardiac movements could be detected from the tenth week onward by this method.[64] Alfred Kratochwil undertook similar work in Vienna. However, both the Danish and the Austrian procedures were cumbersome and time-consuming, because the operator had to search a large part of the lower abdomen more or less blindly for possible fetal echoes. It was difficult, under these circumstances, to have confidence in a negative finding, and there was a danger of confusion with pulsations from the maternal circulation.

Using the NE4102, Robinson devised a faster and more accurate method of detecting the fetal heartbeat. The uterus was scanned in B-scan to locate the gestational sac and the fetus within it. Electronic cursors, which appeared on the B-scan image as curved lines, were then placed precisely above and below the fetus. Robinson then shifted his attention to the second screen on which, in A-scan, the cursors appeared as bright dots. Any echoes coming from the area between these dots could be presumed to originate from fetal structures. The NE4102 had a delay facility that allowed the operator to select a region of the image for more detailed visualization. The area between the markers was then carefully searched until rhythmically moving echo spikes appeared on the A-scan screen. Early in pregnancy, the movements of the fetal heart walls may be less than 1 mm in magnitude. Such small displacements would have been very difficult to observe with earlier ultrasound equipment, but with the NE4102, Robinson was able to visualize these tiny oscillations clearly (fig. 8.2).

Once he was sure that he had found echoes from the fetal heart in A-scan, Robinson switched the image on the first screen from B-scan to M-mode. The oscillating echoes now appeared as regular, sinusoidal traces, revealing the motion of the fetal heart. This identification would be confirmed by noting the frequency of oscillation—the fetal heart rate is normally much faster than the maternal heart rate. With experience, Robinson was able to detect fetal heartbeats reliably from seven weeks of amenorrhea and sometimes from as

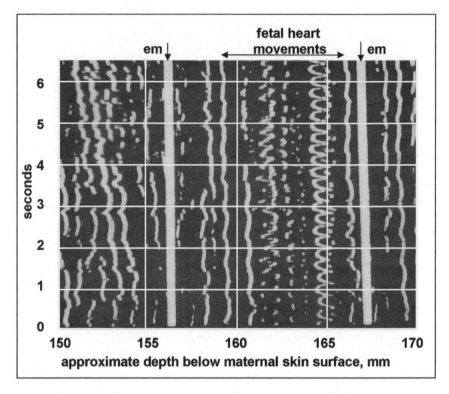

Figure 8.2. NE4102 M-mode trace, showing fetal heart valve and wall movements; gestational age is 9 weeks 4 days; heart rate is 208 beats/minute. The two thick vertical lines are electronic markers (em); these were positioned on a B-scan image and indicate the region of the fetal heart. *Adapted by John Fleming from a Polaroid recording kindly supplied by Dr. H. P. Robinson in 1975*

early as six weeks. Detection of fetal life so early with such confidence was unprecedented.

With its use of electronic markers and rapid switching between different display modes, Robinson's technique for locating the fetal heart was similar to Stuart Campbell's method of cephalometry. And, like fetal cephalometry, it required, even with the refinements of the NE4102, considerable dexterity and rapid and assured reading of ultrasound images.[65] Nevertheless, once he had perfected the procedure, Robinson was normally able to locate the heartbeat within five minutes, often less. Prolonged searches of the entirety of the lower abdomen were no longer required.

The identification of movement within the gestational sac was, of course, absolute confirmation that a living fetus was present. The woman could be immediately reassured that she was indeed pregnant. If a heartbeat was not initially detected, a meticulous search was undertaken throughout the whole volume of the gestational sac. If a heartbeat was still not found, Robinson was sufficiently confident in his method to conclude that no living fetus was present. The patient could be advised accordingly and, usually, was offered a prompt uterine evacuation.

As noted above, Robinson had undertaken an earlier investigation of the clinical value of ultrasonic examination of patients with a history of bleeding in the first trimester. Useful as he had found the procedure, he was aware that, when compared with the precise laboratory methods being introduced in other fields of medicine, the ultrasonic techniques used in early pregnancy were either subjective in nature or had less than optimal limits of accuracy. In particular, he was concerned that, often, no definitive statement could be made as to whether or not a fetus was still alive. Robinson regarded this uncertainty as unsatisfactory from both the clinician's and the patient's point of view. Once the fetal heartbeat could be reliably detected in early pregnancy, many clinical decisions could be based on a single ultrasound examination. Robinson's elegant technique represented a considerable step toward more objective, clearcut diagnoses. The serial scannings cautiously undertaken over ten days or more by MacVicar and Donald under similar clinical circumstances were, in many cases, no longer required.

In the presentation of his results, Robinson employed the fourfold classification of early pregnancy failure, as devised by Donald and Morley. His investigations indicated that live abortions were much less frequent than the other forms of failure and that their natural history was very different from that of missed abortion or blighted ovum. But, to a large extent, the classification of failed pregnancies was now a matter of academic rather than clinical importance. The only crucial issue was whether or not a heartbeat could be detected. If it could, the pregnancy was continuing; if it could not, a living fetus was not present. Robinson noted that it might sometimes be difficult to distinguish a small hydatidiform mole from a long-standing missed abortion in which the placenta had undergone hydropic degeneration. But such confusion made little difference to clinical management—the patient would be offered a uterine evacuation in either case. While still dependent on the skill of the operator, ultrasonic diagnosis was becoming more objective and quantitative, and less a form of clinical natural history. Robinson's work, like Willocks's, was a key stage in this transition.

The newfound ability to identify the fetal heartbeat removed major sources of doubt in the management of early pregnancy. Patients were less likely to be subjected to unnecessary interventions. For instance, a woman with a history of recurrent early abortion, on becoming pregnant again, would often be offered cervical suturing. Her medical attendants could now confirm that she was indeed carrying a viable fetus, before embarking on an otherwise futile procedure. If, on the other hand, a fetus had died, most women found undergoing an elective D&C less distressing than waiting an unpredictable period of time for a miscarriage to occur. The diagnosis of multiple pregnancy was also improved—the detection of two fetal heartbeats being an indubitable indication of the presence of twins.

Robinson also introduced a new quantitative method of assessing gestational age: measurement of the crown-rump length (CRL), the distance between the top of the fetus's head and the end of its spine.[66] In the development of this technique, Robinson worked in close cooperation with Fleming, who devised a method of determining errors inherent in the ultrasound images, such as those caused by the width of the ultrasound beam. CRL measurement proved a more accurate indication of fetal maturity in the early months than any other available technique. Subjective assessments of the appearance and relative size of the uterus and the gestational sac, as employed by Donald and MacVicar, were now largely superseded.

More accurate estimation of gestational age improved the detection of fetal abnormalities. In the Queen Mother's Hospital, by the mid-1970s, all obstetric patients were offered a blood test to measure levels of alpha fetoprotein (AFP) in the maternal blood. If it was high, the amniotic fluid was sampled. A substantially elevated level of AFP in the amniotic fluid resulted in a presumptive diagnosis of neural tube defect. But determination of amniotic AFP levels was useful only if maturity was known exactly, since the levels vary greatly as the fetus develops. In this respect, Robinson's correlation of CRL with gestational age complemented Donald and Abdulla's work on placental localization.[67] Knowledge of the position of the placenta rendered the diagnosis of spina bifida, for example, by amniocentesis, a less daunting undertaking.

As well as its clinical payoff, Robinson's work was of considerable scientific interest. For example, the improved sensitivity of his technique allowed, for the first time, investigation of the fetal heart rate in the early months. He determined that, between six and nine weeks' gestation, the mean rate increased from 125 to 175 beats per minute. Robinson cooperated with John Shaw-Dunn, of the Anatomy Department of Glasgow University, in a study of the developmental changes in the structure of the fetal heart associated with these alterations in heart rate.[68] Robinson also found that twin pregnancies were more common than had previously been thought, with one or both twins often dying in the early weeks.

Thus, by the mid-1970s, with the work of the team of clinicians and engineers led by Donald, the fetus had become a clinical presence in its own right, for the first time in its history. The medical gaze had breached the "iron curtain of the maternal wall": the pregnant woman was no longer the chief arbiter of the condition of her fetus, at any stage of her pregnancy. Her testimony regarding her menstrual dates was no longer crucial in estimating fetal age, her experience of quickening no longer the significant marker of fetal life. Robinson stressed the authority of an objective, quantitative, technologically mediated technique.

> The emphasis of this . . . study was to define criteria by which a non-continuing pregnancy might be diagnosed by ultrasound and for such a diagnosis to be independent of any knowledge of the clinical or menstrual history. This latter caveat was considered important if clinical action is to be taken on the basis of the ultrasound findings, for the potential unreliability of menstrual dates . . . leaves open the possibility of ascribing a "small for dates" gestation sac to a non-continuing pregnancy rather than to a less advanced but viable pregnancy.[69]

Ability to determine the age of the fetus accurately in the first trimester encouraged a more interventionist approach at the other end of pregnancy. Confident that a fetus was mature, obstetricians felt more inclined to induce labor at a time of their choosing. Elective induction, to obviate the effects of placental degeneration or forestall the hazards of postmaturity, became more common. The combination of obstetric ultrasound and new pharmacological agents with which to initiate uterine contractions ensured that birth became more actively managed and medically controlled.

By 1967, Donald had put any remaining doubts about the real and lasting value of obstetric ultrasound behind him. He was sanguine that the innovations he and his colleagues had pioneered represented the bright, confident future of their specialty.

I must say I like doing obstetrics this way and removing as much of the traditional guesswork from our subject as possible. I like to know how well a baby is growing. I like a better estimate of maturity than is often available. I like to know exactly where the placenta is in antepartum haemorrhage and in unstable lie and before employing amniocentesis. I like to be able to diagnose twins early and safely and to know if the second head is larger than the first. I like to know why an abdomen may be too large for the dates. I like to know whether bleeding in pregnancy is associated with a live or a dead baby or a hydatidiform mole and, above all, I find it fascinating to watch a well nidated foetus growing at a time when, today, so many would wish to abort it.[70]

The last sentence is doubly significant. As we shall see, passage of the Abortion Act in 1966 politicized Donald and was to awaken in him serious misgivings about the long-term impact of his ultrasound research.

CHAPTER NINE

Diffusion, Controversy, and Commodification

By the late 1960s, the diagnostic potential of ultrasound scanning was becoming widely accepted. The Queen Mother's Hospital, in Glasgow, was the nationally and internationally acknowledged center for research into obstetric ultrasound. A steady stream of visitors—clinicians, radiologists, and engineers—traveled to Glasgow to learn the new technique for which Ian Donald had become recognized as a world authority. Patients came, too, in substantial numbers as, increasingly frequently, obstetricians and gynecologists chose to refer their problematic cases to the Queen Mother's. In 1967, 562 patients were referred to Donald's Ultrasound Unit, mostly from clinics in Glasgow and the surrounding area, but also from throughout Scotland and as far south as London and Bristol.[1]

Despite this growing interest, the wider adoption of ultrasound imaging was slow, at least initially. By the time Smiths Industries ceased production in 1966, only twelve Diasonographs had been sold. Four were purchased by the U.K. Department of Health as part of an official investigation of ultrasound's clinical potential. The department lent one of these machines to University College Hospital in London and another to Bristol General Hospital, where research into several applications was already underway.[2] The senior medical physicist involved in the Bristol research was Peter Wells. As well as evaluating the Diasonograph, Wells devised a new articulated scanning arm, adapting a design he had encountered in Denver. He hoped that this would improve the versatility of the Diasonograph for hepatic and cardiac applications. Wells also looked for ways to drive the rocking motion of the transducer by an electric motor, thus minimizing "the limitations of . . . operator variability."[3]

Bristol's goal of motorizing the transducer was not pursued for long. The imposition of a high level of standardization on the scanning process was a typical aspiration for an engineer. It had been the reason why Brown had built the Automatic Scanner, but control over scanning had now effectively passed into the hands of clinicians, who wanted practical diagnostic information and were much less troubled about how precisely it was obtained. Moreover, in diagnostic use, moving the probe by hand provided the operator with valuable feedback, aiding his or her active conceptualization of the underlying structures. Thus manual control of the probe was retained.

Although the Bristol researchers were becoming important innovators in their own right, they were not independent of their Glasgow counterparts. "Of course we had lots and lots of trouble with the stability of the Diasonograph electronics," Wells recollected, "and it was only because of our firm friendship with Tom Brown, Angus Hall and John Fleming, that we were able to keep this going. I remember making pilgrimages to Glasgow and people from Glasgow came down to help us as well."[4] Ernest Kohorn, who worked with the Diasonograph given to University College Hospital, also came to Glasgow to learn how to use it.

(((((The first Scottish hospital outside the Glasgow area to acquire a scanner was Aberdeen Maternity Hospital. The initiative behind the acquisition of this equipment came largely from Ian McGillivray, Professor and Head of the Department of Obstetrics and Gynaecology. Appointed in 1964 following the retirement of Sir Dugald Baird, McGillivray was keen to make his mark by modernizing his department. In 1965, he made several trips to the Queen Mother's Hospital, then the most up-to-date obstetric facility in Scotland, in the course of which he became convinced that Aberdeen should acquire its own ultrasound service.

To assist his efforts to convince the local Hospital Board to support the purchase of a scanner, McGillivray enlisted the help of John Mallard, who had arrived in Aberdeen in 1965 to take up the university's newly established Chair of Medical Physics. Mallard had worked on radioisotope imaging at the Hammersmith Hospital and, in this capacity, been engaged by Nuclear Enterprises as a consultant. He would shortly begin work on development of another medical imaging modality, what would become known as magnetic resonance imaging.[5] Mallard knew of Donald's work on ultrasound and duly supported McGillivray's application.

Having obtained a grant from the Medical Research Council, McGillivray took delivery of an NE4101 early in 1967.[6] However, it did not come into service for several months, owing to the difficulties of accommodating such a large and heavy piece of equipment. A dedicated suite of rooms had to be specially refurbished and equipped with a reinforced floor. These modifications had to await further financing from the Maternity Hospital's Endowment Fund.

Developments in the use of the scanner in Aberdeen closely paralleled those in Glasgow. McGillivray enlisted one of his registrars, Dr. Alexander McIntosh, who was looking for a subject for his MD thesis, to build up a program of ultrasound research. Mallard set out to recruit a physicist to work closely with the clinicians. He chose Alexander Christie, a lecturer in electronics at Bath College of Science and Technology. Christie had made his first contact with ultrasound through a colleague who used industrial flaw detectors in the metallurgy laboratory. Learning of the medical applications being pursued in the Bristol hospitals, Christie got in touch with Wells.

> Peter told me about Ian Donald and all the rest of it and I thought it sounded to me just quite fascinating—just one of those things you hear and you think, "that's interesting" and so I started looking into it. Then I contacted, I think I wrote to Ian Donald about it and that is when he invited me to come up. And I didn't know anything about it. I don't think I had ever been in a hospital, well, apart from when I was born![7]

Donald's willingness to invest time and effort to nurture such a naive and casual expression of interest, from someone with a background in neither medicine nor medical physics, vividly exemplifies his determination to proselytize for his diagnostic innovation. And it is a telling indication of the immaturity of the professional structures surrounding diagnostic ultrasound that a few days of informal instruction at the Queen Mother's Hospital was deemed sufficient experience to secure Christie his post in charge of the scanner in the Aberdeen Maternity Hospital. Christie's most important advantage was that everyone else in Aberdeen knew even less that he did: "I was unique in that nobody, when I started up in Aberdeen, nobody knew what ultrasound was, they couldn't spell it . . . For that reason they just had to sort of say, 'Well, okay, you have to do it.'"[8] Just before his scanner came into service, McGillivray paid another visit to Glasgow, accompanied by "a radiologist and two physicists," one of the latter being Christie. Donald was on vacation, but Campbell and Fleming gave their guests a swift introduction to the NE4101.[9]

McIntosh and Christie initially concentrated on simply learning how to use the machine and trying to achieve coherent interpretations of the images they obtained, as Christie recalls.

We didn't know at that time what we were looking at! We looked at it and we saw something and I remember Sandy [McIntosh] said, "Oh look," he said, "There's a round thing there," he says, "I wonder if that could be a head?" And that more or less illustrates what we were trying to do at the time. We were looking at shapes and trying to relate them to some form of basic anatomy, very basic, so we were thrilled to bits if we . . . could actually see and recognise a head or something that moved . . . And then it was sort of, "Oh well, if that's how we get a head . . . where's the body?" And then we'd try to put the body and the head together.[10]

At this stage in his education as an ultrasonologist, Christie was grateful for Donald's continued help and forbearance: "I used to ring him up and I used to send him pictures and things like that and he would send me little notes saying 'Well done, I agree the diagnosis, that's definitely a head.'" It is understandable that McIntosh and Christie's confidence in their diagnostic ability grew only slowly. On starting to scan their first patient, Christie remembers, "the thought that went through my head was, 'You've bitten off more that you can chew this time, son!' I remember that very clearly, I thought, 'What am I doing?'"[11]

Eventually, McIntosh felt able to embark on an investigation of the utility of ultrasound as a means of localizing the placenta. He and Christie scanned nearly a thousand pregnant women, a hundred of whom went on to have cesarean sections, allowing the position of the placenta to be definitively ascertained. The level of agreement between the ultrasonic prediction and the confirmed location was reassuringly high. Their study was, in effect, an extended corroboration of Donald and Abdulla's earlier work. Christie and McIntosh presented their results at the first World Congress on Ultrasonic Diagnostics in Medicine, in Vienna in 1969, a meeting at which Abdulla also spoke.[12] By late 1970, the demand for scanning in Aberdeen was such that the one unit was overwhelmed, and McGillivray initiated the purchase of a second machine.

Relations between McIntosh and Christie and their colleagues in the Department of Radiology in Aberdeen were, on occasion, uneasy.[13] The obstetrician and the physicist felt that the radiologists were not prepared to exert themselves to appreciate the differences between ultrasound and the diagnostic modalities with which they were more familiar. Accustomed to transmission images, the radiologists sometimes misunderstood the planar sections produced by the ultrasound scanner. Also more used to interpreting images taken for them by radiographers, they did not readily appreciate the essentially interactive nature of the ultrasonic diagnostic process. As McIntosh recalled:

> Sandy [Christie] and I could actually cook a picture to make it look like anything we wanted to and then laugh if they got it all wrong. You could manufacture a placenta on a picture if you wanted to just by twiddling the machine a bit. A still image like that is only part of the total scan . . . with ultrasound . . . it's a dynamic process and the diagnosis is made at the time you do the scan by the person doing the scan.[14]

As we have seen, in Glasgow, Donald labored to maintain good relations with his radiologist colleagues. From the late 1950s onward, much of the radiological service for Donald's gynecological clinic in the Western Infirmary and his obstetric clinic in the Royal Maternity Hospital was undertaken by Ellis Barnett. Barnett had been a registrar at the Hammersmith Hospital and had worked closely there with Donald's former colleague and collaborator Robert Steiner.[15] Donald made sure that Barnett was kept fully up-to-date with the latest developments in diagnostic ultrasound. As Donald appreciated, it would considerably assist the general acceptance of the new technology if its worth could be proven beyond the confines of his own field. Barnett responded positively to Donald's encouragement and set out to acquire expertise in the use of the ultrasound scanner. When Donald's Obstetric Unit was relocated to the Queen Mother's Hospital in 1964, Barnett was able to take over much of the obstetric ultrasound diagnostic work at Rottenrow.

The Department of Radiology in the Western Infirmary inherited the Automatic Scanner after Donald took delivery of the first Diasonograph. We described in chapter 8 how Barnett and his colleague Patricia Morley collaborated with Donald in a detailed ultrasonic characterization of blighted ovum, published in 1972.[16] From the early 1970s onward, Morley and Barnett undertook a systematic investigation of the pathological ultrasonic appearances of the kidney, liver, and urinary tract. Important papers appeared steadily, culminating in the publication in 1983 of a remarkable atlas, *Ultrasonic Sectional Anatomy*, of which Morley was the senior editor. Barnett and Morley were also responsible for one of the first comprehensive textbooks on diagnostic ultrasound, *Clinical Diagnostic Ultrasound*, published in 1985.[17] Donald derived much satisfaction from the considerable achievements of his radiologist colleagues.[18]

Donald would provide a short introduction to ultrasonic diagnostics for just about anyone interested enough to make the trip to his clinic. In one four-month period, Donald received twenty-seven visitors on this basis, some staying for half a day, some for several weeks.[19] Proud of the achievements of his team, and not a modest man, Donald doubtless enjoyed these occasions, showing off the latest equipment and conjuring virtuoso feats of diagnosis. Nevertheless, such engagements took up time in what was already the very busy personal schedule of a man in less than perfect health. Given that Glasgow was the place to come to learn ultrasonic diagnosis, there was an evident need for education and training in the modality to be more formally organized.

The arrangements for teaching medical physics at Glasgow University were somewhat unusual. The Western Regional Hospital Board, which administered the hospitals of Glasgow and the surrounding area, supported its own Department of Clinical Physics. Under its charismatic and energetic director, Dr. John Lenihan, this department had, by the 1960s, established itself as one of the most important centers for medical physics in Europe.[20] It was largely independent of, but had close links with, the university's Faculty of Medicine. Its senior staff members were honorary lecturers in the Faculty, where they were largely responsible for the teaching of medical physics. The Department of Clinical Physics also participated in collaborative research with a number of professorial units.

Relations between Donald and Lenihan had been strained by Donald's rejection of the advice from Lenihan and his colleague Ron Greer in the aftermath of the seismic impact of Tom Brown's arrival in the Western Infirmary. The rift had been partially but not entirely healed by the success of the work on fetal cephalometry, undertaken collaboratively by Willocks and Duggan, a member of Lenihan's department. Lenihan realized, however, that the now widespread recognition of Glasgow University as the leading center of an important new diagnostic technology afforded his own department with an opportunity.[21] In September 1967, he wrote to Donald suggesting that a formal training course in diagnostic ultrasound be set up, run by the Department of Clinical Physics in cooperation with Donald's Department of Midwifery. Lenihan's staff would provide lectures and laboratory classes, which would be complemented by clinical demonstrations at the Queen Mother's Hospital and the Western Infirmary. Donald responded with enthusiasm. The following month, the two men traveled to London to meet Dr. A. J. Eley at the Department of Health. As already noted, the department was undertaking an assessment of diagnostic ultrasound, and its support would be crucial to the success of any training initiative. Eley assured Lenihan and Donald that "there is general acceptance of ultrasound as a method of diagnosis and a general determination to continue."[22]

By early 1968, Norman McDicken, who had recently completed a PhD in nuclear physics, was appointed to teach the new course. The intensive, two-week program ran for the first time in January 1970.[23] One of the original students was Donald himself. He booked his place in 1968 by writing to Lenihan, "I would like to have the honour of being one of the first students. It is about time I learned something about this subject." The professor's presence in the class was somewhat daunting for McDicken, but Donald's report to Lenihan was extremely positive: "I think McDicken's stuff was simply magnificent."[24] Barnett and Morley also attended the course in its early years. Later, they undertook some of the clinical demonstrations. Building on the success of the two-week course, a three-day course for radiographers was later offered, as well as a one-day introductory session. In 1974, McDicken left to take up the Chair of Medical Physics at the University of Edinburgh. The teaching continued, successfully taken over by Duggan.

The courses in diagnostic ultrasound organized by the Department of Clinical Physics in Glasgow were the first to be formally taught anywhere in the world. They attracted large numbers of obstetricians, physicians, and radiologists from Britain and abroad and played a major part in ensuring the successful diffusion of the technology to new centers. Meanwhile, Nuclear Enterprises consolidated its position as the world's leading manufacturer of ultrasound scanners. By the early 1970s, there were several other manufacturers in the marketplace, Siemens in Germany, Kretztechnic in Austria, and Picker in the United States, as well as some Japanese companies. However, the more expensive products of Nuclear Enterprises were still generally preferred for advanced clinical applications and for research. The company's sales were also assisted by the fact that most of the clinical teaching in the Glasgow courses was done with its equipment.

In 1972, the Western Regional Hospital Board recognized that an ultrasonic diagnostic service had sprung up, unplanned and uncoordinated, within its area of administration. A working group was set up, chaired by Lenihan, to look at "arrangements for ultrasonic diagnostics services and future policy."[25] Its report affirmed the central place of ultrasound diagnosis within the Hospital Board's provision and made recommendations on purchasing arrangements, training, and maintenance. The working group appreciated that ultrasound scanners were complicated instruments that required regular attention from trained technicians. It also recognized that the market for scanners was now expanding rapidly and that the manufacturers, preoccupied with competing for new business, were not providing an adequate maintenance and repair service. (This would remain true until the late 1970s.) As long as the maintenance issue remained unresolved, the development of a clinical service would be hindered. Lenihan's committee made the radical proposal that the Hospital Board should take over from the manufacturers the maintenance of the machines in its area. Accordingly, in 1973, the Greater Glasgow Health Board (as it had become) appointed Rowland Eadie to service the ten machines installed in Glasgow hospitals. Eadie also acted as a peripatetic tutor in the use of the scanners. The Health Board's support thus effectively underwrote the continued development of the ultrasonic diagnostic service in the Glasgow area.

Many of those who visited Donald at the Queen Mother's Hospital or attended one of McDicken's or Duggan's courses were subsequently instrumental in establishing the technique in their home institutions. For example, in March 1970, Dr. Florence Fraser, a New Zealand obstetrician working at the Perivale Maternity Hospital in Middlesex, wrote to Donald asking to come to Glasgow "for the opportunity to learn a technique not yet used in New Zealand but hoped for in the near future."[26] Donald provided her with residential accommodation in the Queen Mother's, and she stayed in Glasgow for six weeks, attending McDicken's course. She shortly returned to New Zealand to work in the National Women's Hospital in Auckland. By early 1973, that hospital had decided to buy a scanner, and the Radiology Department was advocating the purchase of a Picker machine, one of which they had on loan from the American manufacturer.[27] Fraser, however, persuaded the Auckland Medical School's professor of obstetrics to lobby for the purchase of the more expensive Nuclear Enterprises instrument, which she had worked with in Glasgow. An order was duly placed, and by December 1973, Fraser was corresponding with Donald about unusual cases.[28] Similar sequences of events preceded the purchase of NE scanners by other maternity hospitals, including ones in Dublin, in Winnipeg and Halifax in Canada, in New York and Saint Louis in the United States, and in Bellville, South Africa.[29]

The technology was also disseminated by the outward migration of members of the Glasgow team. John MacVicar, for instance, became Professor of Obstetrics and Gynaecology at the University of Leicester in 1974 and led the setting-up of an ultrasound service for the Leicester maternity hospitals. In 1978, Hugh Robinson moved to the Department of Obstetrics and Gynaecology at the University of Melbourne and played an important role in establishing an ultrasound service in that city.

When recruiting ultrasound researchers, Donald often enlisted registrars who were looking for topics for their MD theses. While this strategy was, as earlier chapters exemplify, often outstandingly successful, it had an inherent weakness. A young doctor who takes up research in pursuit of an MD may equally well abandon the interest once the degree—and a consultant's post—is obtained. Willocks, for example, undertook virtually no further ultrasound research after being appointed consultant obstetrician to the Queen Mother's Hospital in 1966, though he continued to rely on the technology diagnostically. The same was true of Robinson after his move to Australia, though he remained an active and respected clinical user of ultrasound. There were, however, exceptions to this pattern among Donald's protégés. Stuart Campbell, for instance, would sustain an active involvement in ultrasound research throughout his career.

(((((In 1968, Campbell became senior registrar at Queen Charlotte's Maternity Hospital in London. He was chosen for this post because of the expertise he had acquired under Donald's tutelage.

> The reason why Professor Dewhurst appointed me was because of my work with ultrasound . . . in fact it was really unheard of for a Scotsman from Glasgow to get a job in Queen Charlotte's and when I applied for the job there I got an instant reply "No, sorry, there is no place for you," from the Chief Executive of the Hospital . . . I just accepted it, never mind, worth trying, then two days later I got a phone call from Professor Dewhurst to say "Forget that letter you got. Are you interested in the job?"[30]

When Campbell arrived at Queen Charlotte's, the hospital did not have an ultrasound scanner. He was determined, however, to offer an ultrasound service to his patients.

> So I made contact with Ernest Kohorn . . . at the University College Hospital . . . So I used to take these women from Queen Charlotte's. Usually they had bleeding, so we wanted to know where the placenta was. We put this red blanket round them and got them in my little MGB sports car and drove across London to University College Hospital, and put it in a car park that was 500 yards from the Hospital . . . and then walk with the woman into . . . the bowels of the

Hospital, [I] did my placentography, [then we would] get in the car and drive back again. That was a ritual for about a year.[31]

The staff at University College Hospital were having difficulties maintaining their machine and did not yet offer a full clinical service,[32] but Campbell shortly began a research project, in collaboration with Kohorn, on localization of the placenta.[33] Suitable A-scan capability was not available, so he could not continue his research into measurement of the fetal biparietal diameter. Nevertheless, it is an indication of the clinical importance of placenta previa at this time that the first research programs undertaken by the pioneers of ultrasound in both Aberdeen and London focused on placental localization.

Somewhat to Campbell's surprise, neither Dewhurst nor the administrators at Queen Charlotte's were actively trying to secure a scanner for the hospital. "And then the Department of Health wrote me a letter saying, 'I understand you are interested in ultrasound. Would you like us to loan you a machine [Diasonograph], for evaluation?' So I wrote back and said 'Yes, Yes!'"[34] Campbell's ultrasound research could now resume in earnest. As well as recommencing his work on the BPD, Campbell began to measure the fetal abdominal circumference. This project arose in response to a growing awareness that Willocks's method of assessing gestational age by measuring the BPD was occasionally inaccurate. The problem was that some healthy fetuses had skulls that were longer and narrower than the norm on which Willocks's estimates were based. Measurement of the BPD in these fetuses often underestimated their degree of maturity.[35] To eliminate these inaccuracies, Campbell sought to find an alternative developmental yardstick.

Campbell knew that other researchers, Thompson in Denver and Hansmann in Germany, had published measurements of the fetal chest.[36] Campbell recalls:

They sort of measured the thorax and I felt that, the thorax being cone-shaped, it wasn't good enough . . . I was always very careful to get a very reproducible plane and a very reproducible set of markers to guide you so you could give precise measurements . . . but you could never see exactly where they [Thompson and Hansmann] were in the body—no marker there. So I used to scan around the abdomen and eventually I decided that the umbilical vein in the liver was the thing to use as a marker, very reproducible thing to see. So I used to line that [up] . . . to get a nice cross-section.[37]

The ratio of head size to abdominal size gave a good "indication of how starved the baby was of nutrient."[38]

Together with his colleague Donald Wilkins, Campbell developed a technique based on identification of the umbilical vein as it passed under the fetal liver.[39] This soon became generally adopted as the best means of standardizing cross-sectional measurements of the fetal trunk.[40] The fetus, however, did not always accommodate itself to the technique. In about one in twenty cases, the fetus lies with its spine closely proximate to the maternal abdominal wall, meaning that, with Campbell's equipment, the ultrasonic beam could not be directed at right angles to the course of the umbilical vein. Under these circumstances, the vein could not be identified with certainty and, instead, the operator had to use the edge of the fetal stomach, a less precisely determined location.

By the early 1970s, some American hospitals were beginning to equip themselves with ultrasound scanners. But the most commonly purchased machine, the Picker, while cheaper and less bulky than the NE equivalent, did not produce such clear images. Moreover, the heavy gantries of the Diasonograph and the NE4101 and 4102 provided a more stable scanning frame. The obstetrician could set the machine to scan at a chosen angle to the abdomen and could be confident that subsequent scans would be taken at exactly the same angle. This was a significant advantage when making precise measurements of the fetus.

Campbell ascribed his preoccupation with accurate, reproducible measurement partly to the rigor of the training he had received in Glasgow and partly to the technical superiority of the Diasonograph. "When I came down to London," he recalls, "I found myself travelling to America so often, because my pictures were just better than theirs, and that is just lucky. I just happened to have Ian Donald's machine."[41] The quality of the instrument at his disposal, coupled with his confidence in his ability to use it, gave Campbell a head start over his rivals in other centers.

It was difficult to learn to use the machine . . . and you needed a lot of skills, and once you have learned . . . you knew that no one else was going to catch up with you, there was nobody else going to develop these skills very easily. So you had a lovely era when everything that you did, you knew that some sneaky person wasn't going to catch up with you and do it before you.[42]

By moving south, Campbell had acquired a further advantage not enjoyed by his Glasgow colleagues. Many more terminations of pregnancy were undertaken at Queen Charlotte's than in the units under Donald's control. This more liberal policy provided Campbell with a research opportunity, since he could immediately compare measurements of the BPD and abdominal circumference taken in utero with those of the aborted fetus. At Queen Charlotte's, moreover, with the consultants often preoccupied with their private practices and less interested in research, senior registrars such as Campbell had greater autonomy to define and pursue their own programs of investigation. As we saw in chapter 8, the application to the fetus of standardized growth charts, similar to those long used by pediatricians, was begun by Willocks. Campbell's work extended this process of imposing objective criteria on the fetus. Its growth and development were quantified more fully than ever before.

Campbell became senior lecturer at Queen Charlotte's in 1973 and subsequently held chairs at three London hospitals: Queen Charlotte's, King's and St. George's. He was central to achieving recognition for the new diagnostic technique in the capital, a process vital to its general acceptance within British medicine. His triumph of successfully diagnosing and uneventfully managing the Hanson quintuplet pregnancy attracted considerable media attention.[43] Campbell's ultrasound unit began to attract many international visitors, much as did Donald's unit in the Queen Mother's Hospital. It became quite common for those wanting to improve their knowledge of diagnostic ultrasound to travel to both Glasgow and London.

Management of multiple births revealed another benefit of accurate placental localization. In the case of the Hanson quintuplets, Campbell had ascertained, by ultrasound, that one or more placentas lay against the anterior uterine wall. This information proved of considerable value to the obstetrician when undertaking the cesarean section. Alerted in advance that the uterine incision might cause the placenta to bleed, he had prepared for a speedy delivery, to obviate the risk of severe hemorrhage. Campbell regarded this precaution as a key factor in the survival of all five babies.

Up to the early 1970s, major fetal abnormalities had been detected by ultrasound only late in pregnancy. Donald and Brown identified hydrocephalus in the third trimester.[44] Sundén recognized anencephaly at thirty-one weeks—too late to make an effective difference to management of the case. In 1970, an Australian team made the remarkable prenatal diagnosis of polycystic kidney disease, but again, at thirty-one weeks.[45] Campbell thus regarded it as a substantial breakthrough when, in 1972, he and his colleagues at Queen Charlotte's were able to identify anencephaly in a fetus of less then twenty weeks' gestation.[46] This was early enough for the woman to be offered a termination, which she accepted.

Gradually, Campbell accumulated sufficient experience to reliably diagnose a number of abnormalities, notably hydrocephalus, spina bifida and encephalocele.[47] As described in chapter 8, the standard method of identifying neural tube defects was by determining the level of alpha fetoprotein in the amniotic fluid. A substantially elevated level of AFP resulted in a presumptive diagnosis of neural tube defect. One of Campbell's first publications on spina bifida reported three false-positive diagnoses based on amniotic fluid AFP levels, resulting in the termination of pregnancies with four normal fetuses (there was one set of twins). No anomaly had been found by ultrasound in any of these cases, but the ultrasound evidence was ignored in favor of the biochemical results. Gradually, following recognition of the importance of Campbell's work, ultrasound came to be accepted as providing, at least in expert hands, a more reliable means of diagnosing spina bifida and related conditions. Not coincidentally, it was also in the mid-1970s that the term *prenatal diagnosis* began to be accepted into the vocabulary of obstetricians and pediatricians.[48] The fetus was becoming the focus of hitherto unprecedented medical scrutiny. A more dependable means of making intrauterine diagnoses, coupled with the freer availability of therapeutic abortion should a major abnormality be detected, was changing its clinical status. The fetus was not quite a patient as yet, since the possibilities for direct therapeutic intervention in utero remained negligible. But it was gaining an increasingly important presence within clinical decision making.

The nature of what could be accepted as a valid knowledge claim about the fetus was also changing. For example, one might consider the fate of Dr. W. G. Mills's suggestion of "fetal hibernation."[49] In 1970, Mills proposed that fetal development could become suspended for an interval of some weeks, after which normal progress might be resumed. The hypothesis was offered as an explanation for some of the apparent discrepancies between fetal maturity assessed clinically and the duration of amenorrhea. Mills based his theory on his "twenty years personal experience of antenatal care," impressions gained by abdominal palpation, and mothers' reports of fetal movement. Such an evidential basis was not good enough for Campbell, who responded that "a hypothesis of fetal hibernation . . . cannot be considered seriously," because sustained ultrasonic scrutiny of the fetus revealed no such temporary interruptions in its development. Moreover, studies with the scanner "stress how unreliable uterine palpation is in estimation of fetal growth, size and maturity."[50] In other words, ultrasonic diagnosis had set a new standard for authoritative statements about the fetus. The subjective opinions of the palpating obstetrician, not to mention those of the pregnant woman, were not yet wholly discounted, but they now had a status secondary to the testimony of the machine.

(((((Donald followed Campbell's work with great interest and was not too proud to learn from it, especially because the ultrasonic recognition of major fetal abnormalities was also being attempted in Glasgow. In September 1969, Donald was asked by a pediatrician in Yorkshire who was responsible for the care of a microcephalic child whether ultrasound might be of use in identifying microcephaly early enough in pregnancy to allow a termination to be offered.[51] Donald replied that he had considered the possible value of serial ultrasound measurements in the diagnosis of the condition but had had only equivocal success in the one trial he had conducted. He offered, however, to try to assess any patient that the pediatrician cared to refer to him. A year later, the mother of the microcephalic child was pregnant again and was duly referred to Donald's clinic. The correspondence between Donald and her pediatrician is revealing of the process of clinical decision making that was evolving around the novel possibilities of prenatal diagnosis. Donald wrote:

> I examined this interesting patient of yours . . . who had the previous microcephalic baby, by sonar this morning. She gave her dates as 15½ weeks, a period at which there should be no difficulty in demonstrating the fetal head but I was very dismayed at only being able to find a most indefinite affair. Even allowing for the fact that she may have possibly a 38-day menstrual cycle which would put her back to 14 weeks, the picture was still a poor 14-week effort . . . All these things together make me feel somewhat pessimistic although I hope I betrayed none of it to the patient.

The pediatrician replied:

> I note that you will be re-examining Mrs . . . in 4 weeks . . . if there is still no clear evidence of a normal foetal head, would you regard this as sufficiently definite to justify termination of a fairly advanced pregnancy?

Donald's response was unequivocal.

If the second examination of this patient shows an unsatisfactory state of cephalic growth, I think we would have to confirm matters by radiography and if the result were positive I personally would not have the slightest hesitation in terminating the pregnancy despite my opposition to abortion on more liberal grounds.

The findings of the second scan were more encouraging.

I was pleased to see this patient again today and even more pleased to find what looks like a very good head measuring 4.69 cms in its biparietal diameter which would put maturity at 18 weeks, although her dates are 19½ weeks. This now makes sense and confirms that the fetal head which showed up so poorly last time was only 14 weeks. This could be accounted for by her prolonged menstrual cycle . . . Within the limits of our technique (and I would be rash not to admit these) I have no present indication of abnormality.

Donald examined the woman again in the thirtieth week, purely "for my own interest," and was "delighted to report what looks at least in ultrasonic terms like a normal vertex presentation, with head measurements which are right up to schedule." The woman was "much reassured and I have given her a copy of one of the ultrasonograms for the baby book." A healthy, normal baby was duly born.[52]

Several other methods of gaining information about the contents of the uterus were being developed at this time, one of which involved the use of radioisotopes to locate the placenta. In print, Campbell offered a studiously even-handed comparison between the ultrasonic and radioisotope techniques.[53] He was prepared to concede that the latter could locate the placenta effectively in many cases. He cautioned that any exposure to ionizing radiation during pregnancy was undesirable but acknowledged that the dose associated with radioisotope localization was much lower than in X-ray placentography. He was, however, careful to point out that the radioisotope method was less effective in defining the lower edge of the placenta, which was the part most likely to cause problems, particularly when it lay posteriorly. Ultrasound imaging also had the great advantage that the placenta and the presenting part of the fetus could be visualized simultaneously, the juxtaposition of the two often being the most clinically significant datum. With this information, the obstetrician might be able to exclude the diagnosis of minor degrees of placenta previa, on which other methods might be equivocal. With these features, Campbell argued, ultrasonic placental localization was, on balance, the method of choice for large obstetric

units. Its only drawback was that considerable experience was required to interpret ultrasound scans accurately. Campbell acknowledged that the radioisotope method might be suitable for hospitals where the technique was used
in other specialties or where staff skilled in the use of ultrasound machines
were not available.

Campbell's ostensive willingness to take a balanced view of a rival technology was, to some extent, a diplomatic front. In private, he and his fellow users
of ultrasound tended to be a lot less polite. Donald wrote to Campbell:

> If some of the recent isotope pictures and scanning pictures in the British Jour-
> nal are anything to go by, I can hardly refrain from vomiting my contempt, in-
> stead of which I shall have to behave myself and suggest that perhaps sonar has a
> little to offer . . . in comparison to the established research of others. This kind
> of technique pays off but may I be forgiven for it.[54]

For his part, Campbell evidently enjoyed providing his old chief with a dispar-
aging account of a symposium on placentography held at Queen Charlotte's.
The meeting, he wrote, was disappointing.

> Robert Percival, who was Chairman . . . discussed soft tissue radiography and
> retrograde arteriography at great length even to the point of saying that the
> most important new development in placental localisation was in filling the pa-
> tient's rectum with air so that on a lateral film the low lying posterior placenta
> would be clearly shown. They really were completely out of touch . . . I gave a
> short talk on ultrasonic placentography illustrated with some of the pictures
> taken at UCH [University College Hospital]. The two other speakers, however,
> just didn't want to know. Mr Percival's last remark was "what we really want is a
> way of demonstrating the lower edge of the placenta." If he had looked at any of
> the slides I had shown he would have seen his dream already realised.[55]

It would seem that Percival's haughty dismissal of ultrasonic localization of the
placenta sprang not so much from active opposition to the modality as from an
inability to interpret the images it provided. The distinguished surgeon was
not alone in this difficulty. On one occasion, the most eminent periodical in
its field, the *American Journal of Obstetrics and Gynaecology*, printed three of
Donald's ultrasonograms upside down and in the wrong order, effectively rendering the captions meaningless.[56]

In the determination of gestational age, the only innovations that threatened
to rival ultrasonic fetal measurement were techniques based on the biochemical

or cytological characteristics of the amniotic fluid.[57] A leading investigator was Thomas Lind, an obstetrician based at the Medical Research Council's Reproduction and Growth Unit in Newcastle. In 1973, Lind and his colleagues explored a number of technical points relating to the accuracy of ultrasonic cephalometry.[58] They argued that the limitations of ultrasonic cephalometry were not sufficiently appreciated and that the technique needed to be "more stringently appraised." They concluded that clinicians should not have confidence in an ultrasonic estimate of the growth rate of the fetal skull unless measurements were taken regularly over a period of not less than three weeks. Lind's colleague John Davidson raised these concerns privately with Campbell.[59] Prior to the Newcastle publication, an editorial in the *British Medical Journal* had made similar comments, concluding that it was unfortunate that ultrasonic measurement of the BPD required "complex and expensive equipment" and "considerable experience," while noting that amniocentesis was now a "relatively safe procedure."[60] The editorial asserted that ultrasonic measurements could be inaccurate in up to 33 percent of cases.

One of the issues raised by Davidson was that ultrasonic measurements of the fetal abdomen or BPD might vary from one operator to another and with the same operator from day to day. Another was that there were physical limits to the precision of the technique, which Campbell's results seemed to have approached. Both these comments irritated Campbell (and Donald), particularly when they were reiterated in a *Lancet* editorial.[61] The first comment Campbell took to imply that he was inconsistent in his use of the Diasonograph; the second, that he had exaggerated the accuracy of his findings. Despite the umbrage taken by Campbell and Donald,[62] other users of ultrasound seemed to have held the view that the points made by the Newcastle team did not seriously compromise the clinical utility of the technique in experienced hands.[63] As ultrasound scanners proliferated and the expertise necessary to use them was disseminated, the reliability of ultrasonic measurements of the fetus became generally accepted, and the more interventionist technique of estimating fetal age by testing the amniotic fluid was not widely adopted.[64]

Apart from this episode, there seems to have been little sustained opposition to the introduction of diagnostic ultrasound within obstetrics and gynecology in Britain, once initial incredulities had passed. By the mid-1970s, the attitude of most leading radiologists had moved from indifference and polite skepticism to professional acquisitiveness. Imaging, it was argued, was the business of radiologists, and they were the specialists who should have control of the ultrasound scanners. In many general hospitals, this was indeed what happened. As more machines were purchased, they tended to be installed in radiology departments and used by radiologists to provide an imaging service for clinicians. But this arrangement was not, by and large, acceptable to obstetricians. Donald was keen for radiologists to use ultrasound, but "we must be careful that they don't corner the market, however desirable it is for them to have a stake in it." He complained in one letter of "an ill-concealed attempt to climb on the bandwagon by radiologists and monopolise all the seats." And in another, "There is clearly a clash of interest developing between radiologist and obstetricians which I thoroughly deplore. Without the clinicians the radiologists would never have started . . . although it is natural enough that they would wake up to the interest now."[65]

Donald was concerned also that "lazy" radiologists would rely on scans made for them by radiographers, thus lessening the amount of information available for clinical consideration. To an obstetrician, ultrasonic diagnosis was, unlike other forms of imaging, essentially interactive: an understanding of the contents of the abdomen emerged in the course of the scan and was the direct product of physical as well as visual inputs. Moreover, clinicians of Donald's background and training sought to retain command of the diagnostic process, as far as possible.

Sufficient friction was generated between the rival camps—obstetricians and gynecologists versus radiologists—for the two relevant Royal Colleges to set up a joint working party, charged with formulating guidelines. On his appointment as the principal representative of the Royal College of Obstetricians and Gynaecologists, Donald emphasized his determination that "our college should retain a dominant role."[66] His influence is readily discerned in the recommendations of the working party. Its report acknowledged that in many contexts it was appropriate for ultrasound scanners to be located in radiology departments, but wherever possible, clinicians were to have free and equal access to the machines, for research and training as well as diagnostic use. In other words, the right of obstetricians to continue scanning their own patients was enshrined in the official compromise.

(((((A more serious obstacle to the rapid diffusion of ultrasonic diagnosis was anxiety about its safety. Donald regularly received inquiries from prospective purchasers of scanners seeking reassurance on this point. As described in earlier chapters, Donald and Brown had been concerned about the safety of ultrasound since their earliest experiments with the modality. All the scanners built by Smiths and by Nuclear Enterprises incorporated Brown's original cautionary principle that the power output should be the minimum consistent with obtaining echoes of sufficient amplitude, with an attenuator interposed between the transmitter and the probe. Ultrasound was known to damage tissue at high power levels, but initial investigations into the potential hazards associated with the levels employed diagnostically had all been reassuring. It is impossible to prove a negative, however, and Donald was aware that it had taken years for the deleterious effects of ionizing radiation on the fetus to be recognized. Moreover, as the medical physicist Christopher Hill put it when reviewing the subject in 1968, "such investigations as have been made of possible damage following medical ultrasonic irradiation of human beings mostly appear somewhat haphazard in comparison with some of the studies of the hazards of ionising radiation."[67]

The first hint of real trouble on the safety front came in 1968, when Donald received news from the Frederiksburg Hospital in Sweden that two babies who had received Doppler ultrasound in utero were born with deformities of the upper limbs. These cases were looked into carefully by the American manufacturer, who concluded that the abnormal limb development must have been present prior to insonation of the fetuses. Then, early in 1970, a rumor spread that scientists at a Canadian university had managed to enhance the growth of certain varieties of poultry by exposing fertilized eggs to ultrasound.[68] There were tales of chickens more than a meter tall—and a patent had been applied for, it was whispered. Donald responded that if the rumors were true, he would take up chicken farming.

Nothing more was heard of the phenomenal fowl. Nevertheless, the circulation of such rumors is testimony to a certain generalized anxiety about the biological effects of ultrasound. These concerns seem to have been particularly prevalent in the United States. In March and April 1970, Donald spent four weeks as visiting professor at the State University Hospital, New York. The issue of safety cropped up regularly in his discussions with medical staff.

Donald had been invited to New York by Louis Hellman, professor of obstetrics and gynecology, who had studied ultrasonic diagnosis in Glasgow and subsequently introduced the technology to the East Coast. In a bid to allay fears, Hellman initiated a retrospective study of the incidence of abnormality among babies whose mothers had been insonated. He gathered data from his own clinic, from Donald's in Glasgow, and from Sundén's in Lund. Analysis was done by independent statisticians. The outcomes of 1,114 pregnancies, all apparently normal at the time of scanning, were recorded. The incidence of abnormality was no greater than in the general population. Indeed, it was slightly lower. Moreover, the pattern of abnormality was the same as that usually seen in obstetric practice, suggesting that ultrasound was not causing a specific type of damage.

Shortly after returning to Scotland, Donald learned about a paper given during his absence to the European Congress of Perinatal Medicine. D. M. Serr and colleagues at the University of Tel Aviv presented a preliminary account of a study of the effects of ultrasound on human fibroblasts obtained from amniotic fluid.[69] They had observed some chromosomal damage and a reduction in mitotic activity. Serr's team was guarded in the conclusions drawn from these results. Nevertheless, Donald regarded the Tel Aviv work as bringing the issue of safety to a head. He wrote to Hellman, urging him to "get your article out at the earliest possible moment. It at least provides a partial and interim answer to a question that is in everyone's mind."[70]

Hellman's paper must already have been in an advanced state of preparedness. It appeared in the *Lancet* on May 30, with Donald and Sundén as coauthors. While admitting that a retrospective study was necessarily unsatisfactory from a statistical point of view, the three authors presented the absence of excess abnormality as reassuring. Considerable emphasis was also given to the results of an early study by M. G. Smyth in which laboratory rats were insonated for long periods before mating and during pregnancy. No abnormalities were produced. In the same issue of the *Lancet*, an editorial, published anonymously but written by Donald, acknowledged that it was possible that deleterious effects existed that had not yet been detected, but it concluded "these hypothetical hazards have to be assessed against the increasing usefulness of sonar in obstetrics."[71]

The situation was shortly to get much worse, however. Early in October 1970, Donald was having lunch with Sir Charles Wilson, principal of Glasgow University and an important patron of Donald's ultrasound work. Wilson shocked Donald by informing him that he had read in the London *Times* that morning that ultrasound was unsafe. Unbeknown to Donald, two researchers at the University of Cape Town, Ian Macintosh and Denis Davey, had published a "preliminary communication" in the *British Medical Journal* describing experiments in which human blood was exposed to continuous wave ultrasound from a Doppler fetal heart monitor. The authors claimed to have observed a significant increase in the number of gross chromosomal and chromatid aberrations in the insonated blood as compared with controls. They explicitly suggested that ultrasound, as employed diagnostically, might be mutagenic.[72]

Macintosh and Davey's results were extensively reported in the British press and caused much alarm. Shortly after the item appeared in the *Times*, Donald was contacted by officials in the Department of Health, seeking advice on the advisability of allowing the continued deployment of ultrasound in National Health Service hospitals. A serious crisis had been provoked. Donald and the other protagonists for ultrasound were forced on the defensive.

Fortunately for Donald, he was able to respond in kind to the Cape Town study, very quickly indeed. By a coincidence, he had already undertaken an experiment similar to that described by Macintosh and Davey. He had not published the results in detail but had briefly outlined them in a paper in 1969.[73] The study sprang from a conversation Donald had had, in 1966, with Malcolm Ferguson-Smith, an eminent medical geneticist. Ferguson-Smith had claimed that chromosomal damage could be readily detected in tissue samples from any woman who had undergone a diagnostic X-ray, even two or three weeks after irradiation. Donald challenged him to find similar effects after exposure to ultrasound. With his colleague Elizabeth Boyd, a cytogeneticist, Ferguson-Smith examined blood cultures from six neonates whose mothers had been exposed to ultrasound during pregnancy. No chromosomal abnormalities were found. The geneticists also insonated tissue cultures, at diagnostic intensity but over a period of hours rather than the few minutes of a normal diagnostic scan. The results were again negative.

Originally, Donald had not thought to publish a negative result, but now, in the changed context created by the appearance of Macintosh and Davey's article, a negative result was a very pertinent finding. The study was hurriedly written up and submitted to the *British Medical Journal*, where it appeared on May 29, 1971. Donald and his co-workers offered the firm conclusion that "if diagnostic ultrasound causes chromosome damage it does so with less frequency than acceptable levels of diagnostic X-irradiation."[74] The contradiction between the Cape Town study and other earlier work was stressed.

In London, Campbell and his colleagues also responded promptly to the challenge posed by the Cape Town study. Under the different policy on terminations of pregnancy that pertained at Queen Charlotte's, they were able to take blood samples from newly aborted fetuses that had been exposed to ultrasound in utero. Again, no increase in the number of chromosomal aberrations was found.[75] Donald and Campbell presented their preliminary results to a meeting at the Department of Health before the end of 1970, and the officials were "dissuaded from interfering with the continued progress of this work."[76]

Anxious to settle the matter, Donald negotiated the appointment of a geneticist, Pat Watts, to Ferguson-Smith's department, to work with Hall and Fleming on the effect of ultrasound on chromosomes. Publishing their results in 1972, they concluded "the suggestion, based on in vitro studies, that diagnostic ultrasound causes chromosome damage is unfounded."[77] By the early 1970s, diagnostic ultrasound was being adopted by an increasing number of centers throughout the developed world, and publication of the Cape Town paper unleashed a spate of similar studies. None confirmed Macintosh and Davey's results. One study reported that significant chromosomal damage was observed but attributed the finding, not to exposure to ultrasound, but to a flaw in the experimental design. The authors suggested a similar explanation might account for the Cape Town results.[78] Eventually, one of the authors of the original paper (Macintosh) issued a public withdrawal of their claim.[79] The observed chromosomal aberrations had been caused, it now appeared, by chemical contaminants that the ultrasound energy had released from the polyethylene membranes used to contain the specimens.

The Tel Aviv study had, by this time, also been generally discounted. In their conference paper, Serr and his colleagues had not included details of their cytogenetic techniques. They had used nonstandard terminology and had not acknowledged the extent to which cultures of fibroblasts from amniotic fluid display abnormalities even without exposure to ultrasound. A more definitive account of their results never appeared. In 1974, Angus Hall analyzed the results of full-scale replications of both the Cape Town and the Tel Aviv studies, in neither of which significant chromosomal abnormalities were observed.[80]

By the mid-1970s, it was widely accepted that ultrasound, at diagnostic power levels, did not damage chromosomes. But the possibility of some other harmful effect remained. Donald readily conceded that more research into safety was required but admitted that it was difficult to know where to begin. Robinson led a somewhat speculative investigation into whether diagnostic ultrasound might disrupt enzyme activity, but again, the findings were negative.[81] Donald wondered whether insonation might affect the fetal ear, and he obtained a list of names of the children in Glasgow schools who were registered as having hearing defects. Mrs. Miller, Donald's first ultrasonographer, was reemployed and delegated to examine the records of deaf children who were born in the Queen Mother's Hospital. Donald wrote to T. S Wilson, Medical Officer of Health for Glasgow.

> I am constantly watching for signs of any kind of disability which might even remotely be laid at the door of ultrasonic insonation during pregnancy . . . I am aware that there are lots of causes of deafness in early childhood but we are simply clutching at straws. More and more of my time is being spent in trying to chase possible hazards before the whole subject becomes out of hand—So far, thank goodness, with reassuringly negative results.[82]

No association was found between hearing impairment and intrauterine exposure to ultrasound.

As already suggested, the key question in the safety debate was: At what dosage might one begin to see deleterious effects? Donald had been, for some time, urging his laboratory colleagues to try to determine where the threshold of biological damage lay. In 1966, he wrote to Roger Warwick, an anatomist at Guy's Hospital who was conducting experiments on the effects of ultrasound on rats: "I think it is urgent that you should be able to step up the dosage progressively until you find a threshold level of damage if, in fact, any such exists and we are all most anxious to hear of your results at the earliest possible moment."[83]

Detailed threshold dosage data for mammalian tissue were first published by Dunn and Fry in 1971. The levels proved to be well above the power outputs of the commercially available diagnostic ultrasound equipment, which had been accurately measured by Hill in 1969.[84] However, it was possible that fetal tissue thresholds might be different and might vary according to the stage of fetal development.

Despite the failure of substantial research efforts to confirm any deleterious effect, the safety concern surrounding obstetric ultrasound was never quite laid to rest. Throughout the years covered by this book—and, indeed, until the time of writing—anxieties about possible hazards continued. Acute scares, similar to that produced by the Cape Town study, occurred periodically. Donald found these episodes exasperating, but he accepted that technological innovation in an area "so emotive as human reproduction" was bound to attract controversy. And of course, even if previous usage were safe, that was no guarantee that harm might not occur in the future. Certainly, it behooved both clinicians and engineers to proceed with caution, minimizing exposure as much as possible.

Donald voiced a particular concern that improvements in the quality of ultrasound imaging, while desirable in themselves, generally entailed an increase in the energy output of the apparatus. Thus the threshold of fetal tissue damage, wherever that might lie, was gradually becoming less remote. He continued to maintain, however, that "in the meantime, the diagnostic benefits of sonar would appear to outweigh [the] hazards."[85]

(((((One of the most important technical improvements of the 1970s in ultrasound scanning was gray-scaling. Many early scanners used "bi-stable" cathode-ray tubes. Echoes above a certain amplitude were displayed as dots of constant brightness; echoes below this threshold were not displayed at all. Some engineers recognized that some form of gray-scaling, whereby the brightness of the dot on the screen was proportional to the amplitude of the echo it represented, would reveal more detail. Indeed, the first Glasgow machines did have a considerable degree of gray-scaling, a consequence of Brown's innovative design of the signal-processing circuits and the photographic integration used to build up the image. Moreover, the cathode-ray tubes used in the Diasonograph were chosen because of their comparatively wide dynamic range. Attempts were made, in Bristol and elsewhere, to enhance gray-scaling by the use of logarithmic compression amplifiers, which increased the dynamic range of the signals that could be processed. A major advance toward gray-scaling was achieved by George Kossoff and his colleagues at the Ultrasonic Institute in Sydney. The Australian research, published in 1973, was immediately acclaimed as an outstanding breakthrough. On viewing the first images, Donald wrote to Kossoff to express his appreciation: "I fairly drooled over some of your pictures."[86] Gray-scaling gave an impression of the internal texture of tissue that was particularly helpful diagnostically. For instance, disorders of the placenta such as those due to rhesus disease or hypertensive infarction could now be confidently recognized on the basis of their ultrasonic appearance. As Kossoff put it, gray-scale "had the shortest transition phase between development and acceptance," because the improvement in the quality and interpretability of the images was truly dramatic.[87]

Good gray-scale images were, however, technically difficult to achieve. Inspired by Kossoff's success and prodded by Donald's enthusiasm, Brian Fraser, at Nuclear Enterprises, set one of his most talented engineers the task of designing a commercial gray-scale system for the NE4102. Alan Cole based his apparatus on the scan converter, a device recently introduced in the broadcasting industry for changing one television format into another. Cole's specially modified converter enabled the signal from the NE4102 to be displayed on a high-quality television monitor. This made many shades of gray available for imaging purposes. The ultrasound machines in the Western Infirmary and the Queen Mother's Hospital were promptly adapted to incorporate Cole's device, and Donald ran some clinical trials.[88] Besides enabling more diagnostic information to be displayed, the use of television monitors altered the experience of being scanned. The older, smaller oscilloscope screens were best viewed in the dark. The new monitors presented larger, brighter displays that could be used with higher levels of ambient illumination. Scanning would henceforth take place in rooms lit almost as brightly as other parts of the hospital. This was another step in the assimilation of ultrasound scanning into the everyday clinical routines of both obstetrician and patient.

Donald and his colleagues did not welcome all innovation as warmly as they greeted gray-scaling. As mentioned in chapter 8, in 1966, the German electronics company Siemens marketed a real-time scanner, the Vidoson. At a conference in Munster early in 1966, Fleming had seen moving pictures taken by a preproduction model and thought them of quite good quality.[89] But he was not sufficiently impressed to pursue the matter further or to encourage his Glasgow colleagues to do so. He remained convinced that, for clinical purposes, static B-scanning was far superior.

Siemen's Vidoson used three transducers, which rotated at the focus of a parabolic mirror, set in a small water bath. The display was refreshed fifteen times per second. This was fast enough for fetal movements to be captured, if somewhat jerkily. Definition was relatively poor, and the Vidoson did not support the sophisticated electronic measurement techniques on which the Glasgow group prided itself. The display was limited to B-scan; A-scan and M-mode were not available. Nor could parts of the image be magnified. Campbell shared Fleming's low opinion: "There was a German machine called the Vidoson, which gave real-time, and I never thought it would catch on. It wasn't a very flattering image."[90]

Nevertheless, throughout the late 1960s, the Vidoson was successfully used in many hospitals in continental Europe. To those who accustomed themselves to working with the real-time scanner, its ability to portray motion was a major advantage, as one commentator observed.

Many doctors, technicians and expectant mothers had, at the time, the moving experience of being able to observe the living fetus. This seems to me to have been a psychological break-through . . . Those who were present in obstetrics departments when this technique was first used soon realized how indispensable it was proving to be in providing a valid means of observation of the fetus and its health, in ascertaining its age and studying its morphology and growth.[91]

In the early 1970s, a number of inventors tried to improve on the scanning mechanism of the Vidoson. Most designs were based on rotating or oscillating transducers. McDicken, working in Edinburgh, for instance, devised a rotating transducer system with membrane-oil coupling, which went into production as the Emisonic 4260. But in Glasgow into the mid-1970s, real-time scanning continued to generate little enthusiasm. Fleming considered that, with the NE4102 converted to gray-scaling, diagnostic ultrasound had evolved as far as it could. (A statement he later much regretted.) Brown and Donald were more optimistic, but both men believed that the future of diagnostic ultrasound lay, not with real-time scanning, but with three-dimensional imaging.

Donald was keenly aware that the diagnosis of multiple pregnancies with compound B-scan was problematic, since it was unlikely that three or more gestational sacs, or fetal heads, could be captured in a single plane. "The diagnosis of triplets," he wrote, "is something that defeats me still and is inevitable as long as we are limited to two dimensions."[92] Accordingly, he took a close interest in attempts to develop three-dimensional imaging. In the late 1960s, Fleming and Hall collaborated with the engineer David Redman in a feasibility study of a holographic method of three-dimensional display.[93] The technique involved the integration, by light holography, of a series of two-dimensional photographic images. The results were crude, however, and the trial was abandoned. Nevertheless, Donald later responded enthusiastically to Dennis Gabor's suggestion of ultrasonic tomography, a combination of ultrasonic data acquisition with holographic optical display.[94] But nothing came of this research, although it continued for several years.

In the early 1970s, working in the Queen Mother's Hospital, Fleming and Powell built a prototype in which a flexible mirror, functioning as a screen, oscillated along an axis perpendicular to the image. If a series of planar sections were displayed in sequence, some impression of depth could be achieved. But again, the technique did not inspire confidence. Brown, meanwhile, had moved from Nuclear Enterprises, first to the Department of Medical Physics at the University of Edinburgh and then to Sonicaid, one of several small ultrasound manufacturers that had sprung up to take advantage of the booming market. The purpose of his move was to lead the development of a prototype three-dimensional scanner, employing a design idea of his own invention.[95] This project occupied Brown's energies for several years but ended in commercial disappointment. He was later to admit that his failure to recognize the advantages that moving images brought to diagnosis was the biggest professional mistake he ever made.[96]

It is ironic that the collective Glaswegian mindset remained so closed to real-time scanning, when one of their number was, in fact, using it successfully. In the early 1970s, Robinson had discovered that if he manually oscillated the transducer rapidly while scanning, he could produce a rough but readable moving image on the short-persistence screen of the NE4102. Using this technique, he could locate the structures he was interested in, particularly the fetal heart, considerably faster than if he waited for a detailed static B-scan to build up on the storage screen. Not only was Robinson producing what was effectively a real-time image, but he was also exploiting one of the important advantages of real-time ultrasonography, its immediacy. Although knowledge of the possibility of producing images in this way became widely disseminated within Glasgow obstetric circles, and several of Robinson's colleagues also employed the technique, no account of it was ever published. It remained merely an aspect of the craft skill of using the NE4102 effectively in the clinic, its more general implications unexplored.

The real advance in the quality of moving ultrasound images came with the development of linear array transducer systems. These were first devised for ophthalmic applications. The eyeball, a hollow structure filled with fluid, is well-suited to ultrasonic examination. However, most patients found it impossible to hold their eyeball still long enough for it to be scanned effectively. In 1964, Werner Buschmann, working in East Berlin in collaboration with the Austrian electronics company Kretztechnik AG, attempted to address this problem by building a probe that was shaped to fit the eye and had ten small transducers arranged in a concave row.[97] Firing each crystal in sequence, the device could rapidly scan the whole of the eye without having to move the probe across its surface. Ten lines of A-scan did not reveal sufficient detail to be of much use to an ophthalmologist, but an unintended feature of the multiple transducer array was that it could detect movement. Both the electronics and the material science of the linear array were complicated, however, and it was not until 1973 that the American company Advanced Diagnostic Research Corporation (ADR), based in Arizona, produced the first commercial real-time scanner that incorporated linear-array technology. For its time, the design of the ADR probe was remarkably sophisticated. It had sixty-four separate transducers, placed side by side in a carefully arranged acoustic configuration, with advanced piezoelectric and electronic components. Image definition was substantially better than in any previous real-time scanner. In Glasgow, nevertheless, real-time scanning continued to be ignored.

This would soon change. In 1975, ADR marketed a further improved model, the 2130. Early in 1976, Donald attended a conference in Dallas, Texas. By this time, ultrasound conferences had become large events, and the academic proceedings were accompanied by exhibitions of equipment, lavishly staged by the manufacturers.[98] Donald was introduced to engineers from ADR, who demonstrated their new scanner. He was, in the words of his wife, Alix, who accompanied him to the meeting, "wildly excited."[99] Learning that Donald's next stop was St. Louis, Missouri, ADR had a 2130 transported to the city's St. Mary's Cathedral Hospital to allow Donald to experiment with it in a clinical setting.

> I certainly saw some interesting stuff which came up very nicely on this machine . . . a partial fetal heartblock at 29 weeks which was demonstrably no artefact and some intrauterine gasping in a 36 year old primigravid diabetic woman . . . I also found a double uterus but with a curious pulsating endometrial lining . . . I managed to follow the fetal spine with increased facility . . . and was able to detect both fetal and maternal pulsations in the placenta—enormous possibilities are going to open up as I see it in real-time scanning.[100]

It was with great reluctance that Donald declined an invitation to travel to Phoenix to play some more with this new toy. But he returned to Glasgow determined to purchase a real-time machine for the Queen Mother's Hospital.

At around the same time, Stuart Campbell was also lecturing in North America. As he recalls:

> I was in Montreal . . . and I went to see round his [Fred Winsberg's] department and I saw this real-time scanner, he had just got it from ADR . . . and there was this image, and I saw the fetus moving and I thought it was so beautiful . . . I phoned up London, and I phoned up the Chief Executive, Medical Director of the hospital, I am just buying a real-time scanner, a real-time scanner is going to

cost you £30,000 and I said could you write a cheque we must have it, it is absolutely essential and so we got it.[101]

Donald now saw real-time scanning as "the development of the future."[102] He was right. Real-time scanners proved to be easier to learn on and to employ clinically than the static B-scanners. The reason for the greater ease of use of the real-time scanner seems to lie largely in the neurophysiology of perception. The human eye and brain are better at interpreting moving images than stationary ones. When one watches a motion picture, cerebral processing integrates the successive frames to provide a richer impression of detail and texture than one would gain from viewing a single frame taken from the same film. Real-time scanners produce this apparent image enhancement. Moreover, the fact that the image on the monitor followed the motion of the probe as it was moved across the abdomen increased the visual and proprioceptive feedback for the operator during the scanning process. Conceptualization of the abdominal contents was thereby facilitated. The need to wait for a photographic image to develop was removed.

Real-time scanners were also lighter and easier to move about. A scanning session generally took less time—advantageous for both patients and obstetricians. Many commentators believed that real-time ultrasound was also more attractive to laypeople, for another reason, as enthusiastically expressed by Campbell.

> A final, perhaps unexpected, benefit of the real-time revolution was that parents on seeing their fetus moving on the screen were informed and delighted and indeed the ultrasound session became a family event. Maternal-fetal bonding was accelerated, health care recommendations more closely adhered to and there was no doubt that parental acceptance of this particular form of high technology was reassuringly high.[103]

For a time, the development of mechanical and linear-array real-time scanners proceeded in parallel. Some mechanical real-time scanners were modified so that rotation of the transducers could be stopped, allowing them to perform as static B-scans when better-quality images and precise measurements were required. However, the arrival of high-quality linear-array scanners coincided with the introduction into medical technology of the electronic computer. With the digitalization of scanned data, linear-array machines could perform the measurements of biparietal diameter, crown-rump length, and so forth, which had been the preserve of the static B-scan.

In the early 1970s, some obstetric units had bought static scanners but were never able to bring them into full clinical service, because the staff could not acquire the necessary skills. Introduction of the real-time scanner made the technology of diagnostic ultrasound available to every clinic that wanted it. It was no longer necessary for the operator to have such a high degree of craft skill. A well-trained technician could now undertake tasks that only recently had required a level of expertise and dexterity that had taken Willocks, Robinson, or Campbell months of endeavor to acquire. Sales staff, moreover, could demonstrate equipment more effectively.

The advent of real-time scanning also radically changed the commercial market for diagnostic ultrasound. Soon, every hospital in the developed world had to provide an ultrasound service. Indeed, before long, most obstetric clinics deployed several machines. In its early years in Glasgow, ultrasound development had been virtually a cottage industry. Engineers could modify a scanner for the specific purposes of individual clinicians. Then, as new models were successively produced by Smiths Industries and Nuclear Enterprises, the scanner became more of a market commodity. The real-time scanner now brought that process to its apotheosis. From the late 1970s onward, ultrasound machines were medical white goods, standardized products in a high-volume global market. In 1972, Nuclear Enterprises had heartily congratulated itself on selling its hundredth machine.[104] Between 1975 and 1979, ADR sold five thousand units of its 2301. In 1981, more than four thousand new ultrasound machines were bought in the United States alone.[105] The market continued to expand exponentially throughout the next two decades. Nuclear Enterprises soon found itself unable to compete in this changing and dynamic marketplace, and the company's reign as the most successful manufacturer in the world was short-lived. Unable to establish itself sufficiently strongly in the crucial North American market, it soon ceased production of ultrasound scanners. By the late 1980s, the market was dominated by the high-volume producers, backed by large electronics corporations, although three smaller Scottish companies, BCF Technology, Diagnostic Sonar, and Dynamic Imaging, all with historical links to Smiths Industries, continued to supply ultrasound equipment.

Real-time scanning did have some disadvantages. It created, for instance, a whole new set of artifacts and spurious images for the operator to guard against. Visualizing "tight corners" of the pelvic cavity was difficult with a linear array, but this was not generally an issue in obstetric usage.[106] Nevertheless, as we have seen, real-time imaging facilitated an unprecedented dissemination of the diagnostic modality. This had one great advantage for obstetricians, with respect to their professional rivals. The radiologists' ambition to control the technology was only realizable when ultrasound scanners were large, capital-intensive pieces of equipment. Smaller and cheaper, both to buy and to operate, than their static predecessors, real-time scanners created greater access to the modality, and thus, in most hospitals, no one specialty could monopolize the equipment. The long-term availability of the technology to clinicians and, in particular, obstetricians was secured.

By the time Donald retired in 1976, diagnostic ultrasound was established as a component of modern clinical routine. The success of the real-time ultrasound machine and the subsequent rapid diffusion of the diagnostic technology throughout the hospital systems of North America, Europe, and Australasia, together with the ever-increasing range of clinical applications, had ended Glasgow's reign as the preeminent center for the development and clinical application of diagnostic ultrasound. Donald was very gratified by the success of his innovation. But his enthusiasm for the real-time scanner did not wholly spring from its diagnostic capabilities, as we explore in the next chapter.

CHAPTER TEN

Ian Donald after Ultrasound

Contraception and Abortion

In his last decade as Regius Professor at the University of Glasgow, Ian Donald continued his work with ultrasound and developed some other technological interests. In 1968, he adopted the "Snake" as a tool to hold surgical instruments in place during intricate procedures, pioneering its application in the new technique of laparoscopic sterilization.[1] Ever eager to make his mark as a technical innovator, he modified the mechanism that secured the Snake to the operating table.[2] In 1970, the manufacturer of a suction amnioscope (a device for sampling amniotic fluid through the vagina) provided him with its latest model to test. Donald wrote back proposing several design modifications and suggesting a novel use for the instrument in the transabdominal aspiration of the contents of "large clearly benign ovarian cysts." He concluded, somewhat insouciantly, "I am about to try this out on an enormous cyst in a child aged 14 tomorrow and will let you know how I get on," then added in a handwritten postscript: "I duly carried out the operation this morning and was able with the help of the suction amnioscope to empty the cyst sufficiently to deliver it through a very small incision and thereby turn what would have been a big operation with a very large incision into a relatively minor affair."[3] This episode illustrates the remarkable freedom of action that Donald enjoyed as a Scottish clinical professor—one of the conditions that enabled his success with the development of ultrasound.

Sometime around 1972, Donald embarked on a fresh research project in reproductive technology. He hoped to develop an electronic device that could detect when ovulation was about to take place. Unlike diagnostic ultrasound, this attempt at innovation failed. This episode is of some interest both because it can be contrasted with his earlier achievements and because it sheds light on the social role that Donald envisaged for technology, including diagnostic ultrasound, in reproductive medicine.

Donald's attitude to the changing sexual mores of the 1960s was a negative one. He disapproved of extramarital sexual activity and feared that easier availability of contraception was contributing to a moral decline: "Contraceptive techniques and family planning, in so far as they make possible responsible parenthood, are among the great boons of our age but in so far as they facilitate licence and abuse then their effect can be socially disruptive."[4] Donald had serious misgivings about the contraceptive pill, fearing that it might cause persistent atrophy of the ovaries. He was also concerned by reports that the incidence of blighted ovum was greater in conceptions occurring within six months of ceasing oral contraception.[5] His major objection was not, however, medical. "My hostility to the contraceptive pill is not based upon its alleged vascular effects nor even possible carcinogenic sequelae," but rather on "the sheer irresponsibility it introduces into sex."[6] Although he was a pioneer of laparoscopic sterilization, it was not a procedure that Donald resorted to readily. He was prepared to sterilize only women who already had several children or those who had bad obstetric histories, and only if other methods of contraception were not feasible.[7] Sterilization was preferable to abortion, however.[8] In 1973, Donald estimated that his team had performed "200 sterilisations for every so-called legalised abortion."[9] He favored a sterilization technique that could be reversed, should the woman's circumstances change, even though his operation could and occasionally did fail to afford complete protection against pregnancy. Donald commended this arrangement to a female colleague as "keeping you half right with the Holy Father."[10]

Despite his equivocal attitude to sterilization, Donald saw it as essential that women should be able to control their fertility. In his view, the provision of a safe and effective means of doing so was one of the great challenges facing late twentieth-century medicine. His preference was for an improvement in the reliability of the rhythm method. Donald believed that a form of contraception based on the timing of intercourse was suitable for women in stable, responsible relationships—who were, in any case, the only group he believed should be using birth control at all. Such a method would also have the enormous advantage that it would be acceptable to the Roman Catholic Church. A device that detected ovulation would also be of use to couples wishing to optimize their chances of conceiving.

Donald dubbed his invention the Ovutector.[11] Its operation was based on the observation that, prior to ovulation, there is an increase in blood supply to the ovary, marking the "intense local activity associated with the final ripening of the Graafian follicle."[12] Ovulation generally takes place from only one ovary in each menstrual cycle. So, if the blood flow to one ovary were to increase markedly compared with the other, that could be taken as an indication that ovulation would soon take place. Donald enlisted technical support from his Department of Ultrasound Technology. Jonathan Powell and a skeptical John Fleming set about undertaking in vitro experiments to simulate the effect of differential blood flow.

These first investigations, which involved the use of thermistors (resistors whose resistance changes predictably with temperature) in a water bath, were in some respects reminiscent of the early experiments with diagnostic ultrasound. Indeed, the Ovutector project sprang directly from Donald's enthusiasm for visualization of the internal structures of the human body. In the course of a gynecological procedure with the laparoscope, he had been lucky enough to observe the "close application of the fimbriae of the [fallopian] tube to the ovarian cortex," as an egg was released.[13] It was this exciting, fortuitous visual insight into its mechanism that inspired him to try to exploit the physiological changes associated with ovulation.

The Ovutector consisted of a probe made from dental acrylic, with two arms, semicircular in cross section and hinged like a pair of scissors. The basic design was modeled on a stretcher for ladies' evening gloves. Perhaps a distant family resemblance to the short-handled obstetric forceps might also be discerned. A small thermistor was fitted into the end of each arm. The arms of the probe could be closed together for insertion into the vagina and then opened out to place the thermistors in the lateral vaginal fornices, on either side of the cervix. Donald was able to check the position in which the thermistors settled in the vagina by ultrasonically scanning a female colleague who volunteered to insert the device.

Before use, the Ovutector was immersed in water at a known temperature. The operating principle was that if one thermistor were nearer to an active ovary, its temperature would change more rapidly than that of its counterpart, owing to the greater blood flow on that side of the pelvic cavity. Donald took considerable delight in showing audiences how the Ovutector worked, by taking out his false teeth and putting one arm of the probe under his tongue and the other between his gum and his cheek. He could usually demonstrate that blood flow under the tongue was greater.[14]

An application to the World Health Organization for a grant to support the development of the Ovutector was turned down, much to Donald's disgust.

But his cause was taken up by the Society of Jesus, which supplied funding to allow biochemical studies to proceed. The purpose of these studies was to correlate the Ovutector readings with hormonal changes in the urine. Powell built a few prototype devices, and Donald recruited some female volunteers, including three Dublin midwives. There was a widespread rumor in Glasgow medical circles—for which, unfortunately, we have found no documentary corroboration—that the Archbishop of Dublin offered to encourage Irish nuns to volunteer their services.[15] Certainly, Donald's work in this area received considerable moral as well as financial backing from the Catholic Church. Thomas Winning, then the auxiliary bishop of Glasgow, also offered his support.[16]

Donald continued work on his electronic contraceptive for several years, but eventually, in the early 1980s, the venture was abandoned. The detection of differential blood flow proved more difficult than Donald had hoped, and its association with ovulation less clear. He was also disappointed that several volunteers found the method aesthetically unacceptable. In contrast to his experience with ultrasound, Donald met with resistances, to use Pickering's term, that he could not overcome.[17] He was unable adequately to make human biology and human agency cooperate with him in this novel technological development. And, again unlike ultrasound, his proposed innovation had to compete with a powerful, well-financed alternative. The Billings method of observing changes in the cervical mucus became the preferred means of detecting the fertile period and improving the precision of rhythm contraception.[18]

Another of Donald's major concerns, as his retirement approached, was securing his legacy in the university's Department of Obstetrics and Gynaecology. In 1975, he made considerable efforts to persuade Sir Charles Wilson, then university principal, to set up an Institute of Sonar, with the aim of ensuring that Glasgow remained a leading center for ultrasound research and clinical application. The dean of medicine, Professor Edward McGirr, was lukewarm about the scheme. While acknowledging the historic magnitude of Donald's achievements, he considered that the set-up at the Queen Mother's Hospital was "no longer at the front of the field."[19] He was also of the opinion that ultrasound scanning was now so established as a routine procedure that "the potential research interest, except for the enthusiast, is probably minor." When the time came to choose the next Regius Professor, the dean and the principal decided that obstetrics and gynecology in the university needed a new direction.[20] Those candidates who proposed to take up Donald's baton in ultrasound research were rejected, and Charles Whitfield, whose research interests lay in the monitoring of labor, was appointed to the Regius Chair. Donald knew and admired Whitfield and respected the university's right to make a strategic change of research leadership. He professed himself satisfied that his successor was not, as he put it, "a permissive bastard."[21] In this context, not being permissive meant not being liberal on abortion.

Donald's attitude to abortion had been a restrictive one throughout his career. Very few terminations were carried out in either the Western Infirmary or the Queen Mother's Hospital during his period of office. Donald generally refused to perform abortion unless the fetus was grossly abnormal. His personal rule on abortion was "only when it is cast-iron clear that the child is so mentally defective as to be incapable of spiritual development."[22] In other words, he was not willing to perform abortions in cases of mild or moderate physical handicap and certainly not for social reasons. Indeed, Donald's interventions in pregnancy tended in the opposite direction, toward the preservation of fetal life. He even went to the length of attempting to save an ectopic fetus by transplanting it to the uterus—a heroic surgical endeavor that ended in failure but might be taken as emblematic of his attitude to the gynecologist's proper role with respect to the fetus.[23]

Prior to the 1967 Abortion Act, the legal situation of abortion in Scotland was different from that south of the border. The 1861 Offences Against the Person Act, which outlawed abortion in England and Wales, did not apply to Scotland. Prosecutions of "back-street" abortionists were usually brought under the common law of unlawful killing rather than more precisely targeted legislation. In effect, as far as the performance of abortion by qualified medical practitioners was concerned, the matter was left to the conscience of individual doctors. It was this lack of a specific legal prohibition that enabled Sir Dugald Baird to operate a liberal abortion policy in Aberdeen for many years before 1967.[24]

Although he appreciated that Baird was acting out of compassion for women burdened by too many pregnancies (and irresponsible husbands), Donald was fundamentally at odds with Baird's acceptance of termination as a remedy for a social ill. "The really fundamental point at issue," Donald wrote, "is whether conceived but unborn life is important—It is a question of respect for it versus the Aberdonian philosophy of the 'tyranny of motherhood.'"[25] Donald was vehemently opposed to David Steel's Medical Termination of Pregnancy Bill (which became the 1967 Abortion Act). On at least one occasion, Donald gathered signatures for an anti-abortion petition from the women in his own ante-natal wards.[26] Only two dared to refuse.

When the Society for the Protection of the Unborn Child (SPUC) was set up to coordinate opposition to Steel's bill, Donald was a founder member.

> I am now losing a good deal of sleep over this hellish Abortion Bill already past its second reading in the House of Commons and now in its Committee stage. Sir Dugald Baird and his cronies of the Abortion Law Reform Association are doing their worst . . . and I am fighting it hard. I even addressed a Mass Meeting at the Free Trade Hall in Manchester three weeks ago.[27]

The campaign against the bill politicized Donald. His appearance at the Manchester public meeting in 1966 may well have been his first venture into the public gaze as a campaigner, but it was a role in which he would become very familiar.

The passage of the 1967 Abortion Act did not change Donald's policy on abortion. In fact, in the year 1968 to 1969, no abortions at all were performed in the Queen Mother's Hospital. General practitioners who were opposed to abortion being carried out for social reasons tended to refer patients requesting terminations to Donald, knowing that he would refuse.[28] Donald condoned and indeed encouraged this pattern of referral.[29] By contrast, at Glasgow Royal Infirmary, the Muirhead Professor, Malcolm MacNaughton, who had trained under Baird in Aberdeen, operated a more liberal policy.[30] Donald would sometimes refer to his professorial colleague as "the abortionist in the East." However, on at least one occasion, when a woman became pregnant following the failure of Donald's method of sterilization, he referred her to MacNaughton for an abortion, rather than undertake the procedure himself.[31]

Donald's championing of ultrasonic imaging was closely linked to his committed stance against the liberalization of abortion. He believed that the ultrasound image demonstrated, unequivocally, the individuality and humanity of the fetus. He was not afraid to use the technology for this purpose when patients were referred to him for abortion. He would sometimes show ultrasound images to women seeking terminations, in a deliberate attempt to deter them from their chosen course of action. As a colleague described it:

> Then of course you would go and have an ultrasound done and show the mother the picture of this baby you weren't to murder. This all happened in a busy clinic

on a Friday afternoon. So it was full of drama, you were pretty sure of having a couple of dramatic scenes in a Friday afternoon clinic.[32]

These scans, it should be emphasized, were organized solely for the purpose of persuading women to continue with their pregnancies.[33] Donald believed, probably rightly, that many women were indeed deterred from proceeding to abortion as a result.[34]

Donald's attitude to abortion was not absolutist, however. His stance was substantially different from that of the Catholic Church, whose opposition to the termination of pregnancy was categorical. On one occasion, giving a public lecture in Dublin, Donald had sufficient moral courage to criticize the Irish obstetric profession for not performing therapeutic terminations frequently enough.[35] The constitution of the Irish Republic forbade abortion for any reason whatsoever. But, as an advocate of ultrasound scanning, Donald asserted that there was little point in having a diagnostic technology that enabled one to detect major congenital abnormalities early in pregnancy if one was not prepared to offer termination selectively to women who were so affected: "One cannot have at one's disposal highly accurate scientific information as is now available by modern techniques of prenatal diagnosis of fetal abnormality and not take the responsibility of making intelligent use of it."[36] Donald was effectively urging Irish obstetricians to challenge the Irish abortion law and to use the evidence provided by the ultrasound scanner in defense of their position.[37]

Donald spoke regularly at meetings of the charity Action for the Crippled Child, and he received a grant from the organization to work on the ultrasound detection and assessment of disabling conditions before birth.[38] He would refuse to put his name to statements by pro-life groups if he considered their attitudes to the abortion of severely impaired or "monstrous" fetuses to be too restrictive.[39] As we saw in chapter 9, Donald was willing to abort microcephalic fetuses, even though an occasional microcephalic child can achieve considerable educational development. His views also reflected the prevailing negative attitudes toward children with Down syndrome.[40] "I spoke to the Edinburgh bunch" of the SPUC, he wrote, "and told them a few home truths about major abnormalities like Mongolism."[41] To Donald, one of the advantages of ultrasound imaging was that it would allow the termination of pregnancy to be decided on, according to appropriate clinical criteria, by medical professionals.

(((((Ian Donald retired from the Regius Chair in September 1976. In October, the Royal College of Obstetricians and Gynaecologists marked the occasion by holding its Scientific Congress in Glasgow. The meeting was entitled "Sonar in Obstetrics and Gynaecology," and Usama Abdulla, Stuart Campbell, John Fleming, Angus Hall, Patricia Morley, and Hugh Robinson all spoke. Afterward, Donald gave the James Simpson Oration. This was a signal honor, because the oration had previously always been given at the Royal College's premises in London. In a rather diffuse and literary talk, Donald took the opportunity to denounce the members of the Royal College not only for their readier resort to abortion for social or trivial reasons but also for their complicity in the moral decay of society as a whole. On another occasion, he described abortion as "the thin end of the wedge that leads to Belsen."[42] It is hardly surprising that these trenchant expressions of his moral indignation provoked, on occasion, equally strong responses. A Birmingham obstetrician apparently took to referring to Donald as "that red-headed bastard from Glasgow."[43] Donald rather gloried in the description.

In retirement, Donald remained greatly in demand as a lecturer on diagnostic ultrasound. He traveled the world, always accompanied by Alix Donald as "cardiac chaperone" to get him home should he fall ill. But his most prominent public role from 1976 onward was that of a moral campaigner.[44] In April 1978, he published a long, polemic article in the *Daily Telegraph*, entitled "After the Pill: Society under Siege."[45] He bemoaned liberal attitudes to premarital sexual activity, contraception, abortion, and divorce, all of which he associated with a decline in respect for authority and established religion.

> There is a certain squalor about multiple disposable sexual relationships, quite apart from the very nasty effects of infection and unwanted pregnancy. Eventual marriage after such a history has little basis for that loyalty and mutual trust without which no marriage can be expected to endure whether fertile or not . . . We should recognise the evildoers for what they are, the pornographers, the advocates of "free love," the drug pushers, the perverts and the exploiters of youth's very natural urges and vulnerable passions.[46]

Donald's jeremiad evidently struck a chord with the readership of the *Telegraph*. He had articulated widely held anxieties about changing social and sexual attitudes and their effect on young people. The resulting correspondence, both to the newspaper and to Donald personally, was voluminous and overwhelmingly supportive. Indeed, Donald received only one letter that expressed dissent from his diagnosis of moral and social crisis. It came, oddly enough, from the Young Conservatives, one of whose office-bearers offered a modest defense of the right to personal freedom on matters of sexual expression.[47] From then on, Donald seems to have been something of a figurehead to those of a conservative (with a small *c*) social persuasion.[48] He was regularly invited to address church and parents' groups, as well as organizations such as the Responsible Society.

In 1984, the Report of the Committee of Enquiry into Human Fertilisation and Embryology (the Warnock Report) recommended that experimentation be allowed on human embryos for up to fourteen days after in vitro fertilization.[49] Donald reacted with horror. He was inspired to produce some of his most acerbic and scathing rhetoric: "a totally secular, irreligious type of report which would satisfy any atheist . . . Christians cannot fail to recognise its passive acceptance of much that is evil or potentially so." He stigmatized experimentation on human embryos as "a sort of scientific cannibalism," motivated by "sheer arrogance . . . to outdo the Almighty that must strike at the very hearts of Christian men and women."[50] The irony that the eggs used for in vitro fertilization were harvested under ultrasonic guidance was not lost on him.

Throughout the anti-abortion campaigns that Donald pursued in his retirement, he routinely employed the ultrasound image of the fetus as a powerful persuasive resource. He regarded moving images as particularly useful in this regard. Indeed, a large part of his enthusiasm for the innovation of real-time ultrasound flowed from a conviction that it conveyed the life of the fetus more vividly than a static image could. Shortly after real-time machines became available in Scotland, Donald filmed a scan of a healthy, normal pregnancy. He regularly showed this film, entitled *Human Development before Birth*, at pro-life meetings.[51] Here is an excerpt from a presentation he gave to such an audience in 1978:

Here's the baby see how he jumps . . . This baby is about a 12 week pregnancy . . . she has only missed two periods. She does not even know she is pregnant. She certainly cannot feel these movements but there is no doubt about the reality, . . . now you see it move its hand up to its face you see his head is up here and his chest is down here then he throws his legs out and his arms . . . You see his hands come up like that. And you see his face here, the back of his head . . . This is the fluid sac in which he is contained. The full bladder is this way . . . It is rather like a child on a trampoline, tremendous strength, energy and vitality.[52]

Donald's commentary moves seamlessly from fetus to pregnant woman and back again, from her lack of awareness of her pregnancy, to the fetus's head, to its fluid sac, to the maternal full bladder. Mother and fetus are conflated, as it were. One gets a strong sense that together they constitute, in Donald's mind, a single clinical entity. And yet, simultaneously, the fetus is also an individual in its own right. Donald conveys a strong sense of the fetus's distinctive personality and identity, with "strength, energy and vitality."

To Donald, pointing to the characteristics of the developing human being in this way was a matter of great pride, a triumphant culmination of his life's work in obstetrics. He also drew from this identifiable individuality of the early fetus a strong moral message.

> Anybody who says this is not alive is talking through his neck. It is a lie, which is intolerable and seeing is believing . . . And one of the things that this film has done if it has done nothing else, is to kill forever the lie of the pro-abortion lobby that there's nothing there just a potential human being, just—oh look at that jump, he bumps his head against the roof nearly, doesn't he—This lie that he is just a potential human being when in fact that baby is as human as an old man . . . the same individual from conception to the grave. And when you destroy a baby by abortion that is what you are destroying. I think you have got to face the fact honestly . . . There can be no argument about it, and if I have done nothing else in my life, I have killed that dirty lie that the foetus is just a nondescript meaningless jelly, disposable at will, something to be got rid of.[53]

Donald's film was broadcast on British and Irish television, where it occasioned widespread comment. He was asked to supply copies to American pro-life groups. But the most dramatic reaction to the film followed its showing in Italy. In 1979, the Italian debate on abortion reform was at its height. Donald was invited to Milan to show his film at a public meeting of the International European Pro-Life Movement. A considerable commotion ensued. Donald received a rapturous reception inside the hall, but he had to be provided with a police escort to protect him from the hostile crowd outside. *Human Development before Birth* was later broadcast on Italian television. In the midst of the turmoil, Donald was invited to a private audience with the Pope, in Rome, a meeting he described as "perhaps the crowning event of my life."[54] Donald was particularly impressed that the Holy Father had copies of his ultrasound papers and appreciated their significance in the recognition of fetal life. He was later to describe John Paul II as "the greatest man on earth."[55] Although he remained an Anglican, Donald frequently expressed his admiration for the firm guidance provided by John Paul II on sexual and reproductive morality.

(((((An irony of the story of obstetric ultrasound is that Donald's program to individualize the fetus produced effects quite different from those he had intended. Ultrasonic scanning certainly gave the fetus a public presence that it could never have had before. The unborn child began to appear in the family photograph albums of thousands, and then hundreds of thousands, of proud parents. It was Donald himself who initiated the practice of giving women copies of their scan photographs. Ultrasound images of fetuses became increasingly common outside the medical domain—for instance, as illustrations for newspaper and magazine articles. Seeing images of the fetus, either their own or those of other women, may indeed have deterred many women from having abortions.[56] But within the technical context of obstetrics research, by far the major impact of the ultrasound image was in precisely the opposite direction.

As we have seen, in the 1970s, ultrasound made possible the detection of many fetal abnormalities and became the essential tool of intrauterine, or prenatal, diagnosis. The delineation of each fetus's individual characteristics led to the increasingly detailed scrutiny of fetal structure for pathology. In this area of its use, ultrasound imaging and abortion were not in contention but were complementary. Indeed, they were mutually dependent, one upon the other. Given that the possibilities of detection far outstripped those of therapy, the only option that could be offered to the majority of women who were presented with a diagnosis of fetal abnormality was termination of the pregnancy. Research into the detection of fetal abnormality would not have proceeded at the pace it did, from the 1970s onward, if that clinical option had not become more readily available. The net effect of the introduction of the ultrasound scanner was the rigorous imposition on the fetus of a reductionist discrimination between the normal and the pathological, which Donald found morally repugnant.

By the late 1970s, Donald was aware of these developments and was appalled by them. He wrote, "My own personal fears are that my researches into early intrauterine life may yet be misused towards its more accurate destruction."[57] And, on another occasion, "I myself would not like to feel that I had contributed to a Huxleyian Brave New World."[58] He mused as to whether, if he were at the beginning of his medical career rather than at its end, he would again choose obstetrics and gynecology as a specialty.[59] His dissatisfaction with obstetrics was that the range of concerns of its practitioners had become mundane and secular.

> Will the gynaecologist of tomorrow, I wonder, be able to withstand the humanist pressure groups, that we may, in the words of a famous Anglican Collect, "So pass through things temporal that we lose not the things that are eternal." Or will we simply fall in with the new philosophy of expediency, to supply contraception without advice, abortion when contraception fails, and a neutral attitude towards the vagaries of human behaviour. Would this be failing the traditional role of guide, philosopher and friend to our patients?[60]

Donald was here expressing sentiments with which he would have been familiar during his training and early career at St. Thomas's. In particular, he was articulating the holistic vision of his distinguished teacher John Shields Fairbairn. As outlined in chapter 3, Fairbairn maintained that the proper discharge of the obstetrician-gynecologist's professional responsibilities involved not only the provision of comprehensive medical care to mother and fetus but also the assumption of leadership in psychological, moral, and social issues.

Donald's views on the issue of abortion coincided precisely with Fairbairn's. In 1927, Fairbairn made it clear that he was uncompromisingly opposed to the termination of pregnancy for social reasons.

> I would advocate that none other than purely medical considerations be allow to weigh . . . Once other than purely medical factors are allowed to count no line can be drawn between criminal and therapeutic abortion . . . It is obvious why all civilised nations protect themselves against abortion-mongering for it is but infanticide anticipated by a few months. The destruction of a pregnancy . . . is the destruction of life and the killing of a potential citizen.[61]

Fairbairn characterized the increased willingness, as he saw it, to "resort to the procuring of abortion," in the absence of "grave danger to the mother," as the consequence of "a slackening of moral standards." Unlike Donald, Fairbairn had no reliable means of assessing the health of the fetus. Many of the maternal diseases that Fairbairn accepted as valid grounds for termination had become manageable by the 1970s. But otherwise, the views of the two men may be regarded as essentially identical.[62]

Forty years or so on from his student days, many aspects of Donald's clinical work were radically different from that of his teachers. He practiced a form of obstetrics that was considerably more technologically mediated and interventionist than that of Fairbairn or Wrigley. Yet his use of technology, especially obstetric ultrasound, was guided by the same social and profession agenda that his teachers at St. Thomas's had championed.

Donald and his generation of obstetricians had secured reductions in the rates of maternal and neonatal mortality and morbidity, which his predecessors could only have dreamed of and which they would undoubtedly have admired as enormous achievements. And yet, at the end of his career, Donald felt that, judged by the criteria central to his and Fairbairn's credo for the specialty, obstetrics and gynecology was in danger of failure.

> The passage of the Abortion Act . . . is only a signpost in the changing world, a result more than a cause . . . I think it is necessary for all of us to take close stock of the effect from all that is happening . . . on ourselves as clinicians who find ourselves willy-nilly at the hub of ethical decisions. The professional status of the gynaecologist is under threat and if we cannot embrace the philosophy and exercise the judgement then we have no right to claim a status much above that of a plumber or a technician.[63]

To Fairbairn, there could have been few fates more disgraceful than being regarded as the equivalent of "a plumber or a technician."[64] He had articulated a form of obstetric discourse that embodied the values of patrician clinical holism, which entailed responsibility for the welfare not merely of women and babies but of society as a whole. A crucial aspect of that elevated position of trust was ensuring that decision making in the termination of pregnancy was based solely on medical criteria. This was a position that Donald heartily endorsed.

This is not, of course, to argue that Donald was wholly a creature of his training at St. Thomas's, or merely a slavish disciple of Fairbairn. He was in many respects his own man, with his own views. Important aspects of his moral outlook—his sympathy with the poor, his disdain for social pretension, his abhorrence of apartheid in South Africa, his rejection of elitist private practice—might be attributed (if an explanation is sought) more to his father's charitable egalitarianism and sense of civic responsibility than to any influence of Fairbairn. Glasgow provided a context for obstetric practice very different in character from the London voluntary hospitals, not to mention Harley Street and Wimpole Street. Nevertheless, the values of clinical holism were the standard under which Donald and his contemporaries had labored to improve the status of obstetrics throughout the 1940s and 1950s. It is hardly surprising that he continued to regard moral judgments as falling centrally within his professional remit in the 1960s and 1970s. And one of the purposes to which he put the ultrasound image of the fetus was the articulation and defense of that moral agenda.

It would be an exaggeration to say that Donald's old age was a bitter one. He enjoyed the warm support of his wife and his family and the consolations of his profound religious faith. Feeling that he had lived a full and active life, he took a great deal of satisfaction from what he had achieved in medicine. He was delighted to be made a Commander of the British Empire in 1973. He received many honorary fellowships from, among others, the American Institute of Ultrasound in Medicine, the American Gynecological Society, the Edinburgh Obstetrical Society, and the American College of Obstetricians and Gynecologists. The universities of London and Glasgow each gave him an honorary DSc. He was awarded the Blair Bell Medal of the Royal Society of Medicine and the Victor Bonney Prize of the Royal College of Surgeons of England. The Ian Donald School of Ultrasound in Dubrovnik was named after him. In 1981, he was nominated for the Nobel Prize, and if a prize had been awarded for the invention of diagnostic ultrasound, he would certainly have had a share of it. He yearned for a knighthood but was fated never to receive one.[65] Although he was put forward for the honor twice, on both occasions the responsible civil servants felt that the award might be interpreted as an official endorsement of his opposition to the Abortion Act.

As Donald frequently acknowledged, he would not have attained any degree of success as a pioneer of diagnostic ultrasound without the "help I got from my Scottish engineering friends [who] made the whole thing possible."[66] As we have seen, among all the engineers he worked with, he owed—and recognized—a special debt to the inventive brilliance of Tom Brown.[67] Brown's later career, however, was problematic. After the commercial failure of the three-dimensional scanner he built with Sonicaid, Brown experienced serious professional difficulties. He had long periods of unemployment, interspersed with short-term contracts in engineering work unrelated to ultrasound. Financial difficulties, compounded with ill health and personal problems, sowed, as he put it, "the seeds of bitterness."[68] He wrote to Donald in 1982:

When I received the programme for the Brighton meeting on ultrasound, with its foreword by the Duke of Edinburgh, and the prominence of the names of so many of the non-contributors I have seen climbing aboard the bandwagon over the years and my own apparently total eclipse—I want to hit out.[69]

Gradually, Brown recovered his health and established himself as a consulting engineer. But financial security took a long time to achieve, and he never worked in product development again. He now lives in retirement in Fife, proud of his achievements in ultrasound, jealous of his place in the history of the subject, but becoming more philosophical about the way in which his career as an ultrasound innovator petered out prematurely.

Brown's contribution to the development of diagnostic ultrasound has not been entirely ignored. In 1984, he and Donald were honored together as the first two Honorary Members of the British Medical Ultrasound Society. Brown's role in the original paper of 1958 is commemorated by the Donald, MacVicar, and Brown Lecture, the keynote address of the BMUS annual meeting. In 1988, Brown was presented with the History of Medical Ultrasound Pioneer Award by the World Federation of Ultrasound in Medicine and Biology, and in 1996, he received the Ian Donald Gold Medal for Technical Merit from the International Society of Obstetrics and Gynecology. In 2007, he was made an honorary Fellow of the Royal College of Obstetricians and Gynaecologists. But even this degree of belated recognition is hardly commensurate with the magnitude of his contribution to the development of diagnostic ultrasound. The contrast with the wealth of tributes showered on Donald is telling. Brown has never, it may be noted, been honored by the University of Glasgow, whose scientific and clinical reputation he did so much to enhance.

One might discern here, in the relative neglect of Brown as compared with Donald, the workings of what has been called the Matthew effect—"For every one that hath shall be given"—in the allocation of academic honors. An individual already eminent is more likely to attract further marks of distinction than a colleague of lower profile. Moreover, when a publication has several authors, "the role of junior collaborators becomes obscured by the brilliance that surrounds their illustrious co-authors."[70] There is also an evident tendency for the medical profession to attract greater social esteem than the engineering profession. It is revealing that when establishment of the BMUS keynote address was first mooted, the original intention was to call it simply the Ian Donald Lecture. Only when John Fleming (himself an engineer) pointed out to the then president of BMUS that the Glaswegian achievement could not reasonably be attributed to Donald alone was the decision made to name the lecture for all three of the original pioneers.

There is another issue here, however. Donald had many of the personal characteristics that often distinguish the outstanding medical or scientific innovator. He was self-assured, self-confident, and tough-minded. He possessed great reserves of fortitude and determination. All in all, he was a charismatic figure. He created what Merton has called "a bright ambience," which is still remembered with some awe and affection by many of his former colleagues in Glasgow.[71] Yet it is striking how few of his junior colleagues went on to follow their chief in the successful and sustained prosecution of important research. Unlike many other charismatic scientific leaders, Donald did not found a major school of investigators, nor did he populate the key positions within his specialty with his protégés. We have noted how both MacVicar and Willocks dropped out of research when they had secured their consultant posts. Robinson, for whom Donald evidently had high hopes, also gradually ceased to be active in research. Only Campbell might be said to have fully emulated Donald's example and acquired a lasting eminence in both clinical medicine and research. It was not that Donald selfishly or illegitimately denied the younger men their fair share of credit. Rather, his personality had a degree of self-absorption that did not equip him to take the care and time necessary to rear and fledge the next generation of researchers in his own image. Possibly Brown was as disadvantaged by this failing, if such it should be termed, as were his clinical colleagues.

Ian Donald died on June 19, 1987, aged seventy-seven. In October, a memorial service was held in the Chapel of the University of Glasgow. James Willocks gave the eulogy. His concluding remarks were: "If you seek Ian Donald's memorial, look around you and in every maternity hospital you will see ultrasound in use."[72] This was a fitting and accurate, indeed a modest, tribute to a great medical innovator. But, as we have observed in this chapter and will explore further in the next, the legacy to which Willocks referred was always to be, in certain aspects at least, a problematic and disputed one.

CHAPTER ELEVEN

Maternity and Technology

At Ian Donald's memorial service, James Willocks suggested that those seeking a memorial to him should look around them in any maternity hospital. But one particular hospital manifested Donald's legacy very directly indeed. The Queen Mother's Hospital was, to a substantial degree, Donald's creation. Situated across Kelvingrove Park from the University of Glasgow and the Western Infirmary, in an impressive position above the confluence of the Rivers Clyde and Kelvin, the QM (as it became known) was planned and built to realize Donald's conception of what good obstetric care should be. It was, in itself, an innovative piece of medical technology. It was also an environment designed specifically to facilitate a form of clinical care in which ultrasonic diagnosis would have a central role. An examination of the character of the QM assists us in analyzing the role of technology, especially ultrasound, in the changing social relations surrounding birth and reproduction in the last decades of the twentieth century.

In 1954, Hector Hetherington, principal of the university, attracted Donald to Glasgow with the promise that a new maternity hospital would be built and that the holder of the Regius Chair of Midwifery would have a major part in its planning. Many obstacles had to be overcome before this plan could be realized. Negotiations with the Health Board were complex, and there was difficulty in finding a suitable site. But eventually, in 1958, work began at Yorkhill, adjacent to the Royal Hospital for Sick Children.

Donald threw himself into the design and planning process with his customary vigor, working closely with the architect, Joseph Lea Gleave. Gleave was a fortunate, if somewhat controversial, choice as leader of the project. On the one hand, he had received considerable praise for his innovative design of the Vale of Leven Hospital in Alexandria, Dunbartonshire, which opened in 1955. On the other hand, he was known to be eccentric and unpredictable in his style of work. However, Gleave and Donald evidently collaborated effectively, the professor valuing his colleague's "original" and "imaginative" responses to the challenges of the project.[1]

The Yorkhill site was not an easy one on which to place a large structure, at least with the financial resources at Gleave's disposal. In the context of National Health Service planning in the late 1950s, economy was always a key consideration. The softness of the subsoil meant that any multistory construction required expensive foundation piling. Accordingly, Gleave built horizontally, as far as the long, narrow, and hilly site would allow. Multistory construction was concentrated in a central "spinal ridge," with a large tower at one end. Despite these constraints, the broad main corridor on the ground floor, glazed from floor to ceiling on one side, gave an impression of spaciousness, and from the first floor there were fine views southwest across the Clyde to Renfrewshire.

Notwithstanding the restrictions under which he and Gleave had worked, Donald was able to say, with evident satisfaction, that he got everything he asked for from the Health Board, save "one lift shaft and a couple of coats of paint."[2] He personally selected many of the staff of the new hospital, including Marjorie Marr as the matron and Winnie Childs as medical almoner. Like Fairbairn, Donald saw the almoner as a key appointee; Childs's provision for unmarried mothers and their babies was central to Donald's restrictive abortion policy. Donald chose the name of the hospital (in honor of his favorite member of the Royal Family) and successfully petitioned for the Queen Mother herself to be invited to perform the official opening (fig. 11.1). Donald's daughters recall the day of the opening ceremony, September 23, 1964, as one of high excitement in their household.

The regime that Donald instigated in the Queen Mother's Hospital was different in several key respects from that of the old Royal Maternity Hospital at Rottenrow. Donald had insisted that the layout of the building be arranged around what he saw as an essential distinction between, on the one hand, physiological labor, in which nature could be allowed to take its course, under supervision and with provision of analgesia, in conditions of normal hospital hygiene, and, on the other hand, labors that required instrumental intervention, which should all, in his opinion, be regarded as surgical cases. The latter were to be undertaken with full aseptic precautions in place. Accordingly, the surgical corridor was strictly demarcated from the rest of the hospital and had a number of arrangements to preserve its aseptic integrity, such as double

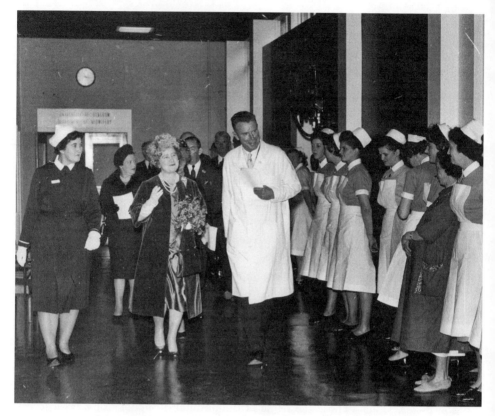

Figure 11.1. Her Majesty The Queen Mother with Professor Ian Donald and Matron Marjorie Marr (*left*) in the main corridor of The Queen Mother's Hospital during the official opening, September 23, 1964. *Reproduced with permission of Yorkhill NHS Archive*

doors and positive-pressure ventilation. The building was designed to allow rapid transfer of patients from the normal labor rooms to the surgical corridor, whenever the need arose. Such transfer happened relatively frequently, since Donald was, by this time, willing to resort to the Wrigley forceps quite promptly if the progress of labor seemed to stall with the baby's head low in the pelvis. Donald also chose to regard all breech presentations as surgical cases requiring the attendance of an anesthetist.

Many other maternity hospitals at this time divided their patients not according to whether they were physiological or surgical cases but whether they were in the first or late stages of labor. As one of Donald's correspondents put it, "This results in a mad scramble to transfer fully dilated patients from a first stage room . . . [to] the delivery theatre . . . There is a relatively high incidence of uncontrolled deliveries beneath the bedclothes as might be predicted."[3] Using the same type of accommodation for every birth, regardless of its circumstances, also meant that all delivery rooms had to be equipped to a level beyond that necessary for normal delivery. Donald believed that the distinction he made between physiological and abnormal labor was more rational and economical and that it could save lives by providing surgical cases with a better standard of care and equipment.[4] Given the criticisms that were to be made of obstetric practice in the following decades, it is ironic that Donald's preferred arrangement embodied an assumption that most births were not to be regarded as pathological events.

Another noteworthy feature of the QM was a self-contained "suspect unit," with its own labor ward and delivery room, which housed all patients considered to be infectious. The rigid segregation of infectious cases from the rest of the patient population enabled Donald to allow a liberal regime in the main parts of the hospital. The layout of the wards was planned to enable mothers to look after their babies themselves, in as relaxed an environment as possible. To encourage mothers to be ambulant shortly after birth, spacious and comfortable day rooms were provided, adjacent to the wards on the ground floor. Visiting hours were long and visitors lightly regulated. In a major departure from his own previous practice, Donald allowed children to come into the wards to visit their mothers and greet their new siblings. In most maternity units at this time, including those at Rottenrow, visiting children were deemed to pose a risk of infection and were rigidly excluded from the postnatal wards. In the QM, moreover, men were encouraged to play an active role in supporting their partners before, after, and, increasingly often, during labor. Overall, Donald's credo was that "the atmosphere to be cultivated must be a breakaway from the traditional penitentiary discipline of the hospital of yesterday." In the "Information for Patients" leaflet that he provided for prospective patients, Donald wrote: "It is your hospital. Every thing has been done to provide the atmosphere of a comfortable hotel rather that a hospital."[5] This may have been something of an overstatement, but the leaflet clearly expressed Donald's aspiration to depart from the utilitarian austerity and authoritarianism of previous hospital regimes. He even undertook to ensure that the armchairs in the day room were comfortable for pregnant women to sit in.

It was not only the physical, organizational, and social aspects of the maternity hospital that Donald sought to reform. In the 1969 edition of his textbook

Practical Obstetric Problems, Donald proudly announced that he had seized "the happy opportunity" offered by the opening of the new hospital "to cast aside much that was useless and traditional in both medical and nursing care."[6] For instance, he minimized the use of enemas, ended the use of nonabsorbable perineal sutures, and strongly discouraged the use of elaborate dressings, which required regular changing and were uncomfortable for the patient.

Among its innovations, the Queen Mother's was probably the first hospital in the world to have rooms allocated specifically for both ultrasound examinations and ultrasound research and development. On occasion, ultrasound played a key role in making the essential distinction between normal and abnormal pregnancy that was central to the organization of the hospital. Overall, the fanfare with which Donald presented the QM, both to its lay constituency and to the fellow members of his specialty, announced that, through the instrument of the new hospital, Scottish obstetrics was to be reformed. The institution would deliver a form of maternity care that was both clinically innovative and humane, both scientifically advanced and patient-centered.[7] To Donald, such dual commitments were a key expression of the hospital's modernity and a measure of the extent to which obstetrics had emancipated itself from the discreditable aspects of its past.[8] The Queen Mother's Hospital was, in many respects, a physical realization of the aspirations for the status of specialty for obstetrics that were articulated by John Shields Fairbairn and his colleagues in the 1930s. Enshrined in a facility like the QM, with the most modern diagnostic and therapeutic apparatus at its disposal, and with fine facilities for research and teaching, obstetrics could now hardly be described as the Cinderella of medicine. It was, the new building proclaimed, the equal of any other medical discipline.

The maternity hospital was linked to the adjacent Sick Children's Hospital by both an enclosed walkway and underground passages. The two hospitals shared their service departments of pathology and radiology as well as a number of other facilities. These arrangements had great advantages in economy, but, for Donald, the proximity of his wards to a pediatric hospital exemplified where the most pressing clinical and research challenges facing his specialty now lay—namely, with the health of the fetus and the neonate. Much of the work of the antenatal department, aided by ultrasound scanning, now focused as much on the well-being of the fetus as that of the pregnant woman. The QM also had its own neonatal facilities, and Donald included a pediatrician, Margaret Kerr, on his staff.

Writing before the building opened, Donald acknowledged that "every battleship, at its launch, is reputed to be already out of date," but he hoped that, owing to the inherent flexibility of its design, the Queen Mother's Hospital would "be able to meet the foreseeable changes in obstetric practice." However, the very scientific modernity that was the flagship principle of the hospital quickly rendered unfounded Donald's optimism about the extent to which he could predict the future of his specialty. He had deliberately designed the rooms for normal deliveries to be quite small, allowing the woman to labor in what he had hoped would be a nonthreatening, relatively private environment. (It might be said that he was, to some extent, making a virtue out of a necessity here, given the spatial and economic constraints that he and Gleave were working under. Many of the staff offices and research spaces were also quite small.) When the labor rooms were planned, Donald had not anticipated that within a few years of the QM receiving its first patient, the medical presence at the bedside would greatly increase, both in personnel and equipment. Donald had worked within the customary pattern of attendance by a midwife or obstetrician, or both, accompanied perhaps by a nurse or a medical or midwifery student. Soon, room beside the bed would be taken up by sophisticated instruments to monitor the fetus and provide improved analgesia for the laboring woman, not to mention the arrival in the 1970s of new, mobile, ultrasound scanners. Space had also to be found, increasingly often, for a neonatal pediatrician and her or his equipment and students. The QM's labor rooms were simply not big enough to contain all the accoutrement of the highly medicalized childbirth of the 1970s and 1980s—an accommodation problem exacerbated by the more frequent presence of the woman's husband or partner at the bedside.[9]

Greater demands on space in the delivery room were not the only changes that Donald did not wholly foresee. In the 1950s, the Royal Maternity Hospital had been so overcrowded that only those women who were deemed to be at some risk of a complicated birth, or whose domestic circumstances were unsuitable for a home delivery, were admitted. Thus the overwhelming majority of Rottenrow's patients were drawn from the working class. Middle-class women entered the institution only in an emergency, normally choosing to give birth either at home or in one of the several private maternity homes that were available in the city. However, since the 1940s, the Royal College of Obstetricians and Gynaecologists had been leading a campaign to encourage more women to give birth in a hospital. In 1959, this policy had been emphatically endorsed by the Montgomery Report on Maternity Services in Scotland.[10] Maternity units should be, the medical establishment increasingly argued, the preferred locus for confinement. In the hospital, high standards of hygiene could be maintained and skilled staff were at hand to provide effective pain relief and whatever other professional assistance might be required.

The opening of the QM facilitated this shift toward hospital birth within its catchment area. In the early 1960s, little more than half of Glasgow's births took place in hospitals, despite a continuing problem of inadequate housing in the city. The new hospital provided 112 additional beds, which constituted a substantial step toward the provision of a comprehensive service. These beds were not taken up solely by the poorly housed, working-class women who had formed the major patient base of Rottenrow. Within a few years of the opening of the QM, the private maternity homes that had previously lined Park Circus, in the West End of the city, began to close, as middle-class women became increasingly willing to accept referrals to the attractive new facility at Yorkhill.[11] Donald was sharply critical of the quality of care in the private nursing homes and encouraged this trend very actively.[12] Despite his personal commitment to the NHS, he would occasionally turn a blind eye to one of his senior colleagues admitting a private patient to a single room in the new hospital.[13]

Thus the Queen Mother's Hospital was a technological instrument not only for the delivery of Donald's chosen form of maternity care but also for advancement of the medicalization of childbirth, which was a defining characteristic of the development of obstetrics in Britain in the quarter-century following establishment of the NHS and in which diagnostic ultrasound played a key part. However, an important consequence of the opening of the QM, together with similar institutions elsewhere in the United Kingdom, was that considerable numbers of the well-educated, articulate women of the middle classes were brought into contact with hospital obstetrics, often for the first time. They did not always like what they encountered. With the availability of pharmacological agents to initiate labor, together with fetal monitoring, obstetricians were now managing childbirth in a more interventionist manner than ever before. By the 1970s, the QM had gained a reputation, both within the specialty and among laypeople, for being at the forefront of the active management of labor, albeit a development led more by Donald's colleagues than by the Regius Professor himself.[14] But even within Donald's relatively conservative practice, nature seemed to need a helping hand from the obstetrician more frequently than had been the case twenty or thirty years previously.[15]

The number of episiotomies performed in the Queen Mother's increased year after year.

Within a decade of its opening, a minority of women were refusing to be referred to the Queen Mother's, preferring instead regimes perceived as less driven by a strict timetable in their management of labor, as in the maternity units at the Southern General Hospital and even at Rottenrow, now renovated and renewed under the leadership of Professor Malcolm MacNaughton. Many women still gave birth in the Queen Mother's, of course, and Donald's correspondence from his last two or three years as Regius Professor in the mid-1970s indicates that most of his patients remained appreciative of the quality of care they received. Nevertheless, less deferential attitudes were also increasingly evident—a circumstance that Donald found perplexing and, on occasion, more than tested his powers of diplomacy.

(((((Donald was, of course, encountering the beginnings of the sustained feminist challenge to the medicalization of childbirth in general, and to the authority of the obstetrician in particular, which developed throughout North America and Western Europe from the 1960s onward. In the context of this critique, the deployment of diagnostic ultrasound in obstetrics has attracted a substantial amount of adverse comment, even frank hostility. Critics have argued, for example, that ultrasonic imaging has assisted in the subjection of the pregnant woman to a professional, predominantly male, hegemony. Submission to technological monitoring, it is said, requires the woman to be a passive, rather than active, participant.[16] It is certainly true, as we have demonstrated, that the ultrasound image has displaced the woman's testimony from the central position it once held in the understanding of the fetus and the development of her pregnancy.[17]

Feminist commentators have also objected to what they see as the arrogant assumption by some advocates of ultrasonography that the fetus has been constituted, de novo, as an object of knowledge by the visualizing technology. An example of the sort of discourse that is objected to may be drawn from a 1982 essay, "Unborn: Historical Perspectives of the Fetus as a Patient," by Michael Harrison, an eminent pioneer of fetal surgery.

> The fetus could not be taken seriously as long as he remained a . . . recluse in the opaque womb; and it was not until the last half of the century that the prying eye of the ultrasonogram rendered the once opaque womb transparent, stripping the

veil of mystery from the dark inner sanctum and letting the light of scientific observation fall on the shy and secretive fetus . . . The sonographic voyeur, spying on the unwary fetus, finds him to be a surprisingly active little creature, and not at all the passive parasite we had imagined.[18]

What was considered objectionable in this mode of discourse was that a woman's sensory awareness of her own fetus, a form of knowledge that, of course, long predates ultrasonography, is here completely ignored. Rosalind Petchesky, a leading writer on obstetrical issues, responded to this passage: "It is naive to imagine a pregnant woman thinking about her fetus this way, whether she longs for a baby or wishes for an abortion." By producing an image of the fetus floating free, apparently independent of the uterus that sustains it, and by constituting the fetus as a patient in its own right, ultrasound has divided, so it is claimed, the fetus from the pregnant woman.[19] The autonomy, even the presence, of the female body in pregnancy and birth has thus been diminished. Some commentators, notably Barbara Duden, assert that this transfer of epistemological authority from the pregnant woman to her medical attendant has adversely affected women's confidence in and enjoyment of their experience of pregnancy.[20] Something of value has been lost in this move from a lived encounter with the fetus to a technologically mediated one. The increasingly refined visual scrutiny of the fetus for abnormality has also, it is argued, contributed to the redefinition of pregnancy as essentially a pathological process and encouraged premature or unnecessary resort to other technological and instrumental interventions.

Another very influential critic of the modern practice of obstetrics is Ann Oakley. Her major books, *Women Confined* and *The Captured Womb*, published in 1980 and 1984, respectively, were formative in feminist opinion with regard to obstetrics in the 1980s and 1990s. In reference to the ultrasonic image, Oakley commented that the "representation of pregnant women as objects of mechanical surveillance rather than recipients of antenatal care is an obvious message of these pictures."[21] Scientific reductionism, she asserted, has ousted more humane considerations.

As already noted, Donald had difficulty dealing sympathetically with lay criticism of his work or that of his junior colleagues. He would often respond to adverse comments either with a blunt appeal to his own status and authority or with mere bluster. However, his attitude to Oakley was interestingly different. Oakley interviewed Donald in the course of her research for the writing of *The Captured Womb*. She sent him part of the manuscript for his comments. Donald responded to her account of his work on the development of ultrasound with evident care and some sensitivity and wit. First, he criticized her title, *The Captured Womb*, by suggesting that it conveyed too passive a notion of the uterus, an organ that he, as an obstetrician, knew to be energetic and powerful. Perhaps, he suggested, the title should be changed to *The Capturing Womb*. It is evident from her reply that Oakley was discomfited at being outflanked by a male obstetrician on the issue of the active agency to be attributed to the female body. Her embarrassment was compounded when she later had to ask Donald if he could send her duplicate copies of some documents she had previously received from him, explaining that the originals had been rendered unreadable by one of her young children. Donald took this opportunity to comment wryly on the general difficulty of controlling the processes of reproduction, making the behavior of Oakley's offspring a metaphor for the unruliness of the agencies of fetus, neonate, and infant and implicitly making a sly comparison between her domestic challenges and his professional ones. Occasional failures in both spheres, he implied, had to be expected.[22] It is telling that Donald, together with Dugald Baird, is one of the few obstetricians that Oakley treats with obvious respect in her major books.

It might be said that Donald and Oakley recognized one another as being genuinely concerned with the welfare of pregnant women, despite their different perspectives on the matter. To Donald, as a result of his training at St. Thomas's and his acute awareness of what had passed for obstetric medicine earlier in the century, a woman's best hope for the preservation of her own health and that of her baby lay in trusting herself to the care of a well-trained obstetrician with the full paraphernalia of modern technological medicine at his disposal. (Even in the early 1980s, obstetricians and gynecologists were still overwhelmingly male.) Oakley saw that, in obstetrics as elsewhere, the unregulated exercise of male hegemony and power could be inimical to female agency and personhood. She also feared that a narrowly technocratic attitude toward pregnancy and labor would dehumanize. But unlike some other feminist critics, Oakley did not seek to abandon scientific medicine or wholly banish men and their technologies from the birthing room. By the same token, enthusiast for scientific medicine that he was, Donald was by no means unresponsive, as we have seen, to the need for maternity clinics to provide an environment in which women felt comfortable and emotionally fulfilled. Oakley and Donald would have agreed that there was a balance to be sought in the provision of maternity care, even if they approached that balance point from opposite directions—Oakley prioritizing the active engagement of pregnant women in determining the character of their care, Donald giving precedence to what he saw as the expertise and experience of the obstetrician.

Concerns have also regularly been raised about the safety of obstetric ultrasound,[23] as we have discussed in earlier chapters. It is, of course, impossible to prove a negative. But millions of fetuses have now been insonated in utero, and many extensive trawls for adverse effects have yielded no convincing evidence of harm. Surely, then, the pulse-echo modality may be cautiously regarded as reasonably safe—at least in the manner it has been employed for diagnostic purposes so far—given that a certain level of risk is inherent in virtually every medical procedure.[24] Thus, as far as the safety of ultrasound is concerned, it is hard to take the anxieties surrounding the issue entirely at face value. The role played by the issue of the safety of ultrasound in the feminist critique of obstetrics would seem to be a symbolic one. Raising the possibility of danger allows the expression of deeper disquiets about the encroachment of technology into the realms of pregnancy and birth.

(((((The questions regarding the value of obstetric ultrasound in routine antenatal care, posed by Oakley and others, do merit being carefully addressed. It is certainly the case, as Donald's mentor, A. J. Wrigley, eloquently pointed out in the 1930s, that the effectiveness of antenatal care is crucially dependent on the accuracy of its diagnostic procedures.[25] False positives increase anxiety, at the very least, and false negatives may be actually dangerous. The advocates of ultrasonic imaging in obstetrics would assert that the ability to visualize the fetus has greatly increased the accuracy of diagnosis and thus has enhanced the efficacy of antenatal care. Skeptics would counter that proper cost-benefit analyses have never been undertaken.[26]

Ultrasound is employed in many different ways by obstetricians, but, roughly speaking, three broad categories of use can be distinguished. Scans may be undertaken when frank clinical symptoms appear that require further investigation. This may happen at any stage of pregnancy but especially in the second and third trimesters. Few would dispute that a reliable imaging technology has a valuable role to play under these circumstances. The remaining two types of scan are performed without direct clinical indications and are thus considered routine. The booking scan is usually undertaken at around ten or twelve weeks, the fetal anomaly scan at around twenty weeks. Some clinics offer both scans, some only the former. A minority of obstetricians scan still more fre-quently.[27] Booking scans allow the ultrasonographer to check for the presence of a live fetus (eliminating blighted ovum and so forth), to confirm the dura-tion of gestation, and to identify multiple pregnancies. Since twins are at con-siderably increased risk for almost every complication of pregnancy and labor, many obstetricians believe it is good clinical practice to distinguish those preg-nancies as early as possible. They offer this consideration as, in itself, sufficient justification for the routine scanning of women whose pregnancies are appar-ently normal, at ten or twelve weeks.[28] However, for some women at least, this introduces a new worry into the first weeks of pregnancy, a time that might otherwise be joyful, as the outcome of the booking scan is anxiously awaited.[29]

In the course of our research into the history of ultrasound, we collected the testimony of a dozen or so women regarding their experience with the technology. Most of the interviewees said they had found their booking scans greatly reassuring, but perhaps they would have been less anxious, and thus in less need of reassurance, during the early part of their pregnancies if they had not had the outcome of the booking scan to fear. Of course, some women went for their booking scans and found they were not reassured—found that all was not well with their fetuses. But most of the women we interviewed said they would prefer knowledge to ignorance, as far as the condition of their pregnan-cies was concerned. The more they knew, the better they felt they could pre-pare for whatever was to transpire. And several said they would prefer prob-lems such as blighted ovum to be identified and dealt with promptly. We can make no claim, however, that our interview sample was a representative one. Also, all interviews were conducted some time after the event.

The situation regarding the pros and cons of the fetal anomaly scan seems to be somewhat more problematic. The improvement in the quality of the ultra-sonic image achieved in the late 1970s and 1980s allowed, for the first time, characterization of the soft tissue of the major fetal organs. Considerable en-thusiasm was accordingly engendered about the possibility of using ultrasound to detect a wide variety of fetal abnormalities early in gestation. Many mater-nity units began to offer routine scans at around twenty weeks, often in addi-tion to an earlier booking scan, with this aim in view. Whether the benefits of the fetal abnormality scan outweigh the costs and the disadvantages, however, is uncertain.[30] Often, the results of the anomaly scan are equivocal. Additional investigations may then be embarked upon—a situation that invokes severe anxiety, often needlessly. Moreover, a resort to interventionist diagnostic procedures, such as amniocentesis or sampling of the chorionic villi, carries significant risks for a normal fetus. A false positive, even when later discounted, may adversely affect the mother's peace of mind and may even impair the quality of her relationship with her child long after birth.[31] If it is indeed confirmed that something is seriously wrong with the fetus, there is often nothing that can be done, other than offering the woman the option of an abortion. These circumstances add weight to the charge made by some feminist observers that ultrasound imaging can "spoil the experience of pregnancy."

Such practical considerations about the utility of obstetric ultrasound, however, miss a very important point—as do the "second-wave" feminist critics such as Duden. The ultrasound image of the fetus is now so centrally embedded in our culture that criteria of cost-benefit analysis can no longer be meaningfully applied to it. As Eugenia Georges argues, to fully grasp the significance of the ultrasound image at the end of the twentieth century, "it is necessary to put aside common-sense notions of efficacy."[32] Whether or not ultrasonic imaging produces a quantifiable improvement in perinatal outcomes is substantially irrelevant.[33] The status now granted to the ultrasound image as the primary source of "objective" knowledge about the fetus is unassailable. It may well be, as Wagner maintains, that scanning provides no more accurate a measure of gestation, in most cases, than asking the woman about her last menstrual period.[34] But obstetricians are not going to take the mother's word for something they can now determine for themselves. In 1967, Donald wrote, with respect to the place of ultrasonography in his practice, "I must say I like doing obstetrics this way and removing as much of the traditional guesswork from our subject as possible. I like to know how well a baby is growing."[35] Four decades later, to practice obstetrics in any other way has become unthinkable. The ultrasound scanner has become as important to the professional identity of the obstetrician as the stethoscope has long been to the general physician. It symbolizes modern, scientific, good-quality obstetric practice, as exemplified by its centrality to the provision of care in the Queen Mother's Hospital.

Many expectant women broadly agree with the professionals on this point. Even though obstetricians and pregnant women often bring radically divergent interests to the clinical encounter, a considerable consensus surrounds the deployment of the ultrasound scanner. Our interviewees voiced general acceptance of the need for their booking scans. They did not express anxiety about the safety of the equipment and did not seem to regard themselves as passive victims of the imaging process. As several commentators have noted, many pregnant women not only expect that their fetuses will be imaged but would be aggrieved if they were not.[36] If denied an ultrasound scan, they would feel they had not received the best care that modern technological medicine can provide. Indeed, the experience of being scanned may be a very positive one, as Petchesky describes:

> Far from feeling victimised or pacified, they [pregnant women] frequently express a sense of elation at their direct participation in the imaging process, claiming it "makes the baby more real," "more a baby," that visualizing the fetus creates a feeling of intimacy and belonging, as well as a reassuring sense of predictability and control . . . Some women even talk about themselves as having "bonded" with the fetus through viewing its image on the screen . . . [and] ultrasound imaging in pregnancy seems to evoke in many women a sense of greater control and self-empowerment.[37]

The prospect of being scanned may well provoke anxiety. But pregnancy has always been unpredictable, and the credence granted to the technology has the power to rapidly assuage feelings of uncertainty.

As Georges points out, the ultrasound image compellingly combines what are held to be the two most potent sources of authoritative knowledge in Western culture: the visual and the scientific. Obstetrics is here participating in a larger trend within modern medicine. Many other specialties became more intensively visual in the latter half of the twentieth century, as the CT scanner, the MRI machine, and other imaging devices were introduced. Diagnostic imaging and scientific medicine are now inseparable.

Moreover, as Donna Haraway eloquently argues, it is not the case that women (or men) can counterpoise the natural against the artificial, our intuitive, direct knowledge of our own bodies against the alien information derived from a machine. Rather, our experience of our bodies is now, like our experience of the rest of the material world, irreducibly mediated through technology. We aid and improve our senses with technology. We observe distant places and participate in distant events via technology—they are present in our living rooms. We travel in machines; we build technological apparatuses in which to be born—the Queen Mother's Hospital, for instance—in which to live, and in which to die. Technology constructs us as we construct it. Haraway uses the term *cyborg* to denote this inseparable union of the human body with the made environment. The recent acquisition of social status by the fetus is a good illustration of the processes Haraway describes—the fetus owes its public presence entirely to the mediation of a technology, yet it has come to be accepted as both a patient and an individual. That the fetus is now a cyborg, in Haraway's sense, has been compellingly expounded by Eugenia Georges and Lisa Mitchell.[38]

It is not surprising, therefore, that the ultrasound image has been accepted as a virtually unchallengeable source of authoritative knowledge about the fetus, by professionals and laypeople alike. Indeed, adoption of the image by the laity happened very early in the history of imaging technology. As noted in earlier chapters, it was Donald himself who first began the practice of giving pregnant women an ultrasound image of their fetus to take home with them. Most mothers and fathers were, of course, unable to understand exactly what the picture conveyed. But there is no doubt that many parents were reassured and comforted by learning that the scan showed all was well and were proud to put the ultrasound print into the family album.

As we explored in chapter 9, introduction of the real-time, as opposed to the static, scanner greatly intensified the social presence of the fetus, in the consultative encounter as elsewhere. Seeing her fetus move on a screen made scanning a more immediate and more emotional experience for the pregnant woman. Gradually, ultrasound images have become easier to read, and lay viewers more skilled at reading them. Women who were of child-bearing age in the last decades of the twentieth century, having grown up with television, were accustomed to relating confidently to visual technologies. We live in a society that accords special epistemological status to the visual sense. The visual is the real—and the moving image conveys reality to us in a particularly convincing manner.

As Petchesky and Georges both document, for many women in the twenty-first century, the moment they become really convinced that they are pregnant is when they first see their fetus move on the screen of the real-time ultrasound scanner, an event that can only occur via the technology of an antenatal clinic. For younger women, this experience often elicits the same emotions that quickening did for previous generations of mothers. Ultrasound also enables fathers to relate to the fetus more directly than ever before.

Barbara Katz Rothman, on the other hand, argues that the impact of reproductive technologies on pregnant women has been to delay, rather than accelerate, affective responses to the fetus.[39] She describes the "tentative pregnancy." Given that it is many weeks after conception before the various tests for fetal abnormality can be performed, Rothman argues that women postpone emotional bonding with their fetuses until they have received an assurance from their obstetricians, via the technology, that all is well. This may well be the case for women who feel themselves to be at high risk for fetal abnormality or noncontinuance of pregnancy. But the general point we made above still holds true. The power of the ultrasound scanner to condition an emotional response to the fetus is as clearly evident in Rothman's uncertain cases as it is in the happier scenarios discussed by Georges or Petchesky.

An uncritical acceptance of the ultrasound image as the unproblematic conveyor of reality can be found in the most unexpected quarters. One of the feminist commentators most hostile to modern technocratic obstetrics is the radical midwife Jo Murphy-Lawless. Murphy-Lawless regards male obstetricians as incompetent to manage labor, by reason of the incapacity for empathy intrinsic to their gender, as well as their scientific arrogance and technological alienation from the lived experience of women's bodies. Yet, without any apparent awareness of the irony inherent in her position, she regularly points to the evidence provided by the ultrasound image whenever conclusive proof is required of the misdeeds and miscomprehensions of obstetricians.[40] In effect, Murphy-Lawless grants as much epistemological status to the technologically mediated fetal image as Ian Donald ever did.

If Murphy-Lawless might be said to be at one end of a spectrum of female opinion around the turn of the century, then Ann Widdecombe, Conservative Member of Parliament, devout Catholic, and campaigner against abortion, might be said to be at the other. But she, too, appeals to the ultrasound image as the unequivocal arbiter of reality. Indeed, Widdecombe has made the intriguing suggestion that the ultrasound scanner has fundamentally changed the way women conceptualize the first trimester of pregnancy.[41] She contends that previously, in the interval between conception and quickening, pregnant women imagined the contents of their uteruses to be disorganized collections of cells. But educated by the ultrasound image, they now envisage the fetus, even in the early months, as having a definite structure and the characteristics of a living thing. The similarity between Widdecombe's view and the discourse of Michael Harrison, quoted above, is striking, given their different backgrounds. Both Catholic politician and fetal surgeon accept that a technologically mediated image has radically changed how we think of the contents of the gravid uterus.

In whatever way the fetus was imagined before it was imaged, it is undoubtedly true that development of the ultrasound scanner has enabled women and men to make links with their unborn children in ways once unimaginable. This is true even of parents who can derive little reassurance, no assuaging of anxiety, from what the scan reveals. A senior obstetrician recounted to us the following case.

> A patient who had screening was discovered to have a fetus with no kidneys, a case of renal agenesis. Now there is just no hope in that situation and this was diagnosed at around 20 weeks. Many people at that stage would choose, since there is no good outcome, to abort the pregnancy. This couple was R[oman] C[atholic] and strongly believed that abortion was wrong and they wished to continue with the pregnancy. Now I couldn't offer her anything in terms of being upbeat about the pregnancy but she wanted to come for scans on a regular basis and it was the only way her husband actually saw the baby, well she saw it too but she as a mother was able to feel it. But that couple came monthly over the next 20 weeks and she finally went into labour and delivered. Because we knew it was a case of renal agenesis there were no great attempts at resuscitation, she was able to quietly hold the baby in her arms and the baby died within an hour or so. That couple were able, because they knew that the baby wasn't going [to] survive, they poured 40/50 years of love into 20 weeks of pregnancy and I have never ever experienced a couple who just gave so much to their pregnancy.[42]

Here, obstetric ultrasound had an application that truly transcends considerations of cost and benefit. Its value in these circumstances is beyond any quantification, yet it was crucial to the support provided to loving, grieving parents by a sensitive and caring obstetrician. It would be very crass indeed to argue that this couple's experience of their child was diminished by its being largely mediated by a machine. Rather, the ultrasound scanner enabled a novel yet profound expression of human love.

The medium of ultrasound has not merely created an objectified image of the fetus. The fetus has become, simultaneously, the subject of scientific objectification and of increased emotional attachment. These two processes have readily coexisted throughout the history of the imaging technology. Donald, MacVicar, and Brown did not anticipate, when ultrasound transducers were first applied to the abdomen of elderly women to try to distinguish between solid and cystic tumors, that the new imaging technique would radically change not only the practice of obstetrics and gynecology but also the emotional and bodily experiences of pregnancy. But those have been its effects. Donald himself, although eager to see the fetus objectified as an aid to clinical decision making, also enthusiastically invested the fetal image with meanings that were affective, ethical, and religious rather than narrowly diagnostic. John Fleming can personally vouch that even many years of quantitative mapping of fetal characteristics in charts of crown-rump length or biparietal diameter, and the analysis of thousands of fetal images, do not diminish the response to the death of a particular fetus, when that fetus is one's own grandchild.[43]

As we hope we have made clear in this book, the ultrasound scanner does not reveal the fetus directly or unproblematically. What is portrayed is not a one-to-one representation of the whole structure of the fetus but a rather unusual signal received from particular interfaces within it. The gathering of information by pulse-echo has many peculiarities and technical limitations; much of the character of the final image depends on the form of display that is chosen. As Brian Fraser put it, the ultrasound image is an "illusion."[44] But it has become, in our culture, a uniquely powerful illusion.

Notes

CHAPTER ONE: Introduction: Historiographies of Obstetrics

1. See S. Blume, *Insight and Industry: On the Dynamics of Technological Change in Medicine* (Cambridge, MA: MIT Press, 1992); B. H. Kevles, *Naked to the Bone: Medical Imaging in the Twentieth Century* (New Brunswick, NJ: Rutgers University Press, 1997); B. Pasveer, "Knowledge of Shadows: The Introduction of X-ray Images in Medicine," *Sociology of Health and Illness* 11 (1989): 360–81.

2. For example, A. B. Wolbarst, *Looking Within: How X-ray, CT, MRI, Ultrasound, and Other Medical Images Are Created* (Berkeley: University of California Press, 1999); S. Webb, *From the Watching of Shadows: The Origins of Radiological Tomography* (Bristol, UK: Hilger, 1990).

3. J. S. Taylor, "The Public Fetus and the Family Car: From Abortion Politics to a Volvo Advertisement," *Public Culture* 3 (1992): 67–80. For the job advertisement, see M. Nicolson and J. E. E. Fleming, "Scottish Innovations: The Case Study of Ultrasound," in *Anatomy Acts: How We Come to Know Ourselves*, ed. A. Patrizio and D. Kemp (Edinburgh: Birlinn, 2006), 51–62. In the early 2000s, a television advertisement for the Scottish soft drink Irn Bru featured an ultrasonically imaged fetus apparently drinking the product; www.youtube.com/watch?v=2LZPTZmAveQ (accessed June 2012).

4. R. P. Petchesky, "Fetal Images: The Power of Visual Culture in the Politics of Reproduction," *Feminist Studies* 13 (1987): 263–92.

5. P. A. Sullivan, "Public Perceptions and Politics: When Diagnostic Medical Ultrasound Is Employed as a Nondiagnostic, Nonmedical Tool," *Journal of Diagnostic Medical Sonography* 18 (2002): 211–17; J. S. Taylor, "The Public Life of the Fetal Sonogram and the Work of the Sonographer," *Journal of Diagnostic Medical Sonography* 18 (2002): 367–79.

6. For the historiography of childbirth in the twentieth century, see H. Marland, "Childbirth and Maternity," in *Medicine in the Twentieth Century*, ed. R. Cooter and J. Pickstone (Amsterdam: Harwood Academic, 2000), 559–74; S. Williams, *Women and Childbirth in the Twentieth Century: A History of the National Birthday Trust Fund, 1928–93* (Stroud, UK: Sutton, 1997); J. Garcia, R. Kilpatrick, and M. Richards, eds., *The Politics of Maternity Care: Services for Childbearing Woman in Twentieth-Century Britain* (Oxford: Clarendon Press, 1990).

7. G. Blackwell, *The World Market for Ultrasound Imaging Systems: Clinica Reports* (London: PJB Publications, 1995).

8. P. Rhodes, *A Short History of Clinical Midwifery: The Development of Ideas in the Professional Management of Childbirth* (Hale, UK: Books for Midwives Press, 1995).

9. J. Murphy-Lawless, *Reading Birth and Death: A History of Obstetric Thinking* (Cork: Cork University Press, 1998); see also M. Tew, *Safer Childbirth? A Critical History of Maternity Care* (London: Chapman and Hall, 1990).

10. For the view that ultrasonography is antifeminist, see L. M. Mitchell, *Baby's First Picture: Ultrasound and the Politics of Fetal Subjects* (Toronto: University of Toronto Press, 2001).

11. A. Oakley, *The Captured Womb: A History of the Medical Care of Pregnant Women* (Oxford: Blackwell, 1994).

12. B. L. Beech and J. Robinson, *Ultrasound? Unsound* (London: AIMS, 1994).

13. Blume, *Insight and Industry*, chap. 3; J. Woo, "A Short History of the Development of Ultrasound in Obstetrics and Gynecology," www.ob-ultrasound.net/history1.html (accessed June 2012).

14. For links between the clinico-anatomical method and diagnostic technology, see S. J. Reiser, *Medicine and the Reign of Technology* (Cambridge: Cambridge University Press, 1978); M. Nicolson, "The Introduction of Percussion and Stethoscopy to Early Nineteenth-Century Edinburgh," in *The Five Senses in Medicine*, ed. W. F. Bynum and R. Porter (Cambridge: Cambridge University Press, 1992), 134–54.

15. E. B. Koch, "In the Image of Science? Negotiating the Development of Diagnostic Ultrasound in the Cultures of Surgery and Radiology," *Technology and Culture* 34 (1993): 858-93; E. B. Koch, "The Process of Innovation in Medical Technology: American Research on Ultrasound" (PhD diss., University of Pennsylvania, 1990), chap. 3.

16. R. C. Alexander, *The Inventor of Stereo: The Life and Works of Alan Dower Blumlein* (St. Louis: Focal Press, 1999); R. W. Burns, *The Life and Times of A. D. Blumlein* (London: Institution of Electrical Engineers, 2000).

17. Blume, *Insight and Industry*, 73.

18. In the sociology of technology, a "black box" is a device that is characterized only by its outputs and inputs. Its user need not understand what goes on inside. T. Pinch and W. E. Bijker, "The Social Construction of Facts and Artifacts: Or How the Sociology of Science and the Sociology of Technology Might Benefit Each Other," in *The Social Construction of Technological Systems: New Directions in the Sociology and History of Technology*, ed. W. E. Bijker, T. P. Hughes, and T. Pinch (Cambridge, MA: MIT Press, 1987), 17–50. For analysis of the process of black-boxing, see D. A. MacKenzie, *Inventing Accuracy: A Historical Sociology of Nuclear Missile Guidance* (Cambridge, MA: MIT Press, 1990).

19. Blackwell, *World Market*, chap. 4.

20. D. MacKenzie and J. Wajcman, eds., *The Social Shaping of Technology* (Buckingham, UK: Open University Press, 1999); P. Rosen, "The Social Construction of Mountain Bikes: Technology and Postmodernity in the Cycle Industry," *Social Studies of Science* 23 (1993): 479–513.

21. A. Pickering, *The Cybernetic Brain: Sketches of Another Future* (Chicago: University of Chicago Press, 2010).

22. A. Pickering, *The Mangle of Practice: Time, Agency, and Science* (Chicago: University of Chicago Press, 1995), esp. 9–26.

23. J. V. Pickstone, "Introduction," in *Medical Innovations in Historical Perspective*, ed. J. V. Pickstone (Basingstoke, UK: Macmillan, 1992), 1–16, 16.

24. A. Pickering, "Practice and Posthumanism: Social Theory and a History of Agency," in *The Practice Turn in Contemporary Theory*, ed. T. Schatzki, K. Knorr Cetina, and E. von Savigny (New York: Routledge, 2001), 163–74.

25. D. Haraway, *Simians, Cyborgs, and Women: The Reinvention of Nature* (London: Free Association Press, 1991).

26. Harry Collins critiques the posthumanist program in his "Humans Not Instruments," *Spontaneous Generations* 4 (2010): 138–47. Although we cannot agree with his negative assessment of the methodological value of treating human and nonhuman entities symmetrically, he is certainly correct that emotional responses must be understood as distinctively human phenomena.

CHAPTER TWO: Diagnostic Ultrasound before Thomas Brown

1. Stuart Blume has provided an insightful account of some of the developments described here, to which our indebtedness is evident. S. S. Blume, *Insight and Industry: On the Dynamics of Technological Change in Medicine* (Cambridge, MA: MIT Press, 1992); E. Yoxen, "Seeing with Sound: A Study of the Development of Medical Images," in *The Social Construction of Technological Systems: New Directions in the Sociology and History of Technology*, ed. W. Bijker, T. P. Hughes and T. Pinch (Cambridge, MA: MIT Press, 1987), 281–303.

2. Sonar uses high-frequency sound; radar uses pulses of electromagnetic radiation.

3. Doppler ultrasound works on a different principle. For the physics of the ultrasound scanner, see E. N. Carsen, "Ultrasound Physics for the Physician: A Brief Review," *Journal of Clinical Ultrasound* 3 (1975): 69–75; P. N. T. Wells, *Physical Principles of Ultrasonic Diagnosis* (London: Academic Press, 1969).

4. A transducer converts one form of energy to another, such as electrical energy to sound, and vice versa.

5. By *beam* we mean a narrow, well-defined cylindrical volume in which the ultrasound pulse travels. Frequencies as high as 30 MHz are used to examine small body parts such as eyes or testes.

6. J. W. Strutt, Baron Rayleigh, *The Theory of Sound* (London: MacMillan, 1877).

7. L. F. Richardson, "Patent No. 9423. Apparatus for Warning a Ship of Its Approach to a Large Object in a Fog," in *Collected Papers of Lewis Fry Richardson*, ed. O. M. Ashford, H. Charnock, P. G. Drazin, J. C. R. Hunt, P. Smoker, and I. Sutherland (Cambridge: Cambridge University Press, 1993), 1: 999–1004. Echolocation by sound was not original to Richardson, but his suggestions as to its deployment were more sophisticated than those of his predecessors. H. Charnock, "Echo-ranging: L. F. Richardson's Contribution," *Weather* 36 (1981): 316–22.

8. Quoted in O. M. Ashford, *Prophet or Professor: The Life and Work of L. F. Richardson* (Bristol, UK: Hilger, 1985), 40.

9. W. Hackman, *Seek and Strike: Sonar, Anti-submarine Warfare, and the Royal Navy* (London: HMSO, 1984), 77–78; P. Biquard, "Paul Langevin," *Ultrasonics*, Sept. 1972, 213–14.

10. F. V. Hunt, *Electroacoustics: The Analysis of Transduction and Its Historical Background* (Cambridge, MA: Harvard University Press, 1954), 19–21.

11. W. Thomson, "On the Thermoelastic, Thermomagnetic and Pyroelectric Properties of Matter," *Philosophical Magazine* 5 (1878): 4–27.

12. W. P. Mason, "Piezoelectricity, Its History and Applications," *Journal of Acoustical Society of America* 70 (1981): 1561–66.

13. Hackman, *Seek and Strike*, 81, 82.

14. G. Hartcup, *The War of Invention: Scientific Developments, 1914–1918* (London: Brassey, 1988), 15–21; T. Devereux, *The Messenger Gods of Battle* (London: Brassey, 1990).

15. Hackman, *Seek and Strike*, 97–138, 224.

16. In Britain, piezoelectric research was classified. Civilian echo sounders employed the alternative technology of magnetostriction. B. Carlin, *Ultrasonics* (New York: McGraw-Hill, 1949), 222–42.

17. Hackman, *Seek and Strike*, 231; I. Spencer, J. E. E. Fleming, and M. Nicolson, *A Scan through the History of Ultrasound* (Glasgow: Wellcome Unit for the History of Medicine, 1996), video.

18. "How the Wreck of the *Lusitania* Was Found," *Hydrographic Review* 13 (1936): 165.

19. V. J. Phillips, *Waveforms: A History of Early Oscillography* (Bristol, UK: Hilger, 1987).

20. F. L. Hopwood, "Ultrasonics: Some Properties of Inaudible Sound," *Nature* 128 (1931): 748–51; R. W. Wood and A. L. Loomis, "The Physical and Biological Effects of High-Frequency Sound Waves of Great Intensity," *Philosophical Magazine* 4 (1927): 417–36; E. Newton Harvey, "Biological Aspects of Ultrasonic Waves: A General Survey," *Biological Bulletin* 59 (1930): 306–25.

21. C. R. Hill, "Medical Ultrasonics: A Historical Review," *British Journal of Radiology* 46 (1973): 899–905.

22. J. F. Herrick, "Ultrasound and Medicine: A Survey of Experimental Studies," *Journal of the Acoustical Society of America* 26 (1954): 236–40; "Ultrasonics in Diagnosis" (editorial), *Journal of the American Medical Association* 146 (1951): 1033. Eventually, ultrasonic tissue heating gained a place in orthodox physiotherapy. S. S. Kitchen and C. J. Partridge, "A Review of Therapeutic Ultrasound," *Physiotherapy* 76 (1990): 593–600.

23. K. T. Dussik, untitled typescript, lecture given at Mount Sinai Hospital, 12 Oct. 1951, British Medical Ultrasound Society Historical Collection Papers HB 112, NHS Greater Glasgow and Clyde Health Board Archive (hereafter, BMUS Papers), 2/7/4.

24. D. N. White, "The Early Development of Neurosonology I: Echoencephalography in Adults," *Ultrasound in Medicine and Biology* 18 (1992): 112–65.

25. Dussik, untitled typescript.

26. Ibid.

27. J. Krautkramer and H. Krautkramer, *Ultrasonic Testing of Materials* (London: Allen and Unwin, 1969).

28. Yoxen, "Seeing with Sound," 284.

29. K. T. Dussik, F. Dussik, and L. Wyt, "Auf dem Wege Zur Hyperphonographie des Gehirnes," *Wiener Medizinische Wochenschrift* 97 (1947): 425–29; K. T. Dussik, "Ultraschall diagnostik, in besondere bei gehirnerkrankungen, mittels Hyperphonographie," *Zeitschrift für Physikalische Medizin* 1 (1948): 140–45; K. T. Dussik, "Zum heutigen stand der medizinischen Ultraschallforschung," *Wiener Klinische Wochen-*

schrift 61 (1949): 246–48. Hyperphonographs are reproduced in K. T. Dussik, "The Ultrasonic Field as a Medical Tool," *American Journal of Physical Medicine* 33 (1954): 5–20. It is difficult for the uninitiated to interpret the image in the manner suggested.

30. A. Dénier, "Les ultra-sons. Leurs applications au diagnostic: Ultra-sonoscopie, et a la therapeutique: Ultra-sonotherapie," *Journal de Radiologie* 27 (1946): 481–87, 483, our translation; A. Dénier, "Essai de détection de mass tumorale du cerveau par ultra-sonoscopie," *Compts-Rendu de la Société de Biologie* 140 (1946): 763–64. For illustrations of his apparatus, see A. Dénier, *Les Ultra-Sons Appliques á la Medicine* (n.p.: L'Expansion Scientifique Francaise, 1952), 62–64.

31. Pohlman invented the ultrasonic dosimeter and a means of visualizing ultrasonic shadows. T. F. Hueter, "Foundations and Trends in the 1950s," in W. Nyborg, "Biological Effects of Ultrasound: Development of Safety Guidelines. Part 1: Personal Histories," *Ultrasound in Medicine and Biology* 26 (2000): 937–38.

32. R. Sharpe, "1996—An Anniversary Year for British Ultrasonics," *Insight* 38 (1996): 330–34.

33. C. H. Desch, D. O. Sproule, and W. J. Dawson, "The Detection of Cracks in Steel by Means of Supersonic Waves," *Journal of the Iron and Steel Institute* 153 (1946): 319–53; J. Nutting, "Desch, Cecil Henry (1874–1958)," *Oxford Dictionary of National Biography* (Oxford: Oxford University Press, 2004), www.oxforddnb.com/view/article /37355. The term *supersonics* was used for industrial applications of ultrasound in the 1940s and 1950s.

34. B. Carlin, *Ultrasonics*, 2nd ed. (New York: McGraw-Hill, 1960), 176–78.

35. Desch, Sproule, and Dawson, "Detection of Cracks," 324; D. O. Sproule, *The Supersonic Flaw Detector: An Equipment Capable of Detecting Flaws in Opaque Solids* (Barkingside, UK: Henry Hughes Ltd., ca. 1946), 1–2.

36. J. F. Hinsley, *Non-destructive Testing* (London: Macdonald and Evans, 1959), 171.

37. To detect a 1 mm crack, a frequency of about 3 MHz is required.

38. O. S. Puckle, *Time-Bases* (London: Chapman and Hall, 1945).

39. T. Soller, M. A. Starr, and G. E. Valley, *Cathode-Ray Tube Displays*, M.I.T. Radiation Laboratory Series, vol. 22 (New York: McGraw-Hill, 1948).

40. For comparison of the instruments, see Carlin, *Ultrasonics*, 216–18.

41. F. A. Firestone, "The Supersonic Reflectoscope, an Instrument for Inspecting the Interior of Solid Parts by Means of Sound Waves," *Journal of the Acoustical Society of America* 17 (1945): 287–99; F. A. Firestone, "The Supersonic Reflectoscope for Interior Inspection," *Metal Progress* 48 (1945): 505–12; Desch, Sproule, and Dawson, "Detection of Cracks."

42. E. N. Simons, "The Supersonic Flaw Detector," *Metal Progress* 48 (1945): 513–16; Sharpe, "1996—Anniversary Year." In 1961, the company's name was changed to Kelvin Hughes; www.kelvinhughes.co.uk/history (accessed June 2012).

43. W. P. Mason, "Fifty Years of Ferroelectricity," *Journal of Acoustical Society of America* 50 (1971): 1281–98; B. Jaffe, H. Jaffe, and W. R. Cook, *Piezoelectric Ceramics* (London: Academic Press, 1990).

44. B. Carlin, interview, interviewer unknown, undated transcript, BMUS Papers, 2/7/4. Carlin worked with Firestone in the mid-1940s and later designed the Sonomedic, one of the first ultrasound scanners to be marketed in the United States.

45. Untitled, undated Eppendorf company publicity sheet, BMUS Papers, 2/7/1.

46. S. Young White, "Applications of Ultrasonics to Biology," *Audio Engineering* 32 (1948): 30–45.

47. Ibid., 43–45.

48. M. B. W. Graham, *RCA and the VideoDisc: The Business of Research* (Cambridge: Cambridge University Press, 1986), 68–72; R. P. McLoughlin and G. N. Guastivino, "LUPAM: Localizador ultrasonoscopico para aplicaciones medicas," *Revista Asociacion Medica Argentina*, Sept. 1949, 421–35.

49. R. Buderi, *The Invention That Changed the World: How a Small Group of Radar Pioneers Won the Second World War and Launched a Technological Revolution* (New York: Simon and Schuster, 1996), 78.

50. Soller, Starr, and Valley, *Cathode-Ray Tube Displays.*

51. Hackman, *Seek and Strike*, 291.

52. By 1950, RCA was closely following similar developments in the United States. J. H. Holmes, D. H. Howry, G. J. Posakony, and C. R. Cushman, "The Ultrasonic Visualization of Soft Tissue Structures in the Human Body," *Transactions of the American Clinical and Climatological Association* 66 (1954): 208–25.

53. J. E. Burchard, *Q.E.D.: MIT in World War II* (New York: John Wiley, 1948).

54. Buderi, *Invention*, 100–134.

55. D. Cardwell, *The Fontana History of Technology* (London: Fontana, 1994), 479.

56. Devereux, *Messenger Gods*; G. Hartcup, *The Effect of Science on the Second World War* (Basingstoke, UK: Macmillan, 2000).

57. H. T. Ballantine, R. H. Bolt, T. F Hueter, and G. D. Ludwig, "On the Detection of Intracranial Pathology by Ultrasound," *Science* 112 (1950): 525–28.

58. Hueter, "Foundations and Trends."

59. G. D. Ludwig and F. W. Struthers, "Detecting Gallstones with Ultrasonic Echoes," *Electronics* 23 (1950): 172–78.

60. G. D. Ludwig, "The Velocity of Sound through Tissues and the Acoustic Impedance of Tissues," *Journal of the Acoustical Society of America* 22 (1950): 862–66; Ludwig and Struthers, "Detecting Gallstones."

61. Ludwig and Struthers, "Detecting Gallstones."

62. Ludwig, "Velocity of Sound."

63. Hueter, "Foundations and Trends."

64. Yoxen, "Seeing with Sound."

65. Hueter, "Foundations and Trends," 937.

66. Sproule quoted in Desch, Sproule, and Dawson, "Detection of Cracks," 322.

67. In 1950, having achieved good results with fixed brains in vitro, Bolt estimated that his team was "a few months" away from clinical trials and "two or three years" from clinical application. H. T. Ballantine, G. D. Ludwig, R. H. Bolt, and T. F. Hueter, "Ultrasonic Localisation of the Cerebral Ventricles," *Transactions of the American Neurological Association* 51 (1950): 38–41, 41.

68. Yoxen, "Seeing with Sound," 288.

69. G. D. Ludwig, R. H. Bolt, T. F. Hueter, and H. T. Ballantine, "Factors Influencing the Use of Ultrasound as a Diagnostic Aid," *Transactions of the American Neurological Association* 51 (1950): 225–28.

70. W. Güttner, G. Fielder, and J. Pätzold, "Über Ultraschallabbildungem am Menschlichen Schädel," *Acustica* 2 (1953): 148–56.

71. H. T. Ballantine, T. F. Hueter, and R. H. Bolt, "On the Use of Ultrasound for Tumour Detection," *Journal of the Acoustical Society of America* 26 (1954): 581.

72. United States Atomic Energy Commission, *Studies in Methods and Instruments to Improve the Localization of Radioactive Materials in the Body with Special Reference to the Diagnosis of Brain Tumors and the Use of Ultrasonic Techniques* (Oak Ridge, TN: AEC V-3012 Technical Information Service, 1955).

73. Güttner, Fielder, and Pätzold, "Über ultraschallabbildungem."

74. H. T. Ballantine, T. F. Hueter, W. J. H. Naita, and D. M. Sosa, "Focal Destruction of Nervous Tissue by Focussed Ultrasound: Biophysical Factors Influencing Its Application," *Journal of Experimental Medicine* 104 (1956): 337–60; T. F. Hueter, H. T. Ballantine, and W. C. Cotter, "On the Problem of Dosage in Ultrasonic Lesion Making," in *Ultrasound in Biology and Medicine*, ed. E. Kelly (Washington, DC: American Institute of Biological Sciences, 1957), 131–55.

75. K. Kikuchi, K. Tanaka, and R. Uchida, "Detection of Intracranial Anatomical Abnormalities by Ultrasound," *Journal of the Acoustical Society of Japan* 8 (1952): 111, reprinted in D. N. White, "Neurosonology Pioneers," *Ultrasound in Medicine and Biology* 14 (1988): 541–62.

76. Y. Kikuchi, R. Uchida, K. Tanaka, and T. Wagai, "Early Cancer Diagnosis through Ultrasonics," *Journal of the Acoustical Society of America* 29 (1957): 824–33; M. Oka, "Clinical Use of Ultrasonics and Related Biological Research in Japan," *American Journal of Physical Medicine* 37 (1958): 210–18; E. Kelly, ed., *Ultrasound in Biology and Medicine* (Washington, DC: American Institute of Biological Sciences, 1957).

77. R. Ford and J. Ambrose, "Echoencephalography: The Measurement of the Position of Mid-line Structures in the Skull with High Frequency Pulsed Ultrasound," *Brain* 86 (1963): 189–96. For mention of the Japanese work, see D. N. White, "Neurosonology Pioneers," 551–53; B. Goldberg and B. A. Kimmelman, *Medical Diagnostic Ultrasound* (Washington, DC: Eastman Kodak, 1988). An accessible English-language account is J. Woo, "A Short History of the Development of Medical Ultrasonics in Japan," www.ob-ultrasound.net/japan_ultrasonics.html (accessed June 2012).

78. C. R. Hill, "Notes on the Historical Development of Aspects of Medical Ultrasonics," typescript, 1987, BMUS Papers, 2/96.

79. F. W. Spiers, "William Valentine Mayneord," *Biographical Memoirs of the Royal Society* 37 (1991): 341–64.

80. E. O. Backlund, "Lars Leksell—A Portrait by a Friend," *Applied Neurophysiology* 49 (1986): 173.

81. Our account of Leksell's work follows that in D. N. White, "Neurosonology Pioneers."

82. L. Leksell, "Echo-encephalography 1: Detection of Intracranial Complications following Brain Injury," *Acta Chirurgica Scandinavica* 110 (1956): 301–15.

83. D. N. White "Early Development of Neurosonology."

84. L. Edler, "The Diagnostic Use of Ultrasound in Heart Disease," *Acta Medica Scandinavica Supplement* 308 (1955): 32–36. The echo was later realized to be from the anterior leaflet of the mitral valve. L. Edler, "Early Echocardiography," *Ultrasound in Medicine and Biology* 17 (1991): 425–31.

85. L. Edler and C. H. Hertz, "The Use of Ultrasonic Reflectoscope for the Continuous Recording of the Movements of Heart Walls," *Kungliga Fysiografiska Sällskapets i Lund Förhandlingar* 24 (1954): 1–19.

86. This work is documented in the Annual Reports of the British Empire Cancer Campaign, 1950–1961.

87. J. A. Newell, "The Use of Ultrasonics in Medical Diagnosis," *Proceedings of the Third International Conference on Medical Electronics, 1960* (London: Institution of Electrical Engineers, 1961), 422–24; J. C. Taylor, J. A. Newell, and P. Karvounis, "Ultrasonics in the Diagnosis of Intracranial Space-Occupying Lesions," *Lancet* 1 (1961): 1196–99.

88. "Douglass Howry," *Journal of Clinical Ultrasound* 1 (1973): 2–4. For interesting accounts of Howry's research, see E. B. Koch, "In the Image of Science? Negotiating the Development of Diagnostic Ultrasound in the Cultures of Surgery and Radiology," *Technology and Culture* 34 (1993): 858-93; E. B. Koch, "The Process of Innovation in Medical Technology: American Research on Ultrasound" (PhD diss., University of Pennsylvania, 1990), chap. 3.

89. J. H. Holmes, "Diagnostic Ultrasound: Historical Perspective," in *Diagnostic Ultrasound*, ed. D. L. King (St. Louis: Mosby, 1974), 1–15.

90. D. H. Howry and W. R. Bliss, "Ultrasonic Visualization of Soft Tissue Structures of the Body," *Journal of Laboratory and Clinical Medicine* 40 (1952): 579–92, 579.

91. Koch, "Process of Innovation," 116; Blume, *Insight and Industry*, 85.

92. Howry and Bliss, "Ultrasonic Visualization," 579.

93. G. Posansky, quoted in Koch, "Process of Innovation," 147.

94. Howry quoted in ibid., 116; D. H. Howry, G. Posakony, C. R. Cushman, and J. Holmes, "Three-Dimensional and Stereoscopic Observations of Body Structures by Ultrasound," *Journal of Applied Physiology* 9 (1956): 304–6.

95. D. H. Howry, "The Ultrasonic Visualization of Soft Tissue," unpublished report, 1954, BMUS Papers, 2/7/2; Koch, "Process of Innovation," 117.

96. Howry and Bliss, "Ultrasonic Visualization"; D. H. Howry, "The Ultrasonic Visualization of Soft Tissue Structures and Disease Processes," *Journal of Laboratory and Clinical Medicine* 40 (1952): 812–13.

97. The exact relation between the amplitude of the echo and the brightness of the dot depends on the characteristics of the electronic processing and the display unit.

98. Howry and Bliss "Ultrasonic Visualization," 589.

99. D. H. Howry, D. A. Stott, and W. R. Bliss, "The Ultrasonic Visualisation of Cancer of the Breast and Other Soft Tissue Structures," *Cancer* 7 (1954): 354–58, 357.

100. D. H. Howry, J. H. Holmes, C. R. Cushman, and G. J. Posakony, "Ultrasonic Visualisation of Living Organs and Tissues," *Geriatrics* 10 (1955): 123–28.

101. Holmes et al., "Ultrasonic Visualization of Soft Tissue."

102. Greene Engineering Consultants, "Mark IV Somascope Specifications," unpublished report, undated, BMUS Papers, 2/7/2.

103. D. H. Howry, "Techniques Used in Ultrasonic Visualisation of Soft Tissues," in *Ultrasound in Biology and Medicine*, ed. E. Kelly (Washington, DC: American Institute of Biological Sciences, 1957), 49–65, 56. For a lucid explanation of compound scanning, see T. G. Brown, "Direct Contact Ultrasonic Scanning Techniques for the Visualization of Abdominal Masses," in *Medical Electronics: Proceedings of the 2nd International Conference on Medical Electronics, Paris, 1959*, ed. C. N. Smyth (London: Iliffe, 1960), 258–66.

104. J. H. Holmes and D. Howry, "Ultrasonic Visualisation of Edema," *Transactions of the American Clinical and Climatological Association* 70 (1959): 225–35.

105. Greene Engineering Consultants, "Mark IV Somascope," 1.

106. J. H. Holmes, "Diagnostic Ultrasound during the Early Years of A.I.U.M.," *Journal of Clinical Ultrasound* 8 (1980): 299–310, 301; B. H. Kevles, *Naked to the Bone: Medical Imaging in the Twentieth Century* (New Brunswick, NJ: Rutgers University Press, 1997), 238.

107. J. H. Holmes, "Notice to Staff Residents and Interns, February 14, 1956," unpublished memo, BMUS Papers, 2/7/2.

108. "Douglass Howry."

109. W. Coombs, quoted in Koch, "Process of Innovation," 120; W[illiam] W[right], interview, transcript, BMUS Papers, 2/7/4.

110. Holmes and Howry, "Ultrasonic Visualisation of Edema."

111. "Douglass Howry," 4.

112. K. Hill, "John Wild, Obituary," *Guardian*, 1 Oct. 2009, 45.

113. J. J. Wild, interview, Nov. 1998. Transcripts of our interviews are available from the Centre for the History of Medicine, University of Glasgow.

114. M. S. Horner, "'Where There's a Will': How an Enterprising Medical Student Has Developed a Successful Home-made Producer-Gas Outfit," *Motor Cycling*, 7 May 1942, 4–5.

115. J. J. Wild, "Intestinal Aspiration Apparatus," *British Medical Journal* 1 (1944): 815.

116. J. J. Wild and J. Strickler, "Clinical Results of the Use of a Long Intestinal Tube of Improved Design," *Bulletin of the University of Minnesota Hospital and Minnesota Medical Foundation* 20 (1949): 1–40.

117. F. J. Larsen, "Ultrasonic Trainer," *Electronics*, June 1946, 126–29.

118. J. J. Wild and J. M. Reid, "Echographic Tissue Diagnosis," in *Proceedings of the Fourth Annual Conference on Ultrasound Therapy, Detroit* (Philadelphia: American Institute for Ultrasonics in Medicine, 1955), 1–26.

119. J. J. Wild, interview with B. Kimmelman, Sept. 1987, transcript, BMUS Papers, 2/7/4.

120. Ibid.

121. J. J. Wild, "The Use of Ultrasonic Pulses for the Measurement of Biological Tissues and the Detection of Tissue Density Changes," *Surgery* 27 (1950): 183–88.

122. L. A. French, J. J. Wild, and D. Neal, "Detection of Cerebral Tumours by Ultrasonic Pulses," *Cancer* 4 (1950): 705–8. French was head of neurosurgery at the University of Minnesota Medical School.

123. Wild, "Use of Ultrasonic Pulses," 187.

124. J. J. Wild, interview, Nov. 1998.

125. J. J. Wild and D. Neal, "Use of High Frequency Ultrasonic Waves for Detecting Changes in Texture in Living Tissues," *Lancet* 1 (1951): 655–57.

126. V. L. Newhouse, "Introduction to Special Issue in Honor of John M. Reid," *Ultrasound in Medicine and Biology* 20 (1994): 599–600.

127. N. Y. Hoffman, "Minnesota Maverick: Owen H. Wangensteen," *JAMA: The Journal of the American Medical Association* 241 (1979): 1090–95.

128. J. M. Reid, "John Wild and the Early Days of Ultrasound," unpublished paper, ca. 1978. We are grateful to Dr. Wild for providing us with a copy. J. M. Reid and J. J. Wild, "Ultrasonic Ranging for Cancer Diagnosis," *Electronics* 25 (1952): 136–38.

129. In some of Wild's images, the field is bright; the echoes are represented by dark dots.

130. Reid, "John Wild."

131. J. J. Wild and J. M. Reid, "Application of Echo-Ranging Techniques to the Determination of Structure of Biological Tissues," *Science* 115 (1952): 226–30; Howry and Bliss, "Ultrasonic Visualization."

132. J. J. Wild and J. M. Reid, "Further Pilot Echographic Studies on the Histologic Structure of Tumors of the Living Intact Human Breast," *American Journal of Pathology* 28 (1952): 839–54.

133. Quoted in J. J. Wild, "The Use of Ultrasonic Pulses for the Measurement of Biological Tissues and the Detection of Tissue Density Changes: Progress Report for Period, July 14, 1952, to July 1, 1953" (Bethesda, MD: National Cancer Institute, United States Public Health Service, 1953), 3–4. We are grateful to Dr. Wild for copies of his progress reports.

134. J. J. Wild and J. M. Reid, "Echographic Visualization of Lesions in the Living Intact Human Breast," *Cancer Research* 14 (1954): 277–83, 281.

135. Quoted in Wild, "Use of Ultrasonic Pulses," 3–4.

136. Reid, "John Wild," 12.

137. Wild and Reid, "Echographic Visualization." By *craft skill* we mean a form of expertise, learned by experience, that cannot be reduced to a set of rules and is not taught by precept.

138. Reid, "John Wild," 12.

139. Ibid.

140. J. J. Wild, "Clinical Results of Echographic Diagnosis of Living Intact Lesions of the Breast of Primate, *Homo sapiens* (Female): The Use of Ultrasonic Pulses for the Measurement of Biological Tissues and the Detection of Tissue Density Changes; Progress Report for Period, July 1, 1953, to October 31, 1953" (Bethesda, MD: National Cancer Institute, United States Public Health Service, 1953).

141. Koch, "In the Image of Science," 881.

142. "The Scientific Righteousness of Dr Wild: A 63-Year Old Cancer Researcher Keeps Hunting for Justice," *Metropolis* (Minneapolis), 17 May 1977, newspaper cutting, Wild, John J., file, University Archives, University of Minnesota.

143. J. H. Holmes to I. Donald, 7 June 1974, BMUS Papers, 1/1/8.

144. B. J. Culliton, "Grant Termination: Scientist Wins $16 Million for Loss of Support," *Science* 178 (1972): 1177–80.

145. J. J. Wild, "The Origin of Soft-Tissue Ultrasonic Echoing and Early Instrumental Application to Clinical Medicine," in *Inventive Minds: Creativity in Technology*, ed. R. J. Weber and D. N. Perkins (New York: Oxford University Press, 1992), 115–41.

146. V. C. Wild, "Statement about Dr John J. Wild's Relationship with the University of Minnesota," 1998, Wild, John J., file, University Archives, University of Minnesota; "French and American Scientists Awarded 1991 (7th) Japan Prize," *Japan Prize News* 9 (1991): 1–3. Wild died in September 2009.

CHAPTER THREE: Ian Donald before Ultrasound I: St. Thomas's Hospital and the Royal Air Force

1. We are grateful to Dame Alison Munro for permission to use her unpublished essay "The Donalds in South Africa." All unreferenced information is from this source. See also J. Willocks, "Ian Donald (1910–1987)," *Oxford Dictionary of National Biography*

(Oxford: Oxford University Press, 2004), www.oxforddnb.com/view/article/40066; J. Willocks and W. Barr, *Ian Donald: A Memoir* (London: Royal College of Obstetricians and Gynaecologists Press, 2004).

2. "James Turner Donald, L.R.C.S.E" (obituary), *British Medical Journal* 1 (1891): 1412.

3. At the time of her marriage, Mrs. Donald was thirty-six years old. The Donald's first child, Kathleen, died at seven months. Mrs. Donald's second pregnancy ended in miscarriage. Her three youngest children were born when she was over forty years of age. Ian Donald often used the example of his mother's reproductive history to inspire older mothers in his care. I. Donald to Johanna [no surname], Mar. 1981, Prof. Ian Donald Papers, HB 110, NHS Greater Glasgow and Clyde Health Board Archive (hereafter, Donald Papers), 5/10.

4. I. Donald to Louise [no surname], 3 Sept. 1984, Donald Papers, 5/12.

5. R. Read, *My Children, My Children: Life before and after Birth; An Account of Some Recent Developments* (London: BBC, 1977), 58.

6. I. Donald to Adam Fox, undated, BMUS Papers, 1/1/6.

7. This was Donald's own diagnosis. I. Donald, *Practical Obstetric Problems*, 4th ed. (London: Lloyd-Luke, 1969), 108; I. Donald to E. R. Delbridge, 26 Nov. 1975, Donald Papers, 1/1/4A.

8. Ibid.

9. Read, *My Children*, 58. Donald spoke bitterly of this incident for the rest of his life. P. Rhodes, personal communication.

10. For the history of St. Thomas's, see E. M. McInnes, *St. Thomas' Hospital* (London: Allen and Unwin, 1963). In 1946, the legal name of the hospital was changed from "St. Thomas's" to "St. Thomas'"; the Medical School retained the older form. For simplicity, we have adopted "St. Thomas's" throughout.

11. L. P. Le Quesne, "Undergraduate Medical Education in London: The Last 40 Years," *Journal of the Royal Society of Medicine* 80 (1987): 606–10; N. Harte, *The University of London, 1836–1986* (London: Athlone, 1986), 193–94; G. Rivett, *The Development of the London Hospital System, 1823–1982* (London: King Edward's Hospital Fund, 1986); *Report of the Royal Commission on University Education in London: Final Report* (London: HMSO, 1913), 98–102, 297.

12. J. Crofton, interview, Nov. 2001. Sir John Crofton was a student at St. Thomas's, graduating in 1937.

13. This account of the London "greats" is substantially derived from the work of Christopher Lawrence: "Incommunicable Knowledge: Science, Technology and the Clinical Art in Britain, 1850–1914," *Journal of Contemporary History* 20 (1985): 503–20; "Still Incommunicable: Clinical Holists and Medical Knowledge in Interwar Britain," in *Greater Than the Parts: Holism in Biomedicine, 1920–1950*, ed. C. Lawrence and G. Weisz (Oxford: Oxford University Press, 1998), 94–111; and "Edward Jenner's Jockey Boots and the Great Tradition of English Medicine, 1918 to 1939," in *Regenerating England: Science, Medicine, and Culture in Inter-War Britain*, ed. C. Lawrence and A.-K. Mayer (Amsterdam: Rodopi, 2000), 45–62.

14. Lawrence, "Still Incommunicable."

15. "Sir Maurice Cassidy," *British Medical Journal* 2 (1949): 985–86; McInnes, *St. Thomas' Hospital*, 153; H.G.-H., "Sir Henry Tidy, K.B.E., M.D., F.R.C.P.," *British Medical Journal* 2 (1960): 1896–97.

16. R. Hutchison, "Harvey: The Man, His Method, and His Message for Us Today," *British Medical Journal* 2 (1931): 733–39, 737.

17. "Sir Maurice Cassidy"; C. Lawrence, "Moderns and Ancients: The 'New Cardiology' in Britain, 1880–1930," in *The Emergence of Modern Cardiology*, ed. W. F. Bynum, C. Lawrence, and V. Nutton (London: Wellcome Institute, 1985), 1–13.

18. C. M. W. Moran, *The Annual Address Delivered to the Royal College of Physicians of London* (London: Harrison, 1950), 8–10.

19. Hutchison, "Harvey," 737.

20. Lawrence, "Incommunicable."

21. W. D. Foster and J. L. Pinniger, "History of Pathology at St. Thomas's Hospital, London," *Medical History* 7 (1963): 330–47.

22. A[rthur] J[oseph] W[rigley], "Joseph Bamforth," *Lancet* 2 (1967): 453; J. Peel, *The Lives of the Fellows of the Royal College of Obstetricians and Gynaecologists, 1929–1969* (London: Heinneman, 1976), 61; S.Y., "Joseph Bamforth," *Lancet* 1 (1967): 453.

23. H. R. D[ean], "Leonard Stanley Dudgeon, 1876–1938," *Journal of Pathology and Bacteriology* 48 (1939): 231–35.

24. A. St. G. Huggett, "Foetal Blood-Gas Tension and Gas Transfusion through the Placenta of the Goat," *Journal of Physiology* 62 (1927): 373–84; J. B. Leathes, "John Mellanby," *Obituary Notices of Fellows of the Royal Society* 3 (1940): 173–95.

25. The Donalds had four children, Tessa Jacqueline (b. 1939, m. Eide), Alison Caroline (b. 1945, m. Wilkinson), Christina Margaret (b. 1952, m. Sargent), and Margaret Antonia (b. 1959, m. Weston). Mrs. Donald died in 2008.

26. Minute Book, Medical and Surgical Officers, St. Thomas's Hospital, 23 Jan. 1939, HI/ST/A137/2, London Metropolitan Archive.

27. I. Loudon, *Death in Childbirth: An International Study of Maternal Care and Maternal Mortality, 1800–1950* (Oxford: Clarendon Press, 1992), 229; O. Moscucci, *The Science of Woman: Gynaecology and Gender in England, 1800–1929* (Cambridge: Cambridge University Press, 1990).

28. "John Shields Fairbairn," *Lancet* 1 (1944): 199.

29. Loudon, *Death in Childbirth*, 191, 173.

30. W. F. Shaw, *Twenty-Five Years: The Story of the Royal College of Obstetricians and Gynaecologists, 1929–1954* (London: Churchill, 1954); W. F. Shaw, "The Birth of a College," *Journal of Obstetrics and Gynaecology of the British Empire* 57 (1950): 877–90.

31. "Charles James Cullingworth," *British Medical Journal* 1 (1908): 1269–72.

32. G. W. Thoebald, "The Changing Face of Midwifery," *Journal of Obstetrics and Gynaecology of the British Empire* 66 (1959): 1021–22; A. W. Bourne, *A Doctor's Creed: The Memoirs of a Gynaecologist* (London: Gollancz, 1962).

33. Peel, *Lives of the Fellows*, 146–48.

34. J. S. Fairbairn, *Gynaecology with Obstetrics: A Text-Book for Students and Practitioners* (Oxford: Oxford University Press, 1924).

35. J. S. Fairbairn, "Clinical Training in Obstetrics and Gynaecology," *Lancet* 2 (1927): 163–65.

36. J. S. Fairbairn, "Plea for a Wider Outlook in the Teaching of Obstetrics," *Journal of Obstetrics and Gynaecology of the British Empire* 46 (1939): 201–12.

37. Peel, *Lives of the Fellows*, 194–95.

38. Fairbairn, "Clinical Training in Obstetrics."

39. Crofton, interview.

40. Quoted in "John Shields Fairbairn."

41. O. Moscucci, "Holistic Obstetrics: The Origins of 'Natural Childbirth' in Britain," *Postgraduate Medical Journal* 79 (2003): 168–73, 170.

42. J. S. Fairbairn, "The Medical and Psychological Aspects of Gynaecology," *Lancet* 2 (1931); 999–1004, 1004.

43. Ibid., 999, 1004, 1003.

44. J. S. Fairbairn, *Obstetrics* (Oxford: Oxford University Press, 1926), 5.

45. McInnes, *St. Thomas'*, 154.

46. Fairbairn, "Medical and Psychological Aspects," 1003.

47. Fairbairn, "Clinical Training in Obstetrics," 164; Peel, *Lives of the Fellows*, 148.

48. J. S. Fairbairn, "On Abortion," *Lancet* 2 (1927): 217–19.

49. For laywomen's response to this crisis, see A. S. Williams, *Women and Childbirth in the Twentieth Century: A History of the National Birthday Trust Fund, 1928–9* (Thrupp, UK: Sutton, 1997); for obstetricians' reactions, see "Discussion on the Interim Report of the Departmental Committee on Maternal Mortality and Morbidity," *Proceedings of the Royal Society of Medicine* 24 (1931): 401–12.

50. Quoted in W. R. Merrington, *University College Hospital and Its Medical School: A History* (London: Heinemann, 1976), 143.

51. Loudon, *Death in Childbirth*, 542–44.

52. Ibid., 230.

53. Crofton, interview.

54. J. M. Munro Kerr, *Maternal Mortality and Morbidity: A Study of Their Problems* (Edinburgh: Livingstone, 1933), 110.

55. A. L. McIlroy, "Pregnancy and Associated Diseases," in *Historical Review of British Obstetrics and Gynaecology, 1800–1950*, ed. J. M. Munro Kerr, R. W. Johnstone, and M. H. Phillips (Edinburgh: Livingstone, 1954), 168–201, 174; J. Mackenzie, *Heart Disease in Pregnancy* (Oxford: Oxford Medical Publications, 1921).

56. Ministry of Health, *Report of an Investigation into Maternal Mortality* (London: HMSO, 1937), Cmd. 5422.

57. I. Donald, letter, 20 July 1939, name of correspondent withheld, Donald Papers, 1/2A. Donald was addressing a common failing. In 1933, the leading obstetrician, Munro Kerr, wrote that "the misuse of the forceps" was "a disgrace to obstetric practice." Munro Kerr, *Maternal Mortality*, 114; M. D. Crawford, "The Obstetric Forceps and Its Use," *Lancet* 2 (1932): 1239–43.

58. All medical students at St. Thomas's in Donald's time were male.

59. A. Donald, interview, July 1996.

60. I. Donald, "Curriculum Vitae," undated, Donald Papers, 1/4.

61. R. A. Watson-Watt, *Three Steps to Victory* (London: Odhams, 1957).

62. R. Buderi, *The Invention That Changed the World: How a Small Group of Radar Pioneers Won the Second World War and Launched a Technological Revolution* (New York: Simon and Schuster, 1996), 55–59.

63. R. A. Watson-Watt, "The Evolution of Radio Location," *Journal of the Institution of Electrical Engineers* 93 (1946): 11–19.

64. A. (Dame Alison) Munro, interview, Sept. 1996. Mrs. Munro's degree was in PPE (philosophy, politics, and economics). See also Buderi, *Invention*, 174.

65. I. Donald to D. Baird, 24 Apr. 1968, Donald Papers, 5/1.

66. Munro, interview.

67. For the history of 206 Squadron, see www.raf.mod.uk/history/h206to617; www .raf.mod.uk/rakkinloss (both accessed June 2012).

68. C. Barnett, *Engage the Enemy More Closely: The Royal Navy in the Second World War* (London: Hodder and Stoughton, 1991).

69. Buderi, *Invention*, 86–89.

70. "Air of Authority—A History of RAF Organisation," No. 206–210 Squadron Histories, No. 206 Squadron, www.rafweb.org/Sqn206-210.htm (accessed June 2012).

71. T. Devereux, *Messenger Gods of Battle* (London: Brassey, 1990), xxvii.

72. Munro, interview; Buderi, *Invention*, 130; *Air Defence Radar Museum Newsletter*, no. 29 (Oct. 2001).

73. We are grateful to Professor Charles Whitfield for sharing his recollections of conversations with Donald on his wartime involvement with radar.

74. J. Gough, *Watching the Skies: A History of Ground Radar for the Air Defence of the United Kingdom by the Royal Air Force from 1946 to 1975* (London: Stationery Office Books, 1992), 20.

75. R. Pool, *Beyond Engineering: How Society Shapes Technology* (Oxford: Oxford University Press, 1997), 67.

76. S. C. Rexford-Welch, *The Royal Air Force Medical Services*, vol. 2, *Commands* (London: HMSO, 1954–58), 312–17.

77. I. Donald, "Clinical Alarm," *Surgo* 22 (1956): 123–28, 127.

78. Munro, interview.

79. M. G. Gelder, "Hill, Sir (John) Denis Nelson (1913–1982)," *Oxford Dictionary of National Biography* (Oxford: Oxford University Press, 2004), www.oxforddnb.com/view /article/31231; R. Cooper, "Walter, (William) Grey (1910–1977)," *Oxford Dictionary of National Biography* (Oxford: Oxford University Press, 2004), www.oxforddnb.com/view /article/38104; D. Hill, *Psychiatry in Medicine: Retrospect and Prospect* (London: Nuffield Provincial Hospitals Trust, 1969).

80. I. Donald to A. Lewis, 15 Mar. 1946, Donald Papers, 1/1. On Lewis and psychiatry at the Maudsley, see K. Angel, E. Jones, and M. Neve, eds., *European Psychiatry on the Eve of War: Aubrey Lewis, the Maudsley Hospital, and the Rockefeller Foundation in the 1930s*, Medical History Suppl. 22 (London: Wellcome Trust Centre for the History of Medicine, 2003).

81. J. Calnan, *The Hammersmith: 1935–1985: The First Fifty Years of the Royal Postgraduate Medical School at Hammersmith Hospital, 1935–1985* (Lancaster, UK: MTP, 1985), 49.

82. T. Donald, personal communication.

83. Ministry of Health, *Report of the Inter-Departmental Committee on Medical Schools*, The Goodenough Report (London: HMSO, 1944); Harte, *University of London*, 251.

84. S. Sturdy and R. Cooter, "Science, Scientific Management and the Transformation of Medicine in Britain, c. 1870–1950," *History of Science* 36 (1998): 421–66; A. Hull, "Hector's House: Sir Hector Hetherington and the Academicization of Glasgow Hospital Medicine before the NHS," *Medical History* 45 (2001): 207–42.

85. Minute Book, Medical and Surgical Officers, St. Thomas's Hospital, 9 June 1947, HI/ST/A137/2, London Metropolitan Archive.

86. I. Donald to Anna [Dionello], 11 Feb. 1984, Donald Papers, 5/5; I. Donald to J. M. Reid, undated, Donald Papers, 5/18. The Government Ex-Service Specialist Scheme supplemented Donald's income by £1,000 a year from 1947 to 1949.

87. I. Donald to Tessa [Donald], 5 Nov. 1983, Donald Papers, 5/20.

88. A. J. Wrigley, "A Criticism of Ante-natal Work," *British Medical Journal* 1 (1934): 891–94; R. H. Boggon and A. J. Wrigley, "Rupture of Ovarian Blood-Cysts Simulating Acute Appendicitis," *Lancet* 2 (1931): 1068–70.

89. A. J. Wrigley to I. Donald, 11 Apr. 1952, Donald Papers, 1/1; P. R[hodes], "A. J. Wrigley," *British Medical Journal* 1 (1984): 156–57.

90. A. J. Wrigley, "The Forceps Operation," *Lancet* 2 (1939): 702–5.

91. A. J. Wrigley to May [no surname], Apr. 1976, S9/5, Archives, Royal College of Obstetricians and Gynaecologists.

92. We have not been able to trace Donald's MD dissertation but have gained an impression of its contents from family members.

93. P. Rhodes, "The Start of the Academic Department of Obstetrics and Gynaecology at St. Thomas's Medical School," *St. Thomas's Gazette*, spring 1989, 10–13.

94. P. Rhodes to M. Young, 3 Aug. 2001. We are grateful to Professor Young for showing us this letter and to Professor Rhodes for allowing us to quote from it.

95. I. Donald, *Practical Obstetric Problems* (London: Lloyd-Luke, 1955); I. Donald, "Aetiology and Investigation of Vaginal Discharge," *British Medical Journal* 2 (1952): 1223–26. Donald was a mature forty-one when his first research paper appeared.

96. A. J. Wrigley, "Puerperal Infection by the Pathogenic Anaerobic Bacteria," *British Medical Journal* 1 (1930): 1176–77.

97. I. Donald, "Aetiology and Investigation," 1223.

98. McInnes, *St. Thomas'*, 178.

99. Ibid., 177–78.

100. I. Donald, "Resuscitation of the Newborn," *Postgraduate Medical Journal* 29 (1953): 247–53.

101. Loudon, *Death in Childbirth*, chap. 15.

102. P. Rhodes, *A Short History of Clinical Midwifery* (Hale, UK: Books for Midwives Press, 1995), 129–46.

103. R. M. Titmus, *Birth, Poverty, and Wealth: A Study of Infant Mortality* (London: Hamilton, 1943).

104. I. Donald and J. Lord, "Augmented Respiration: Studies in Atelectasis Neonatorum," *Lancet* 1 (1953): 9–17, 13. Machines that assist breathing are now known as ventilators.

105. J. Barcroft, *Researches on Pre-natal Life* (Oxford: Blackwell, 1946); I. M. Young, "Classics Revisited: Researches on Pre-natal Life by Sir Joseph Barcroft," *Placenta* 13 (1992): 607–12. On retirement as professor of physiology at Cambridge, Barcroft was made director of the Animal Physiology Unit, Agricultural Research Council. K. J. Franklin, *Joseph Barcroft, 1872–1947* (Oxford: Blackwell, 1953).

106. I. M. Young, interview, Aug. 2001

107. Barcroft, *Researches*, ix.

108. Young, interview.

109. Donald and Lord, "Augmented Respiration"; I. Donald, "Atelectasis Neonatorum," *Journal of Obstetrics and Gynaecology of the British Empire* 61 (1954): 725–37, 736. We are grateful to the Fleet Air Arm Museum for information on Commander Slater.

110. I. Donald and I. M. Young, "An Automatic Respiratory Amplifier," *Journal of Physiology, Proceedings*, 1952, 41–43.

111. I. Donald, "Uterine Rupture," *Proceedings of the Royal Society of Medicine* 40 (1947): 379–80; I. Donald, "Aetiology and Investigation."

112. Calnan, *Hammersmith.*

113. Minutes of the Council, St. Thomas's Medical School, 5 Feb. 1952, Th/AD/2, St. Thomas's Hospital Medical School Record, King's College London Archives.

CHAPTER FOUR: Ian Donald before Ultrasound II: Hammersmith and Glasgow

1. C. Newman, "A Brief History of the Postgraduate Medical School," *Medical History* 10 (1966); 285–88; J. Calnan, *The Hammersmith: 1935–1985: The First Fifty Years of the Royal Postgraduate Medical School at Hammersmith Hospital, 1935–1985* (Lancaster, UK: MTP, 1985), 34.

2. "Francis Richard Fraser," *Lancet* 2 (1964): 867–69; C. Dollery, "Sir John Mc-Michael," *Biographical Memoirs of Fellows of the Royal Society* 41 (1995): 282–96; O. P. Sharma, *Prof: The Life of Sheila Sherlock, "The Liver Queen"* (London: Royal College of Physicians, 2007).

3. C. C. Booth, "Medical Science and Technology at the Royal Postgraduate Medical School," *British Medical Journal* 2 (1985): 1771–79; H. McLeave, *A Time to Heal: The Life of Ian Aird, the Surgeon* (London: Heinemann, 1964); "John Campbell McClure Browne," *British Medical Journal* 2 (1978): 438.

4. J. Crofton, interview, Nov. 2001.

5. Ibid.

6. Calnan, *Hammersmith*, 62.

7. S. Westaby with C. Bosher, *Landmarks in Cardiac Surgery* (Oxford: Isis Medical Media, 1997), 77.

8. I. Aird, D. G. Melrose, W. P. Cleland, and R. B. Lynn, "Assisted Circulation by Pump Oxygenation during Operative Dilation of the Aortic Valve in Man," *British Medical Journal* 1 (1954): 1284–87.

9. I. Donald to William Blair, 17 Nov. 1975, Donald Papers, 5/3A.

10. A. Macfarlane and M. Mugford, *Birth Counts: Statistics of Pregnancy and Childbirth* (London: HMSO, 2000), 1: 51.

11. I. Donald, "Atelectasis Neonatorum," *Journal of Obstetrics and Gynaecology of the British Empire* 61 (1954): 725–37.

12. Calnan, *Hammersmith*, 53.

13. R. E. Steiner, interview, May 2002.

14. I. Donald and J. Lord, "Augmented Respiration: Studies in Atelectasis Neonatorum," *Lancet* 1 (1953): 9–17.

15. "Atelectasis Neonatorum," *Lancet* 1 (1953): 31–32; D. O'Brien, "Augmented Respiration," *Lancet* 1 (1953): 246; Donald and Lord, "Augmented Respiration."

16. I. Donald, "Resuscitation of the Newborn," *Postgraduate Medical Journal* 29 (1953): 247–53.

17. Ibid., 253.

18. I. Donald, "Augmented Respiration: An Emergency Positive-Pressure Patient-Cycled Respirator," *Lancet* 1 (1954): 895–99.

19. Donald, "Resuscitation of the Newborn," 253.

20. Donald, "Augmented Respiration," 897.

21. McLeave, *Time to Heal*, 195.

22. Calnan, *Hammersmith*, 114.

23. R. A. Risdon, "Albert Edward Claireaux," *British Medical Journal* 2 (1995): 1365; A. E. Claireaux, "Hyaline Membrane in the Neonatal Lung," *Lancet* 2 (1953): 749–53.

24. S. J. Reiser, *Medicine and the Reign of Technology* (Cambridge: Cambridge University Press, 1978).

25. Booth, "Medical Science and Technology."

26. Steiner, interview.

27. Donald, "Resuscitation of the Newborn," 253.

28. Steiner, interview.

29. Ibid.

30. I. Donald and R. E. Steiner, "Radiography in the Diagnosis of Hyaline Membrane," *Lancet* 2 (1953): 846–49.

31. J. Caffey, *Pediatric X-Ray Diagnosis: A Textbook for Students and Practitioners of Pediatrics, Surgery, and Radiology* (Chicago: Year Book Publishers, 1945), 248.

32. R. E. Steiner, "The Radiology of Respiratory Distress in the Newborn," *British Journal of Radiology* 27 (1954): 491–99; I. Donald, "Radiology in Neonatal Respiratory Disorders," *British Journal of Radiology* 27 (1954): 500–503.

33. Steiner, interview.

34. Donald, "Atelectasis Neonatorum."

35. Ibid., 726. The source citation refers to D. Baird, "The Influence of Social and Economic Factors on Stillbirths and Neonatal Deaths," *Journal of Obstetrics and Gynaecology of the British Empire* 52 (1945): 217–34.

36. I. Donald, *Practical Obstetric Problems* (London: Lloyd-Duke, 1955).

37. Ibid., 5. *Iron curtain* might seem an odd, even offensive, term for the female abdominal wall. However, the phrase was originally coined to refer to the fire safety curtains used in theaters and had, by the 1930s, acquired the metaphorical meaning of a barrier to communication. P. Wright, *Iron Curtain: From Stage to Cold War* (Oxford: Oxford University Press, 2007).

38. Donald, *Practical Obstetric Problems*, 167, 211.

39. A. Hull, "Hector's House: Sir Hector Hetherington and the Academicization of Glasgow Hospital Medicine before the NHS," *Medical History* 45 (2001): 207–42; H. Conway and R. T. Hutcheson, "The Glasgow Medical Faculty, 1936–39: A Change of Direction," *Scottish Medical Journal* 41 (1996): 178–79.

40. J. Peel, *The Lives of the Fellows of the Royal College of Obstetricians and Gynaecologists, 1929–1969* (London: Heinneman, 1976), 19–20.

41. J. Jenkinson, M. Moss, and I. Russell, *The Royal: The History of the Glasgow Royal Infirmary, 1794–1994* (Glasgow: Glasgow Royal Infirmary NHS Trust, 1994); L. MacQueen and A. B. Kerr, *The Western Infirmary, 1874–1974* (Glasgow: Horn, 1974).

42. D. A. Dow, *The Rottenrow: The History of the Glasgow Royal Maternity Hospital, 1834–1984* (Carnforth, UK: Parthenon, 1984).

43. J. M. Munro Kerr, R. W. Johnstone, and M. H. Phillips, *Historical Review of British Obstetrics and Gynaecology, 1800–1950* (Edinburgh: Livingstone, 1954), 79.

44. I. Loudon, *Death in Childbirth: An International Study of Maternal Care and Maternal Mortality, 1800–1950* (Oxford: Clarendon Press, 1992), 137.

45. J. M. Munro Kerr, *Operative Midwifery* (London: Baillière, Tindall and Cox, 1908); J. M. Munro Kerr, *Clinical and Operative Gynaecology* (Oxford: Oxford Medical Publications, 1922).

46. H. Hetherington to several correspondents, 1 Mar. 1954, Hetherington Papers, 49.8, 892, Glasgow University Archives (hereafter, Hetherington Papers).

47. W. I. C. Morris to H. Hetherington, 4 Mar. 1954, Hetherington Papers.

48. "T. N. MacGregor" (obituary), *British Medical Journal* 1 (1988): 437.

49. R. J. Kellar to H. Hetherington, 4 Mar. 1954, Hetherington Papers.

50. W. I. C. Morris to H. Hetherington, 4 Mar. 1954, Hetherington Papers.

51. J. H. Dible to H. Hetherington, 2 Mar. 1954, Hetherington Papers.

52. C. Illingworth, *University Statesman: Sir Hector Hetherington* (Glasgow: Outram, 1971), 57.

53. Steiner, interview.

54. I. Donald to J. J. Wild, 28 Feb. 1978, Donald Papers, 5/22. Chassar Moir was interested in placental localization. J. C. Moir, "Fallacies in Soft Tissue Placentography," *American Journal of Obstetrics and Gynecology* 47 (1944): 198–210.

55. J. J. Wild, interview, Nov. 1998.

56. J. J. Wild and D. Neal, "Use of High-Frequency Ultrasonic Waves for Detecting Changes of Texture in Living Tissues," *Lancet* 1 (1951): 655–57.

57. Wild tried to obviate this difficulty by means of transrectal probes, patenting such an obstetric device in 1958. One may speculate how the social significance of the fetal image might have been different if Wild's method of obtaining the pictures had become adopted, rather than Brown's.

58. Wild's University Lecture was not published, but he informed us that it was substantially similar to J. J. Wild and J. M. Reid, "Echographic Tissue Diagnosis," *Proceedings of the Fourth Annual Conference on Ultrasound Therapy, Detroit* (Washington, DC: American Institute of Ultrasound in Medicine, 1955), 1–26.

59. I. Donald to J. J. Wild, 28 Feb. 1978, Donald Papers, 5/22.

60. The reasons for his skepticism are explored in chapter 6.

61. J. R. Greer and I. Donald, "A Volume Controlled Patient-Cycled Respirator for Adults," *British Journal of Anaesthesia* 30 (1958): 32–36.

62. Donald first undertook this procedure at the Hammersmith, having been inspired by the example of Sherlock and McMichael. Donald, "Atelectasis Neonatorum," 727. These experiments resemble ones undertaken on animals by Barcroft.

63. I. Donald, "Neonatal Respiration and Hyaline Membrane," *British Journal of Anaesthesia* 29 (1957): 533–69.

64. A. Stewart, J. Webb, D. Giles, and D. Hewitt, "Malignant Disease in Childhood and Diagnostic Irradiation In Utero," *Lancet* 2 (1956): 447; G. Greene, *The Woman Who Knew Too Much: Alice Stewart and the Secrets of Radiation* (Ann Arbor: University of Michigan Press, 1999).

65. W. M. Court Brown, R. Doll, and A. B. Hill, "Incidence of Leukaemia after Exposure to Diagnostic Radiation In Utero," *British Medical Journal* 2 (1960): 1539–45; T. L. T. Lewis, "Leukaemia in Childhood after Antenatal Exposure to X rays," *British Medical Journal* 2 (1960): 1551–2; I. Donald, *Practical Obstetric Problems*, 4th ed. (London: Lloyd-Luke, 1969), 463; S. Dry, "The Population as Patient: Alice Stewart and the Controversy over Low-Level Radiation in the 1950s," in *The Risks of Medical Innovation:*

Risk Perception and Assessment in Historical Context, ed. T. Schlich and U. Tröhler (London: Routledge, 2006), 116–32.

66. Donald and Lord, "Augmented Respiration," 17.

67. Surfactant therapy became feasible in the mid-1980s. A. Jobe, "Surfactant Treatment for Respiratory Distress Syndrome," *Respiratory Care* 31 (1986): 467–76.

68. Donald, "Neonatal Respiration," 567.

69. R. McAdams, "Learning to Breathe: The History of Newborn Resuscitation, 1929 to 1970" (PhD diss., University of Glasgow, 2008).

CHAPTER FIVE: A-Scope Investigations in Glasgow

1. W. Barr, "Ian Donald," undated typescript, BMUS Papers, 1/1/4.

2. B. Carlin, *Ultrasonics* (New York: McGraw-Hill, 1949).

3. I. Donald, "Medical Sonar—The First 25 years," *Recent Advances in Ultrasound Diagnosis* 2 (1980): 4–20. We have been unable to unearth any information about this machine.

4. Ibid.

5. J. Rennie to J. E. E. Fleming, 25 Oct. 1999, BMUS Papers, 2/19.

6. B. Donnelly, interview, May 1996.

7. Industrial ultrasound technicians still use their thumbs as rough calibration devices. B. Fraser, personal communication. The thumb needs to be wet to facilitate acoustic coupling.

8. Donnelly, interview.

9. Donald, "Medical Sonar," 6.

10. Ibid.

11. W. Barr, interview, Nov. 1995. For Donald's accounts, see his "Ultrasonic Diagnosis: The Story of an Experiment," *Surgo* 22 (1965): 3–6; "On Launching a New Diagnostic Science," *American Journal of Obstetrics and Gynecology* 103 (1969): 609–28; "Apologia: How and Why Medical Sonar Developed," *Annals of the Royal College of Surgeons of England* 54 (1974): 312–40; and "Sonar—The Story of an Experiment," *Ultrasound in Medicine and Biology* 1 (1974): 109–17.

12. No one can recall Babcock's having a "factory artist," but the company would have employed draughtsmen.

13. Having decided to reenact Donald's experiments, we realized that legal, ethical, and public health considerations prevented us filling the trunks of our cars with pathological specimens. Furthermore, we were the victims of ultrasound's success: owing to improved diagnoses, very large ovarian cysts are seldom seen by the modern gynecologist. The solution was to use animal material. Jack Boyd, professor of veterinary anatomy, kindly provided us with fresh solid tumor specimens and a horse ovary with a large Graafian follicle. We were advised, moreover, that the ultrasonic characteristics of a urinary bladder are virtually identical to those of a simple ovarian cyst. We obtained a selection of bovine and canine bladders and filled them with water. In addition to the participants shown in figure 5.2, the following were present: Prof. I. T. Cameron, B. Donnelly, M. Farley, B. W. Fraser, J. R.-B. Powell, R. Service, and D. Smith. For footage of the reenactment, see I. Spencer, J. E. E. Fleming, and M. Nicolson, *A Scan through the History of Ultrasound* (Glasgow: Wellcome Unit for the History of Medicine, 1996), video.

14. See I. Donald, J. MacVicar, and T. G. Brown, "Investigation of Abdominal Masses by Pulsed Ultrasound," *Lancet* 1 (1958): 1188–95.

15. Barr, interview.

16. For techniques of nondestructive testing in the 1950s, see B. Chalmers and A. G. Quarrell, *The Physical Examination of Metals* (London: Arnold, 1960).

17. E. N. Simons, "The Supersonic Flaw Detector," *Metal Progress* 48 (1945): 513–16.

18. Barr, interview.

19. In contrast, during our reenactment, Margaret McNay, using unfamiliar equipment but with years of scanning experience, quickly and confidently showed the difference between a full and empty bladder in vivo (see fig. 5.3F, G).

20. Donald, "Medical Sonar," 18.

21. Some commentators have objected that we denigrate Donald's achievement by emphasizing the importance of chance in the success of these experiments. However, all successful experimenters need luck and must have the ability to exploit their luck. Our point is that how ultrasound would work when applied to cysts and fibroids was not wholly knowable in advance, and certainly was not fully anticipated by Donald.

22. Distortion is the total effect of refraction, absorption, and reverberation.

23. Carlin, *Ultrasonics*, 243–58.

24. Donnelly, interview.

25. A. Stewart, J. Webb, D. Giles, and D. Hewitt, "Malignant Disease in Childhood and Diagnostic Irradiation In Utero," *Lancet* 2 (1956): 447.

26. Donald, "Medical Sonar," 5–6.

27. A solid uterine tumor may also, on occasion, have a malignant origin. This is not mentioned by Donald in his accounts of his early investigations.

28. Donald, "Apologia," 317.

29. D. N. White, "Neurosonology Pioneers," *Ultrasound in Medicine and Biology* 14 (1988): 541–61.

30. Donald, "Sonar—Story of an Experiment," 110.

31. Donald, "Medical Sonar," 7.

32. T. G. Brown, interview, Apr. 2001.

33. Ibid.

34. Ibid.; R. Brownell, D. Nowacek, and K. Ralls, "Hunting Cetaceans with Sound: A Worldwide Review," *Journal of Cetacean Research Management* 10 (2008): 81–88.

35. Alexander Bryce Calder Rankin (1924–1963), a leading member of the Hair-Line Crack Sub-Committee, was the author of many patents on industrial applications of ultrasound.

36. Brown, interview.

37. Ibid. For the U.S. patent, see T. G. Brown, A. B. C. Rankin, and R. G. Haslett, "3,041,872, Apparatus for Ultrasonic Testing of Materials," U.S. Patent Office, 1962.

38. T. Soller, M. A. Starr, and G. E. Valley, *Cathode-Ray Tube Displays* (New York: McGraw-Hill, 1948); B. Chance, V. Hughes, E. F. MacNichol, D. Sayre, and F. C. Williams, eds., *Waveforms* (Lexington, MA: Boston Technical Publications, 1949): J. L. Lawson and G. E. Uhlenbeck, eds., *Threshold Signals* (New York: McGraw-Hill, 1950).

39. This and the following comments by Brown are from Brown, interview.

40. L. Leksell, "Echo-encephalography 1: Detection of Intracranial Complications following Brain Injury," *Acta Chirurgica Scandinavica* 110 (1956): 301–15; D. Gordon,

"Echoencephalography: Ultrasonic Rays in Diagnostic Radiology," *British Medical Journal* 1 (1959): 1500–1504.

41. In 1956, £600 was more than the cost of a family car. Rankin's response was clearly an expression of confidence in Brown.

42. Brown, interview.

43. Ibid.; J. MacVicar, interview, Aug. 1997.

44. T. G. Brown, "Development of Ultrasonic Scanning Techniques in Scotland, 1956–1979," 1999, www.ob-ultrasound.net./brown-on-ultrasound.html (accessed June 2012).

45. The tank is now in the BMUS Historical Collection.

46. MacVicar, interview.

47. Donald, "On Launching a New Diagnostic Science," 613.

48. Donald, MacVicar, and Brown, "Investigation of Abdominal Masses"; J. MacVicar, "Ultrasound as a Diagnostic Aid in Obstetrics and Gynaecology" (MD thesis, University of Glasgow, 1959).

49. Donald, "On Launching a New Diagnostic Science," 613. In fact, the water bath was occasionally used later for testing new equipment or techniques.

50. MacVicar, interview.

51. MacVicar, "Ultrasound as a Diagnostic Aid," 50.

52. Ibid., 55.

53. Ibid., 157.

54. There are several versions of this story, which is an indication of its significance. Donald, "Ultrasonic Diagnosis," 4–5; Donald, MacVicar, and Brown, "Investigation of Abdominal Masses," 1193; Donald, "Sonar—Story of an Experiment," 111; MacVicar, interview. We have made a compound version that seems the most plausible, but nothing hinges on the particular details. In MacVicar's recollection, it was he, not Donald, who was operating the probe.

55. E. M. Tansey and D. A. Christie, eds., *Looking at the Unborn: Historical Aspects of Obstetric Ultrasound* (London: Wellcome Trust, 2000), 20.

56. Donald, "Medical Sonar," 9.

57. T. A. Traill, "Left Atrial Myxoma," in *Oxford Textbook of Medicine*, 2nd ed., ed. D. J. Weatherall, J. G. G. Ledingham, and D. A. Warrell (Oxford: Oxford University Press, 1990), sect. 13.313.

58. Ibid.

59. S. Effert, H. Erkerus, and E. Grosse-Brockhoff, "Ueber die anwendung des ultrashall echoverfahrens in der hersdiagnostick," *Deutsche Medizinische Wochenschrift* 82 (1957): 1253; Donald, Brown, and MacVicar, "Investigation of Abdominal Masses."

60. L. J. Acierno, *The History of Cardiology* (London: Parthenon, 1994), 571–81.

61. Donald, "Sonar—Story of an Experiment," 112.

62. J. J. Wild and J. M. Reid, "Further Pilot Echographic Studies on the Histologic Structure of Tumors of the Living Intact Human Breast," *American Journal of Pathology* 28 (1952): 839–61.

63. Donald, MacVicar, and Brown, "Investigation of Abdominal Masses," 1193–94.

64. Ibid., 1194.

65. MacVicar, interview.

66. American work had indicated that nerve tissue was particularly sensitive to heat coagulation. V. J. Wulff, W. J. Fry, D. Tucker, F. J. Fry, and C. Melton, "Effects of

Ultrasonic Vibrations on Nerve Tissues," *Proceedings of the Society for Experimental Biology and Medicine* 76 (1951): 361–66.

67. J. Willocks, interview, Aug. 1996.

68. MacVicar, "Ultrasound as a Diagnostic Aid," 161.

69. Donald, "Sonar—Story of an Experiment," 112.

70. Obesity makes abdominal palpation difficult; virginity, anxiety, obesity, or absence of consent may preclude vaginal examination.

CHAPTER SIX: The First Contact Scanner

1. I. Donald, "Sonar—The Story of an Experiment," *Ultrasound in Medicine and Biology* 1 (1974): 109–117, 112.

2. T. G. Brown, interview, Apr. 2001.

3. Ibid.

4. R. Buderi, *The Invention That Changed the World: How a Small Group of Radar Pioneers Won the Second World War and Launched a Technological Revolution* (New York: Simon and Schuster, 1996), 78.

5. It is likely that Donald did not have much involvement with radar systems after he left Benbecula in 1943. Hence he may not have been aware of the more sophisticated systems that were developed later.

6. We are grateful to Brown for information on William Slater.

7. Brown, interview.

8. Ibid.

9. I. Donald, "Sonar—Story of an Experiment," 111.

10. T. G. Brown, "Development of Ultrasonic Scanning Techniques in Scotland, 1956–1979: Personal Recollections of T. G. Brown," unpublished typescript, undated, ca. 1989, 10, BMUS Papers, 1/1/40.

11. Meccano is the proprietary name of a construction set, popular with hobbyists from 1930 to the 1960s. A large set was available in the research laboratory at Kelvin and Hughes.

12. For the forms of ultrasound display, see A. B. Wolbarst, *Looking Within: How X-ray, CT, MRI, Ultrasound, and Other Medical Images Are Created* (Berkeley: University of California Press, 1999).

13. T. G. Brown, "Ultrasound in Glasgow," unpublished paper, BMUS Papers, 1/1/40.

14. This aspect of Brown's technique is similar in principle to (if different in practice from) Howry's circular sector scanning.

15. Nicolson is grateful to Wild for a viewing of his cine films.

16. J. J. Wild, interview, Nov. 1998.

17. I. Donald, J. MacVicar, and T. G. Brown, "Investigation of Abdominal Masses by Pulsed Ultrasound," *Lancet* 1 (1985): 1188–95, 1194.

18. J. J. Wild, "The Origin of Soft-tissue Ultrasonic Echoing and Early Instrumental Application to Clinical Medicine," in *Inventive Minds: Creativity in Technology*, ed. R. J. Weber and D. N. Perkins (New York: Oxford University Press, 1992), 115–41, 135; Wild, interview.

19. Donald, MacVicar, and Brown, "Investigation of Abdominal Masses," 1194; J. MacVicar, "Ultrasound as a Diagnostic Aid in Obstetrics and Gynaecology" (MD thesis, University of Glasgow, 1959), 28–29.

20. Brown, interview.

21. Donald was eventually able to arrange for Brown to be excused military service.

22. Brown, interview.

23. Brown, "Ultrasound in Glasgow."

24. E. M. Tansey and D. A. Christie, eds., *Looking at the Unborn: Historical Aspects of Obstetric Ultrasound* (London: Wellcome Trust), 18.

25. T. G. Brown, "Direct Contact Ultrasonic Scanning Techniques for the Visualization of Abdominal Masses," in *Medical Electronics: Proceedings of the 2nd International Conference of Medical Electronics, Paris, 1959,* ed. C. N. Smyth (London: Iliffe, 1960), 258–366.

26. The larger mechanical parts of the scanner were built from Brown's drawings by technicians in the model shop at Hillington. Brown had studied kinematics at Glasgow College of Technology. A vee-roller is so-called because its rolling surface is a V-shaped grove that engages with a guide rail, ensuring precise travel along the rail.

27. Brown, interview.

28. Ibid.

29. Donald, MacVicar, and Brown, "Investigation of Abdominal Masses," 1193–94.

30. The bed-table scanner was acquired by Glasgow Museums and is on long-term loan to the Hunterian Museum, Glasgow University, where it is on public display.

31. Brown, interview.

32. J. MacVicar, interview, Apr. 1997.

33. MacVicar, "Ultrasound as a Diagnostic Aid in Obstetrics."

34. Donald, MacVicar, and Brown, "Investigation of Abdominal Masses," 1192.

35. The interpretation of early X-ray images presented similar difficulties. B. Pasveer, "Knowledge of Shadows: The Introduction of X-ray Images in Medicine," *Sociology of Health and Illness* 11 (1989): 360–81.

36. D. J. Morton, *Manual of Human Cross Section Anatomy,* 2nd ed. (Baltimore: Williams and Wilkins, 1944). Cross-sectional drawings are commonplace in engineering contexts.

37. J. Shaw-Dunn, personal communication. Barr later admitted great embarrassment at his remark; personal communication. In the 1960s, he supported ultrasound research by taking over clinical duties to allow Donald to spend more time on imaging.

38. D. Hamilton, personal communication.

39. I. Donald, "Apologia: How and Why Medical Sonar Developed," *Annals of the Royal College of Surgeons of England* 54 (1974): 132–40, 138; A. Donald, "Vancouver Conference Speech," 13 Oct. 1990, typescript, Donald Papers, 6/8.

40. Illingworth held the Regius Chair; Mackey, the St. Mungo Chair.

41. I. Donald to A. J. Wrigley, undated, Donald Papers, 1/1/21; I. Donald, "Sonar—Story of an Experiment," 112.

42. MacVicar, "Ultrasound as a Diagnostic Aid in Obstetrics," 103, 108.

43. Ibid., 109, 125.

44. Ibid., 116. Hydronephrosis is dilation of the kidney secondary to urinary tract obstruction. In pyelography, the renal pelvis and ureter are filled with a radio-opaque fluid for imaging.

45. Ibid., 130.

46. MacVicar, "Ultrasound as a Diagnostic Aid in Obstetrics," 127–29.

47. Donald used *cystic cavity* to refer to the gravid uterus in Donald, MacVicar, and Brown, "Investigation of Abdominal Masses," 1192. For a discussion between Nicolson and Brown regarding the significance of the early polyhydramnios images, see Tansey and Christie, *Looking at the Unborn*, 10. Nicolson now considers that he should retract his retraction.

48. As stated by Donald, MacVicar, and Brown, "Our apparatus . . . combines B-scope and P.P.I. presentation," which imperfectly captures the sophistication of Brown's imaging technique. Donald, MacVicar, and Brown, "Investigation of Abdominal Masses," 1190.

49. Ibid., 1191, 1192.

50. Ibid., 1194.

51. MacVicar, "Ultrasound as a Diagnostic Aid," 162.

52. J. J. Wild and J. M. Reid, "Progress in the Techniques of Soft Tissue Examination by 15MC Pulsed Ultrasound," in *Ultrasound in Biology and Medicine*, ed. E. Kelly (Washington, DC: American Institute of Biological Science, 1957), 30–48, 46.

53. MacVicar, "Ultrasound as a Diagnostic Aid," 162.

CHAPTER SEVEN: The Automatic Scanner and the Diasonograph

1. I. Donald, J. MacVicar, and T. G. Brown, "Investigation of Abdominal Masses by Pulsed Ultrasound," *Lancet* 1 (1958): 1188–95.

2. J. MacVicar, interview, Aug. 1997. All those who operated the bed-table scanner were male.

3. T. G. Brown, personal communication.

4. T. G. Brown, "Development of Ultrasonic Scanning Techniques in Scotland, 1956–1979: Personal Recollections of T. G. Brown," unpublished typescript, ca. 1989, 23, BMUS Papers, 1/1/40.

5. Ibid, 23, 24.

6. For examples of scientific claims gaining credibility by being decoupled from their originators, see H. Collins, *Changing Order: Replication and Induction in Scientific Practice* (London: Sage, 1985), 145–52.

7. T. G. Brown, interview, Apr. 2001.

8. This technique was used by astronomers. A. A. Hoag and W. C. Miller, "Application of Photographic Materials in Astronomy," *Applied Optics* 8 (1969): 2417–30.

9. Hundreds of cards are preserved in the BMUS Papers.

10. For technologies of record keeping, see S. J. Reiser, "Creating Form out of Mass: The Development of the Medical Record," in *Transformation and the Sciences: Essays in Honor of I. Bernard Cohen*, ed. E. Mendelsohn (Cambridge: Cambridge University Press, 1984), 303–16; G. C. Bowker and S. Leigh Star, *Sorting Things Out: Classification and Its Consequences* (Cambridge, MA: MIT Press, 1999).

11. D. O. Sproule, *The Supersonic Flaw Detector: An Equipment Capable of Detecting Flaws in Opaque Solids* (Barkingside: Henry Hughes Ltd, ca. 1946).

12. Brown, "Development of Ultrasonic Scanning," 17.

13. Ibid., 19.

14. Ibid.

15. Brown, interview. Woods was based at Barkingside.

16. Ibid.

17. R. Steiner, personal communication.

18. W. N. McDicken, *Diagnostic Ultrasonics: Principles and Use of Instruments* (London: Crosby Lockwood Staples, 1976), 253–56.

19. Brown, interview.

20. I. Donald, "Sonar—The Story of an Experiment," *Ultrasound in Medicine and Biology* 1 (1974): 109–117, 113; I. Donald, "Medical Sonar—the First 25 years," *Recent Advances in Ultrasound Diagnosis* 2 (1980): 4–20. Donald's fifteen-year estimate turned out to be accurate.

21. I. Donald to W. Blair, 17 Nov. 1975, Donald Papers, 5/3A.

22. It is perhaps difficult to appreciate the magnitude of these sums in the context of the early 1960s. A revealing comparator might be that John Fleming's salary when he joined Smiths Industries as a project engineer in 1962, aged twenty-eight, was £1,400 per annum.

23. J. Erskine to A. Donald, July 1987, Donald Papers, C/7.

24. J. MacVicar and I. Donald, "Sonar in the Diagnosis of Early Pregnancy and Its Complications," *Journal of Obstetrics and Gynaecology of the British Commonwealth* 70 (1963): 387–95.

25. Brown, "Development of Ultrasonic Techniques," 25.

26. The resulting images are recognizable by the overlapping arcs that define the skin surface. I. Donald and T. G. Brown, "Demonstration of Tissue Interfaces within the Body by Ultrasonic Echo Sounding," *British Journal of Radiology* 34 (1961): 539–45.

27. Brown, interview.

28. I. Donald and T. G. Brown, "Diagnostic Applications of Ultrasound," in *Proceedings of the Third International Conference on Medical Electronics* (London: Institution of Electrical Engineers, 1961), 458.

29. Brown, interview; D. H. Howry "A Survey of the Diagnostic Use of Ultrasound," in *Proceedings of the Third International Conference on Medical Electronics* (London: Institution of Electrical Engineers, 1961), 459.

30. Brown, interview.

31. In the craft mode of production, goods are produced by a single worker or a small team of workers who undertake a number of different tasks. This contrasts with mass production, in which tasks are divided between workers, often on a conveyor-belt system.

32. I. Donald, "Laparoscopy," *Bulletin of the Geisinger Medical Centre* 22 (1968): 162; I. Donald, G. D. Green, and W. H. Bain, "'Snake' Flexible Arm," *British Medical Journal* 4 (1968): 170.

33. B. Sundén, interview, May 1998.

34. Ibid. For the Krautkramer instrument, see www.ob-ultrasound.net/kraut.html (accessed June 2012).

35. Brown, interview.

36. J. E. E. Fleming, interviewed by Ian Spencer, Nov. 1998.

37. On Grey Walter and his tortoises, see A. Pickering, *The Cybernetic Brain: Sketches of Another Future* (Chicago: University of Chicago Press, 2010), 37–51.

38. Brown, interview.

39. A. Hall, in E. M. Tansey and D. A. Christie, eds., *Looking at the Unborn: Historical Aspects of Obstetric Ultrasound* (London: Wellcome Trust, 2000), 10, 12, 20–23, 29, 49–50.

40. Ausonics Ltd. marketed a semiautomatic scanner in the 1970s.

41. The clinical developments achieved with the Automatic Scanner are described in chapter 8.

42. D. Cameron, interview, Sept. 1997; see also Tansey and Christie, *Looking at the Unborn*, 21–29.

43. The Lund machine could also display in M-mode, a recognition of the work of Edler and Hertz on echocardiology.

44. J. MacVicar, interview, Aug. 1997; C. Ross, "Installation of Medical Ultrasonic Apparatus at Lund University Hospital, Sweden," unpublished report, undated, BMUS Papers, 2/203.

45. B. Sundén, "On the Diagnostic Value of Ultrasound in Obstetrics and Gynaecology," *Acta Obstetrica et Gynecologica Scandinavica* 43, suppl. 6 (1964): 1–191.

46. J. E. E. Fleming, "Mr J. E. E. Fleming's Visit to Lund, Sweden, March 1964," unpublished report, 1964, BMUS Papers, 2/203.

47. Brown, interview.

48. Fleming, interview.

49. J. M. L Wood, "The New Mk 7 Ultrasonic Flaw Detector," *Pulse* 3 (1961): 10–13.

50. I. Donald, "Clinical Report for 1964–65," unpublished typescript, 1965, Donald Papers, 1/1/41.

51. Brown, interview; Tansey and Christie, *Looking at the Unborn*, 23.

52. Brown, interview.

53. Fleming, interview.

54. D. Cameron, in Tansey and Christie, *Looking at the Unborn*, 22.

55. Donald, "Sonar—Story of an Experiment," 116.

56. I. Donald to J. H. Holmes, 14 June 1974, BMUS Papers, 2/98. Miller's assistance was acknowledged in several of Donald's later papers. She was invited to address the BMA's Board of Science and Education, an achievement Donald regarded as unprecedented for someone with no qualifications in medicine or a related field. I. Donald to Whom It May Concern, 27 Mar. 1975, Donald Papers, 5/13.

57. Donald employed another doctor's wife, Mrs. Naftalin, to help with ultrasound record keeping. I. Donald to W. F. Freundlich, 4 Dec. 1967, BMUS Papers, 1/1/6.

58. I. Donald, "Opatija speech," unpublished typescript, 1978, Donald Papers, 3/14.

59. I. Donald to W. R. Chatfield, 22 Mar. 1974, Donald Papers, 5/4.

60. Brown, interview.

61. Donald, "Sonar—Story of an Experiment," 116.

62. Ibid.

63. J. E. E. Fleming and A. J. Hall, "Two Dimensional Compound Scanning Effects of Maladjustment and Calibration," *Ultrasonics* 6 (1968): 160–66.

64. Fleming, interview.

65. Ibid.

66. B. Fraser, interview, July 1997.

67. Ibid.

68. Fleming, interview.

69. Nuclear Enterprises sold its hundredth machine in November 1972. I. Donald to W. T. Slater, 19 Nov. 1972, BMUS Papers, 1/1/18. For development of the market for ultrasound scanners, see P. Coste, "An Historical Examination of the Strategic

Issues Which Influenced Technologically Entrepreneurial Firms Serving the Medical Diagnostic Ultrasound Market" (PhD diss., Claremont Graduate School, California, 1989).

CHAPTER EIGHT: Behind the Iron Curtain: Ultrasound and the Fetus

1. I. Donald, J. MacVicar, and T. G. Brown, "Investigation of Abdominal Masses by Pulsed Ultrasound," *Lancet* 1 (1958): 1188–95, 1192.

2. J. MacVicar and I. Donald, "Sonar in the Diagnosis of Early Pregnancy and Its Complications," *Journal of Obstetrics and Gynaecology of the British Commonwealth* 70 (1963): 387–95.

3. Ibid. Obstetricians date pregnancy from the beginning of the last menstrual period.

4. Donald favored the Aschheim-Zondek test, but he documented a case in which four such tests gave negative results but an ultrasonic diagnosis of continuing pregnancy proved to be correct. Ibid., 394.

5. In "missed abortion," the fetus dies in utero but is not expelled for a period of time.

6. Anonymous, personal communication.

7. MacVicar and Donald, "Sonar in the Diagnosis."

8. A-scans of hydatidiform mole previously appeared in A. Shih, W. Tao-Hsin, A. Shin-Yuan, C. Shih-Liang, W. Hsiang-Huei, H. Chih-Chang, and Y. Kuo-Juei, "The Use of Pulsed Ultrasound in Clinical Diagnosis," *Chinese Medical Journal* 81 (1962): 313–25. This paper is in English, but there is no evidence that Donald had read it.

9. J. MacVicar, "Illustrative Examples of Ultrasonic Echograms," *Proceedings of the Royal Society of Medicine* 55 (1961): 2–4.

10. MacVicar and Donald, "Sonar in the Diagnosis."

11. I. Donald, "Transcript of Symposium on Ultrasound Given by Professor Ian Donald at Smith Kline Precision Company, February 21, 1963," unpublished typescript, Donald Papers, 2/2.

12. I. Donald, "Ultrasonography in Two Dimensions," *Medical and Biological Illustration* 14 (1964): 216–24.

13. I. Donald, "Sonar Examination of the Abdomen," *Ultrasonics*, July 1966, 119–24.

14. J. MacVicar, interview, Apr. 1997.

15. I. Donald, "Use of Ultrasonics in Diagnosis of Abdominal Swellings," *British Medical Journal* 2 (1963): 1154–55.

16. MacVicar and Donald, "Sonar in the Diagnosis," 393–94.

17. I. Donald, "Ultrasonic Echo Sounding in Obstetrical and Gynaecological Diagnosis," *American Journal of Obstetrics and Gynecology* 93 (1965): 935–41.

18. I. Donald, "Diagnostic Uses of Sonar in Obstetrics and Gynaecology," *Journal of Obstetrics and Gynaecology of the British Commonwealth* 72 (1965): 907–19.

19. M. W. Skippen, "Obstetric Practice and Cephalopelvic Disproportion in Glasgow between 1840 and 1900" (PhD diss., University of Glasgow, 2009).

20. D. Crichton, "The Accuracy and Value of Cephalo-pelvimetry," *Journal of Obstetrics and Gynaecology of the British Commonwealth* 69 (1962): 366–78.

21. I. Donald, *Practical Obstetric Problems*, 3rd ed. (London: Lloyd-Luke, 1964), 732.

22. T. C. Duggan, interview, Aug. 2001.

23. T. C. Duggan, "Foetal Cephalometry," unpublished paper, undated, BMUS Papers, 2/41.

24. T. Kilburn and L. S. Piggott, "Frederic Calland Williams, 1911–1977," *Biographical Memoirs of Fellows of the Royal Society* 24 (1978): 583–604.

25. T. C. Duggan, interview.

26. G. D. Ludwig, "The Velocity of Sound through Tissues and the Acoustic Impedance of Tissues," *Journal of the Acoustical Society of America* 22 (1950): 862–66; I. Edler, A. Gustafson, T. Karlefors, and B. Christensson, "Ultrasound Cardiography," *Acta Medica Scandinavica* 107, suppl. 370 (1961): 5–123; H. Theismann and F. Pfander, "Uber die Durchlassigkeit des Knochens fur Ultraschall," *Strahlentherapie* 80 (1949): 607–10; W. J. Fry and F. Dunn, "Ultrasound: Analysis and Experimental Methods in Biological Research," in *Physical Techniques in Biological Research*, ed. W. L. Nastuk (New York: Academic Press, 1962), 4: 261–394.

27. For contemporary velocity data, see R. J. Parry and R. C. Chivers, "Data of the Velocity and Attenuation of Ultrasound in Mammalian Tissue, a Survey," in *Ultrasonic Tissue Characterisation II*, ed. M. Linzer (Washington, DC: NBS Special Publications, 1979), 343–60.

28. Thus the effective velocity is 800 m s^{-1}; that is, calculated for travel across the head and back again.

29. Donald, "Ultrasonic Echo Sounding." The time between the echoes from two reflectors corresponds to the time taken for the pulse to travel twice the distance (i.e., there and back). This is the "time of flight," hence the symbol t_{of}.

30. J. Willocks, I. Donald, T. C. Duggan, and N. Day, "Foetal Cephalometry by Ultrasound," *Journal of Obstetrics and Gynaecology of the British Commonwealth* 71 (1964): 11–20. Day was a statistician.

31. J. Willocks, "Foetal Cephalometry by Ultrasound" (MD thesis, University of Glasgow, 1963), 131.

32. Ibid., 116.

33. N. Butler, "Perinatal Mortality Survey," *British Medical Journal* 2 (1962): 1463–65.

34. I. Donald, "Uses of Ultrasonic Echo Sounding in Obstetrics and Gynaecology," First Annual Charles J. Barone Lecture, Magee-Womens Hospital, University of Pittsburgh Health Center, Pittsburgh, 1961, BMUS Papers, 2/2; Donald, "Transcript of Symposium."

35. T. G. Brown, "An Explanation of the Principles of Ultrasonic Echo Sounding," *Proceedings of the Royal Society of Medicine* 55 (1962): 637; I. Donald, "Sonar: A New Diagnostic Echo-Sounding Technique in Obstetrics and Gynaecology," *Proceedings of the Royal Society of Medicine* 55 (1962): 637–38; MacVicar, "Illustrative Examples"; J. Willocks, "The Use of Ultrasonic Cephalometry," *Proceedings of the Royal Society of Medicine* 55 (1962): 640.

36. E. M. Tansey and D. A. Christie, eds., *Looking at the Unborn: Historical Aspects of Obstetric Ultrasound* (London: Wellcome Trust, 2000), 53.

37. J. Willocks, interview, Aug. 1996.

38. B. M. Hibbard, "The Diagnosis of Placenta Praevia with Radioactive Isotopes," *Proceedings of the Royal Society of Medicine* 55 (1962): 640–42, 642.

39. J. Willocks, I. Donald, S. Campbell, and I. R. Dunsmore, "Intrauterine Growth Assessed by Ultrasonic Foetal Cephalometry," *Journal of Obstetrics and Gynaecology of the British Commonwealth* 74 (1967): 639–47.

40. S. Campbell, "An Improved Method of Fetal Cephalometry by Ultrasound," *Journal of Obstetrics and Gynaecology of the British Commonwealth* 75 (1968): 568–76; S. Campbell, "The Prediction of Fetal Maturity by Ultrasonic Measurement of the Biparietal Diameter," *Journal of Obstetrics and Gynaecology of the British Commonwealth* 76 (1969): 603–9.

41. I. Donald, "The Interpretation of Abdominal Ultrasonograms," in *Diagnostic Ultrasound: Proceedings of the First International Conference*, ed. C. C. Grossman, J. H. Holmes, C. Joyner, and E. W. Purnell (New York: Plenum Press, 1966), 316–32.

42. Willocks, interview.

43. Donald, "Interpretation."

44. I. Donald, "Presentation Methods of Ultrasonic Echo Sounding Information from Tissue Interfaces," in *Biomechanics and Related Bioengineering Topics*, ed. R. M. Kenedi (Oxford: Pergamon Press, 1965), 44–61.

45. Donald, "Ultrasonic Echo Sounding."

46. I. Donald, "Uses of Ultrasonics in Obstetrical and Gynaecological Diagnosis," in *Fifth World Congress of Gynaecology and Obstetrics*, ed. C. Wood and W. A. W. Walters (Sydney, Australia: Butterworths, 1967), 525–38.

47. I. Donald, "Anthology of Cracks," notebook, undated, Donald Papers, 6/4. Retention of the products of conception can cause troublesome bleeding and infection, and may indeed affect fertility.

48. H. E. Thompson, J. H. Holmes, K. R. Gottesfeld, and E. S. Taylor, "Fetal Development as Determined by Ultrasonic Pulse Echo Techniques," *American Journal of Obstetrics and Gynecology* 92 (1965): 44–50.

49. Willocks, "Foetal Cephalometry," 116; Donald, "Diagnostic Uses of Sonar."

50. K. R. Gottesfeld, H. E. Thompson, J. H. Holmes, and E. S. Taylor, "Ultrasonic Placentography: A New Method for Placental Localisation," *American Journal of Obstetrics and Gynecology* 96 (1966): 538–41.

51. B. Fraser, personal communication. Fleming recalls that the fetal spine, likewise, was not recognized immediately. During the celebrations for Donald's retirement, Fleming and his colleagues made a display of old pictures. They were surprised to find they could confidently identify the spine, which they had missed when the images were first examined.

52. I. Donald and U. Abdulla, "Placentography by Sonar," *British Journal of Obstetrics and Gynaecology* 75 (1968): 993–1006.

53. M. B. McNay, interview, May 1999.

54. D. A. Callaghan, T. C. Rowland, and D. E. Goldman, "Ultrasonic Doppler Observation of a Fetal Heart," *Obstetrics and Gynaecology* 23 (1964): 637; W. L. Johnson, H. F. Stegall, J. N. Lein, and R. F. Rushmer, "Detection of Fetal Life in Early Pregnancy with an Ultrasonic Doppler Flowmeter," *Obstetrics and Gynaecology* 26 (1965): 305–7.

55. Donald and Abdulla, "Placentography by Sonar."

56. W. Krause and R. Soldner, "Ultrasonic Imaging Technique (B scan) with High Image Rate for Medical Diagnosis," *Electromedica* 4 (1965): 1–5.

57. I. Donald, P. Morley, and E. Barnett, "The Diagnosis of Blighted Ovum by Sonar," *Journal of Obstetrics and Gynaecology of the British Commonwealth* 79 (1972): 304–10.

58. H. P. Robinson, "The Evaluation of Early Pregnancy and Its Complications by Diagnostic Ultrasound" (MD thesis, University of Glasgow, 1978), 23.

59. The observational foundation of these rules is beautifully illustrated in ibid., 90–99.

60. L. M. Hellman, M. Kobayashi, L. Fillisti, M. Lavenhar, and E. Cromb, "Growth and Development of the Human Fetus prior to the Twentieth Week of Gestation," *American Journal of Obstetrics and Gynecology* 103 (1969): 789–98.

61. MRC Programme Grant No. G690/684/C, "Sonar: Its Application to Diagnosis in Obstetrics and Gynaecology and Related Fields," BMUS Papers, 2/139.

62. H. P. Robinson, interview, Apr. 1997.

63. Ibid.

64. J. Bang and H. H. Holms, "Ultrasonics in the Demonstration of Fetal Heart Movement," *American Journal of Obstetrics and Gynecology* 102 (1968): 956–60.

65. A cine film of Robinson demonstrating his technique, in the BMUS Historical Collection, vividly reveals the craft skill involved.

66. H. P. Robinson, "Sonar Measurement of Fetal Crown-Rump Length as a Means of Assessing Maturity in the First Trimester of Pregnancy," *British Medical Journal* 2 (1973): 28–31; H. P. Robinson and J. E. E. Fleming, "A Critical Evaluation of Sonar Crown-Rump Length Measurements," *Journal of Obstetrics and Gynaecology of the British Commonwealth* 82 (1975): 702–10.

67. MRC Programme Grant, "Sonar: Its Application."

68. H. P. Robinson and J. Shaw-Dunn, "Fetal Heart Rates as Determined by Sonar in Early Pregnancy," *Journal of Obstetrics and Gynaecology of the British Commonwealth* 80 (1973): 805–9.

69. Robinson, "Evaluation of Early Pregnancy," 128.

70. I. Donald, "Diagnostic Ultrasonic Echo Sounding in Obstetrics and Gynaecology," *Transactions of the College of Physicians, Surgeons, and Gynaecologists of South Africa* 11 (1967): 61–79.

CHAPTER NINE: Diffusion, Controversy, and Commodification

1. I. Donald, "On Launching a New Diagnostic Science," *American Journal of Obstetrics and Gynecology* 103 (1969): 609–28. The Donald Papers contain much referral correspondence.

2. P. N. T. Wells, "Ultrasonics in Clinical Diagnosis," in *The Scientific Basis of Medicine: Annual Reviews* (London: Athlone, 1966), 38–52.

3. C. F. Powell, "Research into the Use of Ultrasonics for Medical Research," MRC Research Application G.962/222/C, 1967, Donald Papers, 5/1.

4. E. M. Tansey and D. A. Christie, eds., *Looking at the Unborn: Historical Aspects of Obstetric Ultrasound* (London: Wellcome Trust, 2000), 31.

5. S. Blume, *Insight and Industry: On the Dynamics of Technological Change in Medicine* (Cambridge, MA: MIT Press, 1992), chap. 6.

6. For the description of events in Aberdeen we are indebted to D. Nicholson, "Secrets of Success: The Development of Obstetric Ultrasound in Scotland, 1963–1990" (PhD diss., University of Glasgow, 2003), 92–110.

7. A. Christie, interview, Aug. 1998.

8. Ibid.

9. W. Barr to I. Donald, 10 Aug. 1967, Donald Papers, 5/3A.

10. Christie, interview.

11. Ibid.

12. U. Abdulla, "Sonar in Very Early Pregnancy," *Ultrasonographia Medica* 3 (1969): 154; A. S. McIntosh and A. Christie, "Ultrasound Location of the Placental Site," *Ultrasonographia Medica* 3 (1969): 164.

13. Nicholson, "Secrets of Success," 108.

14. A. McIntosh, quoted in ibid., 108.

15. R. E. Steiner, interview, May 2002.

16. I. Donald, P. Morley, and E. Barnett, "The Diagnosis of Blighted Ovum by Sonar," *Journal of Obstetrics and Gynaecology of the British Commonwealth* 79 (1972): 304–10.

17. P. Morley, G. Donald, and R. Sanders, eds., *Ultrasonic Sectional Anatomy* (Edinburgh: Churchill Livingstone, 1983); E. Barnett and P. Morley, eds., *Clinical Diagnostic Ultrasound* (Oxford: Blackwell Science, 1985).

18. I. Donald to J. Holmes, 14 June 1976, BMUS Papers, 1/1/18; I. Donald to W. S. McNab, 10 June 1975, Donald Papers, 5/14.

19. I. Donald to J. H. Hutchison, 2 May 1973, BMUS Papers, 1/1/4A.

20. J. McKie, "Clinical Physics in Glasgow," in *Physics and Physic: Essays in Memory of John M. A. Lenihan*, ed. D. B. Wilson and J. Geyer-Kordesch (Glasgow: Wellcome Unit for the History of Medicine, 2001), 19–36.

21. J. E. E. Fleming, "Ultrasound: The Glasgow Factor," in Wilson and Geyer-Kordesch, *Physics and Physic*, 63–70.

22. A. J. Eley to J. M. A. Lenihan, Oct. 1967, quoted in Fleming "Ultrasound," 75.

23. McDicken's course material formed the basis of his textbook. W. N. McDicken, *Diagnostic Ultrasonics: Principles and Use of Instruments* (London: Crosby, Lockwood, Staples, 1975).

24. W. N. McDicken, interview, June 1997; I. Donald to J. M. A. Lenihan, 22 Apr. 1968, Lenihan Papers, HH88, Greater Glasgow Health Board Archives; I. Donald to J. M. A. Lenihan, 6 Nov. 1970, Donald Papers, 1/1/11.

25. Western Regional Hospital Board, *Report of the Working Party on Ultrasonics* (Glasgow: Western Regional Hospital Board, 1971), 2.

26. F. Fraser to I. Donald, 25 Mar. 1970, BMUS Papers, 1/1/6.

27. For Picker's involvement in ultrasound, see www.ob-ultrasound.net/picker.html (accessed June 2012).

28. F. Fraser to I. Donald, 19 Dec. 1973, BMUS Papers, 1/1/6.

29. See, for example, J. J. de Wet to I. Donald, 28 Sept. 1970, BMUS Papers, 1/1/21; I. Donald to D. Cavanagh, 25 Sept. 1974, BMUS Papers, 1/1/3; J. Drumm to I. Donald, 18 Sept. 1974, BMUS Papers, 1/1/4.

30. S. Campbell, interview, Oct. 1997.

31. Ibid.

32. F. Fraser to I. Donald, 27 Dec. 1970, BMUS Papers, 1/1/6.

33. S. Campbell and E. I. Kohorn, "Placental Localisation by Ultrasound Compound Scanning," *Journal of Obstetrics and Gynaecology of the British Commonwealth* 75 (1968): 1007–13.

34. Campbell, interview.

35. S. Campbell to I. Donald, 19 Nov. 1969, BMUS Papers, 1/1/3.

36. H. E. Thompson, "Studies of Fetal Growth by Ultrasound," in *Diagnostic Ultrasound: Proceedings of the First International Conference,* ed. G. C. Grossman, J. Holmes, C. Joyner, and E. Purnell (New York: Plenum Press, 1965), 416–27; M. Hansmann and U. Voight, "Ultrasonic Fetal Thoracometry: An Additional Parameter for Determining Fetal Growth," in *Proceedings of the Second World Congress on Ultrasonics in Medicine,* ed. M. De Vlieger (Rotterdam: Excerpta Medica, 1973), 47.

37. Campbell, interview.

38. Ibid. Obstetricians and neonatologists later modified this view. L. Weaver, personal communication.

39. S. Campbell and D. Wilkins, "Ultrasonic Measurement of Fetal Abdomen Circumference in the Estimation of Fetal Weight," *British Journal of Obstetrics and Gynaecology* 82 (1975): 689–97.

40. Although acknowledging the value of using the umbilical vein as a standardized landmark, Hansmann and his colleagues maintained that Campbell was, in fact, using the same plane of reference, "the lower aperture of the fetal thorax," that they had been recommending since 1971. H. Kugener and M. Hansmann, "Topography of a Reference Plane for Ultrasonic Thoracometry," *Zeitschrift für Geburtshilfe und Perinatologie* 180 (1976): 313–19.

41. Campbell, interview.

42. Ibid.

43. S. Campbell and C. J. Dewhurst, "Quintuplet Pregnancy Diagnosed and Assessed by Ultrasonic Compound Scanning," *Lancet* 1 (1970): 101–3. An ultrasonogram apparently showing five fetal heads was much reproduced in the press; see, for example, *Daily Record* (Glasgow), 20 Dec. 1969. It was, however, a composite, produced by pasting together images obtained from several scans.

44. I. Donald and T. G. Brown, "Demonstration of Tissue Interfaces within the Body by Ultrasonic Echo Sounding," *British Journal of Radiology* 34 (1961): 539–46; B. Sundén, "On the Diagnostic Value of Ultrasound in Obstetrics and Gynaecology," *Acta Obstetrica et Gynecologica Scandinavica* 43, suppl. 6 (1964): 1–191, 121.

45. W. J. Garrett, G. Grunwald, and D. E. Robinson, "Prenatal Diagnosis of Fetal Polycystic Kidney by Ultrasound," *Australian and New Zealand Journal of Obstetrics and Gynaecology* 10 (1970): 7–9.

46. S. Campbell, F. D. Johnstone, E. M. Holt, and P. May, "Anencephaly: Early Ultrasonic Diagnosis and Active Management," *Lancet* 2 (1972): 1226–27.

47. S. Campbell, "Early Prenatal Diagnosis of Neural Tube Defects by Ultrasound," *Clinical Obstetrics and Gynaecology* 4 (1977): 351–59.

48. M. B. McNay and J. E. E. Fleming, "Forty Years of Obstetric Ultrasound 1957–1997: From A-scope to Three Dimensions," *Ultrasound in Medicine and Biology* 25 (1999): 3–56; B. Dixon, "Medicine for the Unborn Baby," *New Scientist,* 26 Nov. 1967, 94–95.

49. W. G. Mills, "Fetal Hibernation," *Lancet* 1 (1970): 335–36.

50. S. Campbell, R. A. Underhill, and J. M. Beazley, "Fetal Hibernation," *Lancet* 1 (1970): 468.

51. The identities of the patient and her pediatrician are withheld to preserve anonymity. The quotations in the text are, accordingly, not individually referenced.

52. The Donald Papers contain several letters from the grateful mother.

53. Campbell and Kohorn, "Placental Localization."

54. I. Donald to S. Campbell, 24 June 1968, BMUS Papers, 1/1/3.

55. S. Campbell to I. Donald, 18 June 1970, BMUS Papers, 1/1/3. Percival was surgeon obstetrician, London Hospital.

56. I. Donald, "On Launching," 616.

57. T. Lind, F. M. Parkin, and G. A. Cheyne, "Biochemical and Cytological Changes in Liquor Amnii with Advancing Gestation" *Journal of Obstetrics and Gynaecology of the British Commonwealth* 76 (1969) 673–83.

58. J. M. Davidson, T. Lind, V. Farr, and T. A. Whittingham, "The Limitations of Ultrasonic Cephalometry," *Journal of Obstetrics and Gynaecology of the British Commonwealth* 80 (1973): 769–75.

59. J. M. Davidson to S. Campbell, 1 Feb. 1974, BMUS Papers, 1/1/3.

60. "Fetal Maturity" (editorial), *British Medical Journal* 2 (1970): 129–30.

61. "Reappraisal of Ultrasonic Fetal Cephalometry" (editorial), *Lancet* 2 (1973): 892.

62. I. Donald to D. Watmough, 17 Jan. 1974, BMUS Papers, 1/1/21; S. Campbell, "Ultrasonic Cephalometry" *Lancet* 2 (1973): 1145.

63. A. D. Christie, "Fetal Cephalometry" *Lancet* 1 (1974): 177–78.

64. R. A. Underhill, J. M. Beazley, and S. Campbell, "Comparison of Ultrasound Cephalometry, Radiology, and Liquor Studies in Patients with Unknown Confinement Dates," *British Medical Journal* 3 (1971): 736–38.

65. I. Donald to D. Cavanagh, 25 May 1976, BMUS Papers, 1/1/3; I. Donald to W. McKinney, 27 May 1975, BMUS Papers, 1/1/12A; I. Donald to J. Warren, 16 June 1976, BMUS Papers, 1/1/21.

66. I. Donald to S. Clayton, 13 Feb. 1974, BMUS Papers, 1/1/3.

67. C. R. Hill, "The Possibility of Hazard in Medical and Industrial Applications of Ultrasound," *British Journal of Radiology* 41 (1968): 561–69.

68. I. Donald to D. Gordon, undated, Donald Papers, 5/8.

69. As far as we can ascertain, this research was never published.

70. I. Donald to L. M. Hellman, May 1970, BMUS Papers, 1/1/8.

71. L. M. Hellman, G. M. Duffus, I. Donald, and B. Sundén, "Safety of Diagnostic Ultrasound in Obstetrics," *Lancet* 1 (1970): 1133–35; M. G. Smyth, "Animal Toxicity Studies at Ultrasonic Diagnostic Power Levels," in *Diagnostic Ultrasound*, ed. C. C. Grossman, J. H. Holmes, C. Joyner, and E. W. Purnell (New York: Plenum Press, 1966), 296–99; [I. Donald], "Safety of Sonar in Obstetrics" (editorial), *Lancet* 1 (1970): 1158–60; there is a draft of the editorial in the Donald Papers.

72. I. J. C. Macintosh and D. A. Davey, "Chromosome Aberrations Induced by an Ultrasonic Fetal Pulse Detector," *British Medical Journal* 4 (1970): 92–93.

73. I. Donald, "On Launching."

74. E. Boyd, U. Abdulla, I. Donald, J. E. E. Fleming, A. J. Hall, and M. A. Ferguson-Smith, "Chromosome Breakage and Ultrasound," *British Medical Journal* 2 (1971): 501–2.

75. U. Abdulla, S. Campbell, C. J. Dewhurst, and D. Talbert, "Effect of Diagnostic Ultrasound on Maternal and Fetal Chromosomes," *Lancet* 2 (1971): 829–31.

76. I. Donald, "On Launching."

77. P. L. Watts, A. J. Hall, and J. E. E. Fleming, "Ultrasound and Chromosome Damage," *British Journal of Radiology* 45 (1972): 335–39.

78. For review, see J. Thacker, "The Possibility of Genetic Hazard from Ultrasonic Radiation," *Current Topics in Radiation Research Quarterly* 8 (1973): 235–58; I. Donald,

"The Biological Effects of Ultrasound," in *The Present and Future of Diagnostic Ultrasound*, ed. I. Donald and S. Levi (Rotterdam: Kooyker, 1976), 20–32.

79. I. J. C. Macintosh, R. C. Brown, and W. T. Coakley, "Ultrasound and In Vitro Chromosome Aberrations," *British Journal of Radiology* 48 (1975): 230–32.

80. C. J. Dewhurst, "The Safety of Ultrasound," *Proceedings of the Royal Society of Medicine* 64 (1971): 996–97; A. J. Hall, "An Investigation into Certain Aspects of the Safety of Diagnostic Ultrasound" (MSc thesis, University of Glasgow, 1974).

81. H. P. Robinson, F. Sharp, I. Donald, A. H. Young, and A. J. Hall, "The Effect of Pulsed and Continuous Wave Ultrasound on the Enzyme Histochemistry of Placental Tissue In Vitro," *Journal of Obstetrics and Gynaecology of the British Commonwealth* 79 (1972): 821–27.

82. I. Donald to T. S. Wilson, 25 Sept. 1973, BMUS Papers, 1/1/21.

83. I. Donald to R. Warwick, 1 Feb. 1966, BMUS Papers, 1/1/21.

84. F. Dunn and F. J. Fry, "Ultrasonic Threshold Dosages for the Central Mammalian Nervous System," *IEEE Transactions of Biomedical Engineering* 18 (1971): 253–56; C. R. Hill, "Acoustic Intensity Measurements on Ultrasonic Diagnostic Devices," *Ultrasonographia Medica* 2 (1969): 21–27; Hall, "Investigation."

85. I. Donald, "Safety of Sonar in Pregnancy," unpublished draft, ca. 1973, Donald Papers, 2/2.

86. G. Kossoff, W. J. Garret, and G. Radovanovich, "Grey Scale Echography in Obstetrics and Gynaecology," Commonwealth Acoustic Laboratories, Report No. 59 (Sydney, Australia, 1973); I. Donald to G. Kossoff, 13 Sept. 1974, BMUS Papers, 1/1/10.

87. G. Kossoff, in J. Woo "A Short History of the Development of Ultrasound in Obstetrics and Gynecology," www.ob-ultrasound.net/history2.html (accessed Nov. 2007).

88. B. Fraser, personal communication.

89. J. E. E. Fleming, "Report on Ultrasonic Conference on Ophthalmology, Munster," 1966, BMUS Papers.

90. Campbell, interview.

91. R. Chef, "Foreword," in *Real-Time Ultrasound in Perinatal Medicine*, ed. R. Chef (Basel: Karger, 1979), i–v, v.

92. I. Donald to J. Drumm, 25 Sept. 1972, BMUS Papers, 1/1/7.

93. R. D. Redman, W. P. Walton, J. E. E. Fleming, and A. J. Hall, "Holographic Display of Data from Ultrasonic Scanning," *Ultrasonics* 7 (1969): 26–29.

94. I. Donald to D. Gabor, 27 Jan. 1970, BMUS Papers, 1/1/7; I. Donald, "Limitations of Present Day Sonar Techniques in Obstetrics and Gynaecology," in *Ultrasonics in Medicine*, ed. M. de Vlieger, D. N. White, and V. R. McCready (Amsterdam: Excerpta Medica, 1973), 7–13. Dennis Gabor won the Nobel Prize in Physics in 1971 for his holography work.

95. For an account of Brown's three-dimensional scanner, see www.ob-ultrasound.net/brown-on-ultrasound.html (accessed May 2012).

96. T. G. Brown, personal communication.

97. J. M. Thijssen, "The History of Ultrasound Techniques in Ophthalmology," *Ultrasound in Medicine and Biology* 19 (1993): 599–618, 606.

98. By 1974, the American Institute of Ultrasound in Medicine had more than a thousand members. J. Holmes to I. Donald, 31 Oct. 1974, BMUS Papers, 1/1/8.

99. A. Donald, interview, July 1996.

100. I. Donald to E. Leask, 27 Aug. 1976, BMUS Papers, 1/1/11.

101. Campbell, interview.

102. I. Donald to E. Leask, 27 Aug. 1976.

103. S. Campbell, "Foreword," *Clinics in Obstetrics and Gynaecology* 10 (1983): 369–70.

104. I. Donald to W. Slater, 19 Nov. 1974, BMUS Papers, 1/1/18.

105. P. Coste, "An Historical Examination of the Strategic Issues Which Influenced Technologically Entrepreneurial Firms Serving the Medical Diagnostic Ultrasound Market" (PhD diss., Claremont Graduate School, California, 1989), 267; G. Blackwell, *The World Market for Ultrasound Imaging Systems* (London: Clinica Reports, PJB Publications, 1995).

106. I. Donald, "The Impact of Real Time Ultrasonic Scanning," unpublished typescript, 1980, Donald Papers, 3/26.

CHAPTER TEN: Ian Donald after Ultrasound: Contraception and Abortion

1. I. Donald, G. D. Green, and W. H. Bain, "'Snake' Flexible Arm," *British Medical Journal* 4 (1968): 170; A. C. Davidson and I. Donald, "Female Sterilisation," *Scottish Medical Journal* 17 (1972): 210–13.

2. I. Donald to G. D Green, 3 Apr. 1968, BMUS Papers, 1/1/12A.

3. I. Donald to B. D. Muddell, 9 July 1970, Donald Papers, 5/13.

4. I. Donald, "Superfecundity: Simpson Oration; His Problem and Ours," *British Medical Journal* 1 (1977): 555–60.

5. I. Donald to A. Klopper, 20 Feb. 1974, BMUS Papers, 1/1/10; D. H. Carr, "Chromosome Studies in Selected Spontaneous Abortions: 1. Conception after Oral Contraceptives," *Canadian Medical Association Journal* 103 (1970): 343–48.

6. I. Donald, "Naught for Your Comfort," *Journal of the Irish Medical Association* 65 (1972): 279–89.

7. I. Donald, *Practical Obstetric Problems*, 4th ed. (London: Lloyd-Luke, 1969), 328.

8. I. Donald to A. J. Wrigley, 20 Dec. 1970, BMUS Papers, 1/1/21.

9. I. Donald to S. Kullander, 21 Dec. 1973, BMUS Papers, 1/1/15.

10. I. Donald, letter, details withheld.

11. I. Spencer, "The Search for Certainty: The History of an Electronic Contraceptive," unpublished paper, undated, BMUS Papers, 2/200.

12. Donald, "Superfecundity," 559.

13. Ibid.

14. I. Donald, "Prediction of Ovulation," typescript, 1984, Donald Papers, 3/33.

15. The story may well be apocryphal. However, given that a constant theme of this volume has been the importance of the unexpected and the counterintuitive in the development of the ultrasound scanner, we hope it will not be regarded as prurient of us to remark that it would be difficult to imagine any circumstance less intuitively probable, a priori, than that Irish nuns should be actively encouraged, by the Archbishop of Dublin, to insert cylindrical objects into their vaginas. That this story was widely believed is strong support for the view that in historiography as in life itself, context is all.

16. I. Donald to Elizabeth [Ealy], 28 July 1981, Donald Papers, 5/6; T. Winning to I. Donald, 21 Nov. 1973, Donald Papers, 5/22.

17. For Pickering's schema of resistance, modeling, and emergence, see chapter 1.

18. R. A. Hatcher, J. Trussel, F. Stewart, W. Cates, G. K. Stewart, F. Guest, and D. Kowal, *Contraceptive Technology* (New York: Ardent Media, 2000).

19. F. E. McGirr to C. Wilson, 2 July 1975, in "Principal's Notes, 22 May 1975, Medicine, Midwifery," Glasgow University Archives.

20. Papers relating to the appointment are in Glasgow University Archives.

21. *Daily Record* (Glasgow), 26 Jan. 1976, 9.

22. I. Donald, "Does Christianity Help?" (London: Order of Christian Unity, 1977); I. Donald to J. J. Scarisbrick, 23 Mar. 1976, Donald Papers, 1/1/18.

23. S. Campbell, interview, 1997; W. Barr, interview, 1995.

24. D. Baird, "A Fifth Freedom," *British Medical Journal* 2 (1965): 1141–48; G. Davis and R. Davidson, " 'A Fifth Freedom' or 'Hideous Atheistic Expediency'? The Medical Community and Abortion Law Reform in Scotland, c. 1960–1975," *Medical History* 50 (2006): 29–48; G. Davis and R. Davidson, " 'Big White Chief,' 'Pontius Pilate' and the 'Plumber': The Impact of the 1967 Abortion Act on the Scottish Medical Community, c. 1967–1980," *Social History of Medicine* 18 (2005): 283–306.

25. Donald, "Naught for Your Comfort," 288.

26. D. Nicholson, "Secrets of Success: The Development of Obstetric Ultrasound in Scotland, 1963–1990" (PhD diss., University of Glasgow, 2003), 89.

27. I. Donald to D. Charles, 28 Dec. 1966, BMUS Papers, 1/1/3.

28. I. Donald to T. Phillips, 3 Nov. 1971, BMUS Papers, 1/1/15; Donald, "Naught for Your Comfort," 286.

29. We are grateful to Mrs. W. Childs for this information.

30. Davis and Davidson, "Fifth Freedom."

31. M. Macnaughton, interview, July 1996. Glasgow's Royal Infirmary is situated in the East End.

32. W. Childs, interview, July 1996.

33. This was before the booking scan (performed at ten to twelve weeks) became part of routine practice in the Queen Mother's Hospital. Ibid.

34. I. Donald to Peggy [no surname], 15 Aug. 1980, Donald Papers, 5/17.

35. "Selective Abortion Urged in Cases of Foetal Damage," *Irish Times*, 6 Sept. 1978.

36. I. Donald to S. J. Scarisbrick, 23 Mar. 1976, Donald Papers, 1/1/18.

37. I. Donald, "Need for Research," *Irish Times*, 26 Sept. 1978.

38. "Research to Aid the Unborn Child," *Woking News and Mail*, 1978.

39. I. Donald to S. J. Scarisbrick, 23 Mar. 1976, Donald Papers, 1/1/18.

40. I. Donald to S. Kullander, 21 Dec. 1973, Donald Papers, 1/1/10; R. H. Haslam and R. Milner, "The Physician and Down Syndrome: Are Attitudes Changing?" *Journal of Child Neurology* 7 (1992): 304–10.

41. I. Donald to J. S. Scott, 19 June 1974, Donald Papers, 1/1/18.

42. Quoted in *Daily Sketch* (London), 12 Jan. 1967.

43. I. Donald to H. MacLennan, 25 Nov. 1975, Donald Papers, 5/15.

44. For this aspect of Donald's career, see M. Nicolson, "Ian Donald, Diagnostician and Moralist" (Royal College of Physicians of Edinburgh, 2004), website publication, www.rcpe.ac.uk/library/read/people/donald/donald1.php.

45. I. Donald, "After the Pill: Society under Siege," *Daily Telegraph* (London), 10 Apr. 1978.

46. Ibid.

47. Donald Papers, 5/15.

48. B. Nash, "Daughters in Danger," *Mother*, Apr. 1978, 34–36.

49. *Report of the Committee of Inquiry into Human Fertilisation and Embryology* (London: HMSO, 1984).

50. I. Donald, "Problems Raised by Artificial Human Reproduction," *Ethics and Medicine* 1 (1985): 18–21, 19.

51. Donald made two films. The second showed four different fetuses, including one "destined for abortion on demand, the mother being unmarried, who when she saw it dug her toes in and refused the operation." I. Donald to Peggy [no surname], 15 Aug. 1980, Donald Papers, 5/17.

52. Donald, "Prediction of Ovulation."

53. Ibid.

54. I. Donald to Cecil [no surname], 24 May 1979, Donald Papers, 5/4.

55. I. Donald to R. Algranati, 3 May 1979, Donald Papers, 5/2.

56. Some legislators certainly believe this. In Texas, it has recently become a legal requirement that a physician advising a woman who is seeking an abortion must perform an ultrasound scan of the fetus and offer the woman the option of viewing it. Similar legislation is in place in Georgia and South Carolina. Attempts have been made in these states to make it compulsory for the woman to view the ultrasound images. Moiv, "Taking Liberties," 2007, www.texaskaos.com/showDiary,do?diaryId=3149 (accessed May 2007).

57. I. Donald, "Life, Death and Modern Medicine" (London: Order of Christian Unity, 1974), 25.

58. I. Donald, "Hereditary Disease: The Need to Know More," *Action Magazine*, spring 1980, 23–27, 25; Donald, "Does Christianity Help?"

59. I. Donald to R. Fliequer, 13 Jan. 1978, Donald Papers, 4/25.

60. Donald, "Naught for Your Comfort," 289; Donald, "Life, Death and Medicine," 24.

61. J. S. Fairbairn, "An Address on Abortion," *Lancet* 1 (1927): 217–19, 219.

62. Ibid., 218; I. Donald, "Abortion and the Obstetrician," *Lancet* 1 (1971): 1233.

63. Donald, "Naught for Your Comfort," 279.

64. Compare J. S. Fairbairn, "The Medical and Psychological Aspects of Gynaecology," *Lancet* 2 (1931): 999–1004, 1000–1001.

65. It was a poignant moment for Donald when his sister, Mrs. Munro, became Dame Alison in 1985. A. Munro, personal communication.

66. I. Donald to J. Barnes, 1 July 1980, Donald Papers, 5/3A. John Fleming is Scottish by adoption.

67. In 2007, sensationalist newspaper articles appeared implying that Donald had not given Brown due credit for his role in the development of diagnostic ultrasound. See, for example, Y. Bolouri, "The Baby Saviour: Forgotten Genius Who Invented Ultrasound," *Sun* (London), 22 Feb. 2007, 18; A. Dawson, "50 Years On, Meet the *Real* Inventor of Ultrasound Scan," *Daily Mail* (London), 23 Feb. 2007, 39. Brown has published a detailed rebuttal of these claims. T. G. Brown, "Letter to the Editor," *Ultrasound* 15 (2007): 114.

68. T. G. Brown, interview, April 2001.

69. T. G. Brown to I. Donald, 14 Jan. 1982, Donald Papers, 5/3A.

70. R. K. Merton, "The Matthew Effect in Science," *Science* 159 (1968): 56–63, 58.

71. Merton, "Matthew Effect," 60. J. Willocks and W. Barr's *Ian Donald: A Memoir* (London: Royal College of Obstetricians and Gynaecologists Press, 2004) gives an impression of Donald's impact.

72. J. Willocks, "Ian Donald and the Birth of Obstetric Ultrasound," in *Obstetric Ultrasound*, ed. J. P. Neilson and S. E. Chambers (Oxford: Oxford University Press, 1993), 1–18, 18.

CHAPTER ELEVEN: Maternity and Technology

1. J. L. Gleave, "The Planning of a General Hospital, with Particular Reference to the New Alexandria Hospital, Dunbartonshire," *Journal of the Royal Society for the Promotion of Health* 74 (1954): 656–70; "Joseph Lea Gleave," in *Dictionary of Scottish Architects*, 2008, www.scottisharchitects.org.uk/architect_full.php?id=206874 (accessed June 2012); I. Donald, "The New Yorkhill Maternity Hospital," *Scottish Medical Journal* 6 (1961): 164–69, 164.

2. I. Donald to T. Fox, 30 Oct. 1964, Donald Papers, 1/1/6. Gleave's original design was, in fact, substantially modified before completion, doubtless for financial reasons. Presumably, Donald did not see these alterations as adversely affecting his clinical vision for the hospital.

3. D. R. Aickin to I. Donald, 13 June 1973, BMUS Papers, 1/1/1A.

4. I. Donald to D. R. Aickin, June 1973, BMUS Papers, 1/1/1A.

5. Donald, "New Yorkhill Maternity," 166; "The Queen Mother's Hospital—Information for Patients," leaflet, BMUS Papers, 1/1/23.

6. I. Donald, *Practical Obstetric Problems*, 4th ed. (London: Lloyd-Luke, 1969), vi.

7. For the compatibility, or otherwise, of these aims, see W. R. Arney, *Power and the Profession of Obstetrics* (Chicago: University of Chicago Press, 1982), chap. 4.

8. Donald, "New Yorkhill Maternity," 164.

9. The Queen Mother's Hospital closed in 2010, by then obsolete.

10. *Maternity Services in Scotland*, Montgomery Report (Edinburgh: HMSO, 1959).

11. By the 1960s, the middle classes had realized that, provided the facilities were of an acceptable standard, using the NHS could save them money. A. Oakley, *The Captured Womb: A History of the Medical Care of Pregnant Women* (Oxford: Blackwell, 1984), 215.

12. I. Donald, "Clinical Alarm," *Surgo* 22 (1956): 123–28.

13. Anonymous, personal communication.

14. I. Donald to K. A. Harden, 30 May 1975, BMUS Papers, 1/1/8.

15. Comparison of the third and fourth editions of *Practical Obstetric Problems* is instructive here.

16. R. E. Davis-Floyd, "The Technocratic Model of Birth," in *Feminist Theory and the Study of Folklore*, ed. S. T. Holles, L. Pershing, and M. Young (Urbana: University of Illinois Press, 1993), 297–326.

17. S. Kitzinger, *The Politics of Birth* (Edinburgh: Elsevier Butterworth-Heinemann, 2005), 3.

18. M. Harrison, "Unborn: Historical Perspectives of the Fetus as a Patient," *Pharos Alpha Omega Alpha Honor Medical Society* 45 (1982): 19–24, 19.

19. R. P. Petchesky, "Fetal Images: The Power of Visual Culture in the Politics of Reproduction," *Feminist Studies* 13 (1987): 263–92, 277.

20. B. Duden, *Disembodying Women: Perspectives on Pregnancy and the Unborn* (Cambridge, MA: Harvard University Press, 1993).

21. Oakley, *Captured Womb*, 159.

22. Correspondence between Donald and Oakley, Donald Papers, 5/16.

23. B. Beech and J. Robinson, *Ultrasound Unsound* (London: AIMS, 1996).

24. One might, however, urge that Brown's principle of keeping the acoustic energy output to the minimum required for clinical purposes should be strictly adhered to; see remarks by T. A. Whittingham in E. M. Tansey and D. A. Christie, eds., *Looking at the Unborn: Historical Aspects of Obstetric Ultrasound* (London: Wellcome Trust, 2000), 65.

25. A. J. Wrigley, "A Criticism of Ante-natal Work," *British Medical Journal* 1 (1934): 891–94.

26. W. Savage, *Birth and Power: A Savage Enquiry Revisited* (Enfield: Middlesex University Press, 2007), 29; A. M. Vintzileos, C. V. Anath, J. C. Smulian, T. Beazoglou, and R. A. Knuppel, "Routine Second-Trimester Ultrasonography in the United States: A Cost-Benefit Analysis," *American Journal of Obstetrics and Gynecology* 182 (2000): 655–60.

27. We are describing the British practice; frequency of scanning elsewhere varies.

28. M. B. McNay, interview, May 1999.

29. M. Tew, *Safer Childbirth? A Critical History of Maternity Care* (London: Chapman and Hall, 1990), 101–2.

30. This opinion was recently expressed by Hylton Meire, a leading radiologist with extensive experience of obstetric applications of ultrasound. H. B. Meire, "Is Ultrasound as Useful as We Think? The Donald, MacVicar and Brown Lecture, 2006," *Ultrasound* 15 (2007): 177–84.

31. Ibid., 180.

32. E. Georges, "Fetal Ultrasound Imaging and the Production of Authoritative Knowledge in Greece," *Medical Anthropology Quarterly* 10 (1996): 157–75.

33. Some commentators have argued that there is no strong evidence that ultrasound screening results in a statistically significant improvement in perinatal outcome. B. Ewigman, "Effects of Prenatal Ultrasound Screening on Perinatal Outcomes," *New England Journal of Medicine* 329 (1993): 821–27.

34. M. Wagner, *Born in the USA: How a Broken Maternity System Must Be Fixed to Put Mothers and Infants First* (Berkeley: University of California Press, 2006), 40; B. Backie and J. Nackling, "Term Prediction in Routine Ultrasound Practice," *Acta Obstetrica et Gynecologia Scandinavica* 73 (1994): 113–18.

35. A fuller version of Donald's comment is discussed in chapter 8.

36. Georges, "Fetal Ultrasound Imaging."

37. Petchesky, "Fetal Images," 279.

38. D. Haraway, *Simians, Cyborgs, and Women: The Reinvention of Nature* (London: Free Association Press, 1991); E. Georges and L. Mitchell, "Baby's First Picture: The Cyborg Fetus of Ultrasound Imaging," in *Cyborg Babies: From Techno-Sex to Techno-Tots*, ed. R. Davis-Floyd and J. Dumit (New York: Routledge, 1998), 105–124; L. Mitchell, *Baby's First Picture: Ultrasound and the Politics of Fetal Subjects* (Toronto: University of Toronto Press, 2001).

39. B. Katz Rothman, *The Tentative Pregnancy: Prenatal Diagnosis and the Future of Motherhood* (New York: Viking, 1986).

40. J. Murphy-Lawless, *Reading Birth and Death: A History of Obstetric Thinking* (Cork: Cork University Press, 1998), 246–47.

41. A. Widdecombe, "Why Unborn Children Need Our Protection," *Daily Express* (London), 20 Feb. 2008; A. Widdecombe, personal communication.

42. Name of interviewee withheld, with permission.

43. Almuth, Hannah's mother, wishes to record that to her, Hannah was never just a fetus but a baby.

44. S. L. Hagen-Ansent, *Textbook of Diagnostic Ultrasound*, 2nd ed. (St. Louis: C. V. Mosby, 1983), 4–8; B. Fraser, interview, July 1997. For Fraser's role in development of the ultrasound scanner, see chapter 7.

Index